Hand Transplantation

Guest Editors

GERALD BRANDACHER, MD
W.P. ANDREW LEE, MD

HAND CLINICS

www.hand.theclinics.com

November 2011 • Volume 27 • Number 4

SAUNDERS an imprint of ELSEVIER, Inc.

W.B. SAUNDERS COMPANY
A Division of Elsevier Inc.

1600 John F. Kennedy Blvd. ● Suite 1800 ● Philadelphia, Pennsylvania 19103

http://www.theclinics.com

HAND CLINICS Volume 27, Number 4
November 2011 ISSN 0749-0712, ISBN-13: 978-1-4557-7983-3

Editor: David Parsons
Developmental Editor: Donald Mumford

Hand Clinics (ISSN 0749-0712) is published quarterly by Elsevier Inc., 360 Park Avenue South, New York, NY 10010-1710. Months of publication are February, May, August, and November. Business and Editorial Offices: 1600 John F. Kennedy Blvd., Ste. 1800, Philadelphia, PA 19103-2899. Customer Service Office: 3251 Riverport Lane, Maryland Heights, MO 63043. Periodicals postage paid at New York, NY and at additional mailing offices. Subscription price is $338.00 per year (domestic individuals), $540.00 per year (domestic institutions), $169.00 per year (domestic students/residents), $385.00 per year (Canadian individuals), $617.00 per year (Canadian institutions), $459.00 per year (international individuals), $617.00 per year (international institutions), and $223.00 per year (international and Canadian students/residents). Foreign air speed delivery is included in all *Clinics* subscription prices. All prices are subject to change without notice. **POSTMASTER:** Send address changes to *Hand Clinics*, Elsevier Health Sciences Division, Subscription Customer Service, 3251 Riverport Lane, Maryland Heights, MO 63043. Customer Service (orders, claims, online, change of address): Elsevier Health Sciences Division, Subscription Customer Service, 3251 Riverport Lane, Maryland Heights, MO 63043. Tel: 1-800-654-2452 (U.S. and Canada); 314-447-8871 (outside U.S. and Canada). Fax: 314-447-8029. E-mail: journalscustomerservice-usa@elsevier.com (for print support); journalsonlinesupport-usa@elsevier.com (for online support).

Reprints. For copies of 100 or more of articles in this publication, please contact the Commercial Reprints Department, Elsevier Inc., 360 Park Avenue South, New York, New York 10010-1710. Tel.: 212-633-3812; Fax: 212-462-1935; E-mail: reprints@elsevier.com.

Hand Clinics is covered in *MEDLINE/PubMed (Index Medicus)*, *Current Contents/Clinical Medicine*, *EMBASE/Excerpta Medica*, and *ISI/BIOMED*.

Printed and bound by CPI Group (UK) Ltd, Croydon, CR0 4YY

Transferred to Digital Print 2011

Contributors

GUEST EDITORS

GERALD BRANDACHER, MD
Scientific Director, Composite Tissue
Allotransplantation (CTA) Program,
Department of Plastic and Reconstructive
Surgery, Johns Hopkins University School
of Medicine, Baltimore, Maryland

W.P. ANDREW LEE, MD
Department of Plastic and Reconstructive
Surgery, Johns Hopkins University School
of Medicine, Baltimore, Maryland

AUTHORS

LUIS ALFARO, MD
Pathology Division, Hospital Virgen del
Consuelo, Valencia, Spain

KODI K. AZARI, MD
Associate Professor of Surgery, David Geffen
School of Medicine, University of California,
Los Angeles; Department of Orthopedic
Surgery, Los Angeles, California

MARSHALL BALK, MD
Division of Hand and Upper Extremity Surgery,
Department of Orthopedic Surgery, University
of Pittsburgh Medical Center, Pittsburgh,
Pennsylvania

PROSPER BENHAIM, MD
Division of Plastic Surgery, Department of
Orthopedic Surgery, David Geffen School of
Medicine, University of California, Los Angeles,
Los Angeles, California

GERALD BRANDACHER, MD
Scientific Director, Composite Tissue
Allotransplantation (CTA) Program,
Department of Plastic and Reconstructive
Surgery, Johns Hopkins University School
of Medicine, Baltimore, Maryland

WARREN BREIDENBACH, MD
Division of Plastic Surgery, University of
Arizona School of Medicine; Professor of
Surgery, Chief, Division of Reconstructive and
Plastic Surgery, Tuscon, Arizona

FEDERICO CASTRO, MD
Anesthesia Division, Clinica Cavadas,
Valencia, Spain

PEDRO C. CAVADAS, MD, PhD
University Hospital "La Fe"; Reconstructive
Microsurgery, Clinica Cavadas, Valencia,
Spain

JEFF CHANG, MS, MD
Research Fellow, Division of Plastic and
Reconstructive Surgery, Department of
Surgery, University of Washington, Seattle,
Washington

NICOLAS DAUPHIN, MD
Service de Chirurgie Plastique,
Reconstructrice et Esthétique, Centre
Hospitalier de, Luxembourg

ANTHONY J. DEMETRIS, MD
Department of Pathology, Division
of Transplantation, University of Pittsburgh
Medical Center, Pittsburgh, Pennsylvania

ALBERT D. DONNENBERG, PhD
Pittsburgh Cancer Institute, University of
Pittsburgh Medical Center, Pittsburgh,
Pennsylvania

JEAN MICHEL DUBERNARD, MD, PhD
Department of Transplantation, Hopital
Edouard Herriot, Lyon, France

RIVER M. ELLIOTT, MD
Division of Plastic Surgery, University of
Pennsylvania School of Medicine, Philadelphia,
Pennsylvania

TIMM O. ENGELHARDT, MD
Department of Plastic, Reconstructive and
Aesthetic Surgery, Center of Operative
Medicine, Innsbruck Medical University,
Innsbruck, Austria

ABTIN FOROOHAR, MD
Department of Orthopaedic Surgery, University
of Pennsylvania School of Medicine,
Philadelphia, Pennsylvania

MARKUS GABL, MD
Department of Traumatology, Center of
Operative Medicine, Innsbruck Medical
University, Innsbruck, Austria

MIGUEL A. GARCIA-BELLO, MD
Nephrology Division, Dr Negrín University
Hospital of Gran Canaria, Las Palmas De Gran
Canaria, Spain

PEDRO GARCIA-COSMES, MD, PhD
Nephrology Division, University Hospital,
Salamanca, Spain

SIMONE W. GLAUS, MD
Division of Plastic and Reconstructive Surgery,
Washington University School of Medicine,
St Louis, Missouri

ROBERT J. GOITZ, MD
Division of Hand and Upper Extremity Surgery,
Department of Orthopedic Surgery, University
of Pittsburgh Medical Center, Pittsburgh,
Pennsylvania

VIJAY S. GORANTLA, MD, PhD
Associate Professor of Surgery, Administrative
Medical Director, Pittsburgh Reconstructive
Transplant Program, Division of Plastic
Surgery, Department of Surgery, Pittsburgh,
Pennsylvania

TRISTAN L. HARTZELL, MD
Division of Plastic Surgery, Department of
Orthopedic Surgery, David Geffen School of
Medicine, University of California, Los Angeles,
Los Angeles, California

THERESA HAUTZ, MD
Department of Visceral, Transplant and
Thoracic Surgery, Center of Operative
Medicine, Innsbruck Medical University,
Innsbruck, Austria

JAVIER IBAÑEZ, MD
University Hospital "La Fe"; Reconstructive
Microsurgery, Clinica Cavadas, Valencia,
Spain

SUZANNE T. ILDSTAD, MD
Director, Institute for Cellular Therapeutics,
Jewish Hospital Distinguished Professor of
Transplantation, Professor of Surgery,
University of Louisville, Louisville, Kentucky

JOSEPH E. IMBRIGLIA, MD
Division of Hand and Upper Extremity Surgery,
Department of Orthopedic Surgery, University
of Pittsburgh Medical Center, Pittsburgh,
Pennsylvania

JERZY JABŁECKI, MD, PhD
Associate Professor of Surgery and Chief,
Subdepartment of Replantation of Limbs,
St Jadwiga Hospital, Trzebnica; Professor of
Surgery, State Higher Medical Professional
School, Opole, Poland

PHILIP J. JOHNSON, PhD
Division of Plastic and Reconstructive Surgery,
Washington University School of Medicine,
St Louis, Missouri

CHRISTINA L. KAUFMAN, PhD
Christine M. Kleinert Institute for Hand and
Microsurgery, Kleinert Kutz Hand Care Center,
Louisville, Kentucky

TAE WON BENJAMIN KIM, MD
Department of Orthopaedic Surgery, University
of Pennsylvania School of Medicine,
Philadelphia, Pennsylvania

MARTIN KUMNIG, PhD, MSc
Division of Medical Psychology, Department
of Psychiatry and Psychotherapy, Innsbruck
Medical University, Innsbruck, Austria

LUIS LANDIN, MD
University Hospital "La Fe"; Reconstructive
Microsurgery, Clinica Cavadas, Valencia,
Spain

W.P. ANDREW LEE, MD
Department of Plastic and Reconstructive Surgery, Johns Hopkins University School of Medicine, Baltimore, Maryland

L. SCOTT LEVIN, MD, FACS
Department of Orthopaedic Surgery, University of Pennsylvania School of Medicine; Paul B. Magnuson Professor of Orthopaedic Surgery, Chairman, Department of Orthopaedic Surgery, Professor of Surgery, Plastic Surgery, Hospital of the University of Pennsylvania, Philadelphia, Pennsylvania

JOSEPH E. LOSEE, MD
Pittsburgh Reconstructive Transplantation Program, Division of Plastic Surgery, Department of Surgery, Pittsburgh, Pennsylvania

SUSAN E. MACKINNON, MD
Division of Plastic and Reconstructive Surgery, Washington University School of Medicine, St Louis, Missouri

RAIMUND MARGREITER, MD
Department of Visceral, Transplant and Thoracic Surgery, Center of Operative Medicine, Innsbruck Medical University, Innsbruck, Austria

DAVID W. MATHES, MD
Associate Professor of Surgery, Chief of Plastic Surgery Puget Sound VA, Division of Plastic and Reconstructive Surgery, Department of Surgery, University of Washington, Seattle, Washington

CHRISTOPHE L. MATHOULIN, MD
Institut de la Main, Paris, France

SUE V. McDIARMID, MD
Professor of Pediatrics and Surgery, David Geffen School of Medicine, University of California, Los Angeles, Los Angeles, California

SCOTT MITCHELL, MD
Division of Plastic Surgery, Department of Orthopedic Surgery, David Geffen School of Medicine, University of California, Los Angeles, Los Angeles, California

MARINA NINKOVIC, MD
Department of Visceral, Transplant and Thoracic Surgery, Center of Operative Medicine, Innsbruck Medical University, Innsbruck, Austria

PALMINA PETRUZZO, MD
Department of Transplantation, Hopital Edouard Herriot, Lyon, France

GERHARD PIERER, MD
Department of Plastic, Reconstructive and Aesthetic Surgery, Center of Operative Medicine, Innsbruck Medical University, Innsbruck, Austria

HILDEGUNDE PIZA-KATZER, MD
Department of Plastic, Reconstructive and Aesthetic Surgery, Center of Operative Medicine, Innsbruck Medical University, Innsbruck, Austria

JOHANN PRATSCHKE, MD
Department of Visceral, Transplant and Thoracic Surgery, Center of Operative Medicine, Innsbruck Medical University, Innsbruck, Austria

KADIYALA V. RAVINDRA, MD
Department of Surgery, Duke University, Durham, North Carolina

MICHAEL RIEGER, MD
Department of Radiology, Innsbruck Medical University, Innsbruck, Austria

JOSE C. RODRÍGUEZ-PÉREZ, MD, PhD
Nephrology Division, Dr Negrín University Hospital of Gran Canaria, Las Palmas De Gran Canaria, Spain

JOSE D. RODRIGO, MD
Anesthesia Division, Clinica Cavadas, Valencia, Spain

ROEE RUBINSTEIN, MD
Division of Plastic Surgery, Department of Orthopedic Surgery, David Geffen School of Medicine, University of California, Los Angeles, Los Angeles, California

GERHARD RUMPOLD, PhD, MSc
Division of Medical Psychology, Department of Psychiatry and Psychotherapy, Innsbruck Medical University, Innsbruck, Austria

STEFAN SCHNEEBERGER, MD
Department of Plastic and Reconstructive Surgery, Johns Hopkins University School of Medicine, Baltimore, Maryland

ABRAHAM SHAKED, MD, PhD
Division of Transplant Surgery, University of Pennsylvania School of Medicine, Philadelphia, Pennsylvania

JAIMIE T. SHORES, MD
Clinical Director of Hand Transplantation; Assistant Professor, Department of Plastic and Reconstructive Surgery, Johns Hopkins University School of Medicine, Baltimore, Maryland

ALESSANDRO THIONE, MD, PhD
University Hospital "La Fe"; Reconstructive Microsurgery, Clinica Cavadas, Valencia, Spain

FRANCISCO VERA-SEMPERE, MD, PhD
Pathology Division, University Hospital "La Fe", Medical School, Valencia University, Valencia, Spain

ABHIJEET L. WAHEGAONKAR, MBBS, D.Ortho, MCh (Ortho), Diplomate in Hand Surgery
Consultant Upper Extremity, Hand and Microvascular Reconstructive Surgeon, Consultant Brachial Plexus and Peripheral Nerve Surgeon, Department of Upper Extremity, Hand and Microvascular Reconstructive Surgery, Sancheti Institute for Orthopedics and Rehabilitation; Honorary Visiting Hand Surgeon and Clinical Instructor in Orthopedic Surgery, Department of Orthopedics and Traumatology, B.V.D.U. Medical College and Hospitals, Pune, India

ANNEMARIE WEISSENBACHER, MD
Department of Visceral, Transplant and Thoracic Surgery, Center of Operative Medicine, Innsbruck Medical University, Innsbruck, Austria

BETTINA ZELGER, MD
Department of Pathology, Innsbruck Medical University, Innsbruck, Austria

XIN XIAO ZHENG, MD
Pittsburgh Reconstructive Transplantation Program, Division of Plastic Surgery, Department of Surgery, Pittsburgh, Pennsylvania

Contents

Preface: Hand Transplantation   xiii

Gerald Brandacher and W.P. Andrew Lee

The History and Evolution of Hand Transplantation   405

Abtin Foroohar, River M. Elliott, Tae Won Benjamin Kim, Warren Breidenbach,
Abraham Shaked, and L. Scott Levin

> Hand transplantation has proven itself to be a viable treatment option for upper extremity reconstruction. It has grown through advancements in several critical areas: microsurgery, transplant immunology, and hand surgery. The field has also benefited from a global effort with active transplant centers in 3 different continents. The early struggles and breakthroughs of hand transplantation's past have shaped and formed its current state. This article traces the events of the modern era of hand transplantation.

World Experience After More Than a Decade of Clinical Hand Transplantation

**World Experience After More Than a Decade of Clinical Hand Transplantation:
Update on the French Program**   411

Palmina Petruzzo and Jean Michel Dubernard

> The first hand transplantation was realized in Lyon and the results achieved in this case showed the feasibility of the surgical technique, the efficacy of the immunosuppressive protocol, the limited adverse effects and the importance of a patient's compliance and rehabilitation to ensure graft viability and functional recovery. Based on these findings and the positive results achieved in other single hand transplants realized around the world the authors performed also the first double hand transplantation, then followed by other four cases. The recipients received the same immunosuppressive treatment including tacrolimus, prednisone, mycophenolate mofetil and antithymocyte globulins for induction, nevertheless they showed some episodes of acute rejection episodes which reversed after a prompt treatment. All the bilateral hand grafted patients showed a relevant sensorimotor recovery particularly of sensibility and activity of intrinsic muscles. They were able to perform the majority of daily activities and to lead a normal social life. On the basis of the authors' experience the results achieved in hand allotransplantation are very encouraging as major adverse effects due to surgery and immunosuppressive regimen did not occur and patients' quality of life improved considerably.

**World Experience After More Than a Decade of Clinical Hand Transplantation:
Update from the Louisville Hand Transplant Program**   417

Christina L. Kaufman and Warren Breidenbach

> In the last 12 years, the Louisville CTA program has screened more than 600 interested hand transplant candidates and has transplanted 6 patients with 7 hand allografts. The program is a collaborative effort between the surgeons and staff of Kleinert, Kutz and Associates, Jewish Hospital and St. Mary's Healthcare, the Christine M. Kleinert Institute, and the University of Louisville. The functional outcome and long-term results of clinical hand transplantation have exceeded initial expectations both within the program and in the community at large. This report summarizes the

successes and challenges of the Louisville CTA experience in composite tissue allotransplantation.

World Experience After More Than a Decade of Clinical Hand Transplantation: Update on the Innsbruck Program   423

Theresa Hautz, Timm O. Engelhardt, Annemarie Weissenbacher, Martin Kumnig, Bettina Zelger, Michael Rieger, Gerhard Rumpold, Gerhard Pierer, Marina Ninkovic, Markus Gabl, Hildegunde Piza-Katzer, Johann Pratschke, Raimund Margreiter, Gerald Brandacher, and Stefan Schneeberger

Patients who have lost a hand or upper extremity face many challenges in everyday life. For some patients, reconstructive hand transplantation represents a reasonable option for anatomic reconstruction, restoring prehensile function with sensation and allowing them to regain daily living independence. The first clinical case of bilateral hand transplantation at University Hospital Innsbruck was realized on March 17th, 2000. A decade later, a total of 7 hands and forearms were transplanted in 4 patients. This article review the clinical courses of 3 bilateral hand transplant recipients and highlights psychological aspects on reconstructive hand transplantation with special regard to unilateral/bilateral transplantation.

World Experience After More Than a Decade of Clinical Hand Transplantation: Update on the Polish Program   433

Jerzy Jabłecki

It has been demonstrated over the past decade that the generally achieved functional outcomes of patients after hand transplantation (HTx) are better than those of equivalent replantations. However, HTx should be performed in specialized centers with Institutional Review Board–approved transplantation programs. In Poland such requirements are fulfilled by The Subdepartment of Replantation of Limbs of St. Jadwiga Hospital in Trzebnica. A main emphasis of this subdepartment is to make the very involved process of donor recruitment, recipient screening, surgery, and postoperative treatment fully transparent. This article summarizes the experience of this center with HTx over the past 5 years.

The Spanish Experience with Hand, Forearm, and Arm Transplantation   443

Pedro C. Cavadas, Luis Landin, Alessandro Thione, Jose C. Rodríguez-Pérez, Miguel A. Garcia-Bello, Javier Ibañez, Francisco Vera-Sempere, Pedro Garcia-Cosmes, Luis Alfaro, Jose D. Rodrigo, and Federico Castro

This article summarizes the findings from 3 recipients of hand allografts, including a description of the preparatory surgery and the transplant and secondary procedures to enhance the function of the hand, forearm, and arm allografts. The study focuses on the complications and disability reported by each patient, with a minimum follow-up of 2 years. The few complications were controlled successfully with medical treatment. Hand transplantation is a major reconstructive procedure that requires careful medical follow-up. The authors provide the first report of a significant improvement in disabilities of the upper limb as a result of hand allotransplantation.

Functional Outcome after Hand and Forearm Transplantation: What Can Be Achieved?   455

Marina Ninkovic, Annemarie Weissenbacher, Markus Gabl, Gerhard Pierer, Johann Pratschke, Raimund Margreiter, Gerald Brandacher, and Stefan Schneeberger

The first successful hand transplant in the modern era of reconstructive transplantation was performed in 1998. Since then, more than 65 hand and upper limb transplantations have been performed around the globe, with encouraging results. The main goal of all upper limb transplantations is to enhance the patient's quality of life. The transplant must be successfully integrated into the patient's body and self-image and the recipient should be satisfied with the recovery of sensitivity and muscle function of the new limb. To achieve these goals, a proper and thorough design of the rehabilitation regimen is of critical importance.

Immunosuppressive Protocols and Immunological Challenges Related to Hand Transplantation   467

Kadiyala V. Ravindra and Suzanne T. Ildstad

There are many immunological challenges related to hand transplantation. Curbing the immune system's ability to effectively mount an immune response against the graft is the goal. As the various components of the immune response are defined and their mechanisms of action delineated, more specific immunosuppressive agents and protocols have been developed. Complications related to immunosuppression in hand transplant recipients are similar to incidences among solid organ recipients. With longer follow-up, the increased cardiovascular risk factors or the development of a neoplasm will likely cause mortality. Standardizing immunosuppression in hand transplantation with the long-term goal of minimization is critically needed.

Acute and Chronic Rejection in Upper Extremity Transplantation: What Have We Learned?   481

Vijay S. Gorantla and Anthony J. Demetris

To date, 78 upper extremity transplants have been performed in 55 recipients around the world. The purpose of this article is to provide an overview of acute and chronic rejection (CR) and to summarize collective insights in upper extremity transplantation. To date, almost all patients experienced AR that is pathophysiologically similar to that in solid organs. The spectre of chronic rejection is just emerging. Upper extremity transplantation has significant potential as a reconstructive option only if efforts are invested in strategies to reduce risks of prolonged immunosuppression and in approaches to better diagnose, monitor and treat AR and CR.

Clinical Strategies to Enhance Nerve Regeneration in Composite Tissue Allotransplantation   495

Simone W. Glaus, Philip J. Johnson, and Susan E. Mackinnon

Reinnervation of a hand transplant ultimately dictates functional recovery but provides a significant regenerative challenge. This article highlights interventions to enhance nerve regeneration through acceleration of axonal regeneration or augmentation of Schwann cell support and discuss their relevance to composite tissue allotransplantation. Surgical techniques that may be performed at the time of transplantation to optimize intrinsic muscle recovery—including appropriate alignment of ulnar nerve motor and sensory components, transfer of the distal anterior interosseous nerve to the recurrent motor branch of the median nerve, and prophylactic release of potential nerve entrapment points—are also presented.

Favoring the Risk–Benefit Balance for Upper Extremity Transplantation—The Pittsburgh Protocol   511

Vijay S. Gorantla, Gerald Brandacher, Stefan Schneeberger, Xin Xiao Zheng, Albert D. Donnenberg, Joseph E. Losee, and W.P. Andrew Lee

Upper extremity transplantation is an innovative reconstructive strategy with potential of immediate clinical application and the most near-term pay-off for select amputees, allowing reintegration into employment and society. Routine applicability and widespread impact of such strategies for the upper extremity amputees with devastating limb loss could be enabled by implementation of cellular therapies that integrate and unify the concepts of transplant tolerance induction with those of reconstructive transplantation. Such therapies offer the promise of minimizing the risks, maximizing the benefits and optimizing outcomes of these innovative procedures.

Surgical and Technical Aspects of Hand Transplantation: Is it Just Another Replant?   521

Tristan L. Hartzell, Prosper Benhaim, Joseph E. Imbriglia, Jaimie T. Shores,
Robert J. Goitz, Marshall Balk, Scott Mitchell, Roee Rubinstein, Vijay S. Gorantla,
Stefan Schneeberger, Gerald Brandacher, W.P. Andrew Lee, and Kodi K. Azari

The ultimate goal of hand allotransplantation is to achieve graft survival and useful long-term function. To achieve these goals, selection of the appropriate patient, detailed preoperative planning, and precise surgical technique are of paramount importance. Transplantation should be reserved for motivated consenting adults in good general heath, who are psychologically stable and have failed a trial of prosthetic use. While the key surgical steps of transplantation are similar to those of replantation, there are major differences. This article describes the steps in hand allotransplantation, and the importance of patient selection as well as preoperative and postoperative care.

Development of an Upper Extremity Transplant Program   531

Kadiyala V. Ravindra and Vijay S. Gorantla

Starting a hand transplant program poses tremendous challenges. Solid organ transplantation and hand replantation are time-tested procedures and are now standard of care. Hand transplantation is the amalgamation of the scientific principles of reconstructive surgery and the concepts of organ transplantation. Thus, for any hand transplant program to be successful, there must be collaboration within a multidisciplinary team comprising a core group of hand and transplant surgeons. Such a joint effort can overcome the challenges that are inherent in a complex therapeutic option that integrates different disciplines and organizations during the planning, procedural, and posttransplant phases.

Recipient Screening and Selection: Who is the Right Candidate for Hand Transplantation   539

Jaimie T. Shores

Hand transplantation is an elective non–life saving but quality of life–giving surgery for good candidates that is not without risk. Patient screening and selection is the most critical element to successful transplantation outcomes and cannot be overemphasized in terms of importance in the overall scheme of an active composite tissue allotransplantation (CTA) program. This article discusses the various criteria that are important in the selection of patients for CTA.

Donor-Related Issues in Hand Transplantation   545

Sue V. McDiarmid and Kodi K. Azari

The policies and procedures for solid-organ donation, under the auspices of the Organ Procurement and Transplantation Network, currently cannot be applied to hand donation, because a hand allograft is considered a tissue in the United States and is under the jurisdiction of the Food and Drug Administration. Hand transplant centers have developed their own protocols. This article discusses the unique elements of such protocols, including training and education, the consent process, the necessary recipient and donor data, donor management, and operating room procedures. Candidate listing, allocation, and oversight of hand donation in the future are also discussed.

Ethical, Financial, and Policy Considerations in Hand Transplantation   553

Jeff Chang and David W. Mathes

Currently, more than 65 hand transplants have been performed with studies demonstrating favorable cosmetic and functional outcomes and cortical reintegration of the transplanted hand. Due to such favorable outcomes, many view hand transplant as a potential gold standard for treatment of a double amputee. However, ethical debate continues regarding risks and benefits of this nonlifesaving procedure. Clinicians, patients, and society must agree on whether hand transplantation is ethical and affordable. If a decision is made to transplant a hand, this must be performed in a dedicated center that facilitates integration of multiple specialists, ethicists, pharmacists, and rehabilitationists.

Bonus Article: Arthroscopic Dorsal Capsuloligamentous Repair in Chronic Scapholunate Ligament Tears   563

Christophe L. Mathoulin, Nicolas Dauphin, and Abhijeet L. Wahegaonkar
Edited by David J. Slutsky

This article discusses the preliminary results of treatment of chronic scapholunate lesions by arthroscopic dorsal capsuloligamentous repair, which does not require open exposure of the wrist capsule. Thirty six patients underwent arthroscopically assisted dorsal capsuloplasties. Sixteen had percutaneous pinning. Mean follow-up was at 11.4 months. The average arc of motion was 105° preoperatively and 120° postoperatively. The average grip strength attained 92% of the contralateral side. Most of the results were excellent-to-good. Seven professional athletes returned to preinjury level. Arthroscopic dorsal capsuloligamentous repair is a promising option, but a longer follow-up is necessary to confirm these results.

Index   573

Hand Clinics

FORTHCOMING ISSUES

February 2012

Intrinsic Muscles of the Hand
Steven Green, MD, *Guest Editor*

May 2012

Elite Athlete's Hand and Wrist Injury
Michelle Carlson, MD, *Guest Editor*

August 2012

Emerging Technology in Management of Disorders of the Hand
Jeffrey Yao, MD, *Guest Editor*

November 2012

Arthroplasty Around the Wrist
Marwan A. Wehbé, *Guest Editor*

RECENT ISSUES

August 2011

New Advances in Wrist and Small Joint Arthroscopy
David J. Slutsky, MD,
Guest Editor

May 2011

Elbow Arthritis
Julie E. Adams, MD, and
Leonid I. Katolik, MD,
Guest Editors

February 2011

Current Concepts in the Treatment of the Rheumatoid Hand, Wrist and Elbow
Kevin C. Chung, MD, MS, *Guest Editor*

THE CLINICS ARE NOW AVAILABLE ONLINE!

Access your subscription at:
www.theclinics.com

Preface
Hand Transplantation

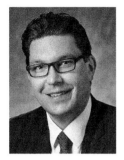 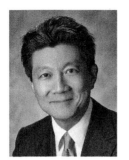

Gerald Brandacher, MD   W.P. Andrew Lee, MD
Guest Editors

Reconstructive transplantation has become a clinical reality over the past decade with more than 70 upper limb transplants performed with highly encouraging graft survival and good to excellent functional outcomes.

This special issue of *Hand Clinics* is devoted to Hand Transplantation. The individual authors are leaders in the field with extensive knowledge and expertise in their particular assignments. The goal for this issue is to cover the various multidisciplinary aspects related to hand transplantation with a focus on clinical and immunological outcomes. This is achieved with a series of articles from some of the leading centers performing hand transplantation in Europe and the United States, providing detailed updates on their experience with hand and forearm transplantation. This cumulative world record substantiates the fact that hand transplantation today is a valuable treatment option for the many patients in need suffering from complex tissue injuries or defects where conventional reconstruction is not feasible.

However, despite the fact that surgical procedures and functional outcomes are largely successful, the need for long-term and high-dose multidrug immunosuppression to enable graft survival still remains a pace-limiting obstacle toward broader application. We therefore devote an entire section to immunosuppressive protocols and immunological challenges related to hand transplantation and to the recognition of acute and chronic rejection mechanisms.

In addition, unlike for solid organs, clinical success in hand transplantation is dictated not only by graft acceptance and survival, but also by nerve regeneration, which determines ultimate functional outcomes. This important topic is dealt with in an article discussing novel strategies and modalities to enhance nerve regeneration. In this regard, several exciting novel therapeutic strategies such as the implementation of cellular and biologic therapies that integrate the concepts of immune regulation with those of nerve regeneration are on the horizon and have shown promising results in experimental models. Such protocols might further optimize functional outcomes and minimize/avoid the need for chronic immunosuppression.

Hand Clin 27 (2011) xiii–xiv
doi:10.1016/j.hcl.2011.08.009

With more and more centers embarking on reconstructive transplantation, logistical aspects, and standardization of the transplant procedure, patient care and postoperative follow-up are of critical importance. Consequently, a sequence of articles are incorporated in this issue to review surgical techniques, establishment of a hand transplant program, criteria for recipient selection, donor-related issues, as well as general ethical, financial, and policy considerations of hand transplantation.

Today we are on the verge of a new era in upper limb transplantation. The constantly improving safety, efficacy, and applicability of these promising reconstructive modalities hold great promise for patients with devastating injuries or deformities that are not amenable to conventional methods of repair.

Gerald Brandacher, MD
Department of Plastic and
Reconstructive Surgery
Johns Hopkins University School of Medicine
Ross Research Building 749D
720 Rutland Avenue
Baltimore, MD 21205, USA

W.P. Andrew Lee, MD
Department of Plastic and
Reconstructive Surgery
Johns Hopkins University School of Medicine
601 North Caroline Street
Baltimore, MD 21287, USA

E-mail addresses:
brandacher@jhmi.edu (G. Brandacher)
WPAL@jhmi.edu (W.P.A. Lee)

The History and Evolution of Hand Transplantation

Abtin Foroohar, MD[a], River M. Elliott, MD[b],
Tae Won Benjamin Kim, MD[a], Warren Breidenbach, MD[c,d],
Abraham Shaked, MD, PhD[e], L. Scott Levin, MD[a,f],*

KEYWORDS

- Hand transplantation • Allotransplant • History

As part of the rapidly expanding vascularized composite allotransplantation (VCA), hand transplantation combines the technical rigors of hand surgery and microsurgery with the complex multidisciplinary care that defines modern solid organ transplantation. Although hand transplantation and solid organ transplantation share a common history characterized by important advances in immunosuppression and surgical technique, hand transplantation has not yet been performed on a scale approaching that of solid organ transplants. The technical demands of hand transplantation, enhanced donor antigen burden of the hand allograft, and complex psychosocial issues pertaining to the recipient account for much of the discrepancy between these 2 related fields. Despite these unique challenges, hand transplantation remains a viable option today for hand amputees and the standard of care for bilateral upper extremity amputees. The early struggles and breakthroughs of hand transplantation's past have shaped and formed its current state.

HAND TRANSPLANTATION AND THE MICROSURGICAL RECONSTRUCTIVE LADDER

The reconstructive ladder refers to a well-known principle of soft tissue reconstruction that places the simplest methods of wound closure at the bottom rung and increases in complexity as one moves upward. Classically, free tissue transfer represented the highest step. Microsurgery and upper extremity surgery, however, have developed over the last half century, leading to functional muscle transfers, nerve transfers, chimeric flaps, flap expansion and prefabrication, perforator flaps, and ultimately VCA. Consequently, free tissue transfer can be expanded into its own reconstructive microsurgical ladder, ascending from simple microsurgical techniques at the bottom rungs to the most complex techniques at the top. The order of progression should be simple vascular and neural repair, followed by interposition nerve and vascular grafts, digital replantation, simple free tissue transfer, composite tissue transfer, functioning muscle transfers, toe to hand transfers, perforator flaps, free style flaps, preexpanded flaps, prefabricated

Disclosure: The authors did not receive any outside funding or grants in support of their research for or preparation of this work. Neither they nor a member of their immediate families received payments or other benefits or a commitment or agreement to provide such benefits from a commercial entity.

[a] Department of Orthopaedic Surgery, University of Pennsylvania School of Medicine, Philadelphia, PA, USA
[b] Division of Plastic Surgery, University of Pennsylvania School of Medicine, Philadelphia, PA, USA
[c] Division of Plastic Surgery, University of Arizona School of Medicine, Tuscon, AZ, USA
[d] Division of Reconstructive and Plastic Surgery, Tuscon, AZ, USA
[e] Division of Transplant Surgery, University of Pennsylvania School of Medicine, Philadelphia, PA, USA
[f] Department of Orthopaedic Surgery, Plastic Surgery Hospital of the University of Pennsylvania, 2 Silverstein, 3400 Spruce Street, Philadelphia, PA 19104, USA
* Corresponding author. Department of Orthopaedic Surgery, Hospital of the University of Pennsylvania, 2 Silverstein, 3400 Spruce Street, Philadelphia, PA 19104.
E-mail address: scott.levin@uphs.upenn.edu

Hand Clin 27 (2011) 405–409
doi:10.1016/j.hcl.2011.07.005
0749-0712/11/$ – see front matter © 2011 Elsevier Inc. All rights reserved.

flaps, and ultimately VCA. Virtually none of these techniques were practiced with any regularity less than 3 decades ago. Now all have taken their place in the upper extremity reconstruction.

EARLY DEVELOPMENTS: THE 1950s AND 1960s

In 1957, Dr Earle E. Peacock Jr, coined the term composite tissue allograft while using cadaveric flexor tendons to treat end-stage tendon incarceration.[1–3] Performed as a salvage operation, flexor tendon units and their synovial sheaths were transplanted without immunosuppression or microanastomosis, relying instead on inosculation. This technique was performed by multiple surgeons and achieved a success rate of 70% in cases in which amputation was the only other choice for salvage. Two-stage tendon reconstruction using silicone rod generated pseudosheaths, and pulley reconstruction eventually replaced this procedure.

In 1964, the first hand transplant was performed in Ecuador by Dr Robert Gilbert.[4] A single hand was transplanted to a bilateral amputee with azathioprine and prednisone used for postoperative immunosuppression. However, the graft was amputated 3 weeks later as a result of acute rejection. This early experience, along with similar failures in animal models, leads researchers to believe that skin-bearing transplants were prohibitively immunogenic. A 30-year period of stagnation followed.

CRITICAL BREAKTHROUGHS: THE 1980s AND 1990s

Significant developments in immunosuppressive drug therapy facilitated the growth of solid organ transplantation in the 1980s and 1990s. In addition to their applications to solid organ transplants, the new medications, such as calcineurin inhibitors, cyclosporine A, tacrolimus, and mycophenolate mofetil (MMF), provided reproducible survival in skin-bearing rat hind limb models.[5] These results were subsequently reproduced in large preclinical animal models[6,7] and completely reinvigorated VCA. Pioneers Jean-Michel Dubernard in Lyon (1998) and Warren Breidenbach in Louisville (1999) performed the next 2 hand transplants, thus starting the modern era of hand transplantation.[8,9]

THE MODERN ERA OF HAND TRANSPLANTATION
Lyon, France

The Lyon group performed the first of the modern era hand transplants in 1998.[9] The patient received a single hand transplant during a 13-hour surgery led by Dubernard. Although the operation was technically successful, the patient proved to be noncompliant with immunosuppression and physical therapy. He left the care of the Lyon group and eventually required an amputation in 2001.[10] This early experience illustrated how psychosocial factors and patient compliance may ultimately affect the survival of the allograft and clearly demonstrated that the psychological ramifications surrounding transplantation of a visible, sensate, and functional part differ greatly from a solid organ transplant.

The Lyon group also conducted the world's first bilateral hand transplant in January, 2000.[11] The patient, a 33-year-old painter, lost his hands when a homemade rocket exploded. This patient represents the first of a series of 5 bilateral hand transplants that addressed the use of hand transplantation in patients with multiple limb amputation.[12] At 6- and 2-year follow-ups, both recipients were able to perform activities of daily living and were satisfied with their transplanted hands.[13]

Louisville, KY, USA

On January 25, 1999, after a 14½-hour surgery, Matthew Scott became the first recipient of a hand transplant in the United States.[11] The patient lost his dominant hand from an M80 explosion. Today, he is the longest surviving successful hand transplant recipient in the world. To date, the Louisville group has performed 5 unilateral and 1 bilateral hand transplants.[14] The recipients are all men, and their ages ranged from 32 to 55 years at the time of transplant. One graft has been amputated because of unmanageable ischemia, possibly because of chronic rejection.[11,14]

Longer-term outcomes have been reported by Breidenbach and colleagues[15] in 2 patients with 8- and 6-year follow-ups. On functional testing, they noted results superior to those expected with prosthesis, including Carroll[16] test scores of 77/99 and 55/99, in comparison with expected prosthetic scores of 20 to 30. Both patients returned to work and reported excellent quality of life. Complications included avascular necrosis of bilateral hips treated with arthroplasty, cytomegalovirus infection, and steroid-induced diabetes.

Pittsburgh, PA, USA

Since March 2009 under the direction of Dr W.P. Andrew Lee, the team at The University of Pittsburgh Medical Center has performed 8 hand transplants (2 single, 3 double), including the first bilateral hand transplant and the first forearm transplant in the United States.[11] Moreover, this group is applying an innovative cell-based immunomodulatory treatment protocol that allows to perform reconstructive transplantation with a single antirejection medication. The initial and emerging data suggest that the protocol is safe, efficacious, and well tolerated and has allowed hand/forearm transplant with low-dose tacrolimus monotherapy while minimizing cumulative risks of immunosuppression.

US Department of Defense

In February 2010, the first hand transplant in a woman in the United States was performed at Wilford Hall Medical Center, Lackland Air Force Base.[11,17] Retired master sergeant Janet McWilliams lost her left hand and suffered severe injuries to her right arm 9 years ago when a package bomb exploded in her office. McWilliams received her new hand from a female donor and is the first patient in whom transplantation was performed by the US Department of Defense. This operation was performed by a team of physicians including Drs William C. Pederson, Dmitry Tuder, and Gregg Martyak.

Other American Experiences

More recently hand transplants have been performed in the University of California, Los Angeles, under Dr Kodi Azari and Emory University under Dr Linda Cendales. The University of Pennsylvania, under Dr L. Scott Levin, has a complete hand transplantation program in place with patients listed for transplantation.

Other European Experience

Based on the work of Drs Breidenbach, Dubinard, Lee, and others globally, hand transplantation has grown tremendously in the last 10 years. The increase in composite tissue allotransplantation has spurred innovative efforts in transplant immunology and enhanced the understanding of the psychosocial barriers facing potential recipients.

In the Italian Institute of Hand Surgery in Monza (Milan, Italy), under Dr Marco Lanzetta, 5 hand transplants have been performed (3 single and 1 double).[11,18] The latest patient is a 52-year-old mother of 2 who suffered quadrimembral amputation as a result of sepsis. She received bilateral hand transplantation in October 2010.

Hand transplants have been conducted in 5 other European centers, including Spain (Dr P. Cavadas, 2 double), Poland (Dr Jeblecki, total 8, 1 double hand, 2 arm), Austria (Dr R. Margreiter, 3 doubles, 1 single), Belgium (Dr van Holder and Shuind, 1 single), and Paris (Drs P. Dumontier

and L. Lantierri, combined face and double hand).[11,18] In 2008, Drs Edgar Biemer and Christoph Hoehnke performed successfully the first double arm transplant in a farmer who suffered bilateral above-elbow amputations from a farming accident.[11,18] With intensive physiotherapy, the patient has learned to open doors and switch on/off lights.

Asian Experience

Hand transplantation in Asia started in 1999 when 2 single hand transplants were performed in Guangzhou, China.[11,18] Shortly thereafter, 2 single hand transplants were performed in Guangxi, China. These transplants were followed by the first arm and hand transplant in Malaysia in 2000 in a 1-month old baby with a severely deformed limb.[18] Performed by Dr Pathmanathan, the limb was taken from a deceased identical twin sibling, thereby obviating postoperative immunosuppression. There is also a subset of early patients from China who lost allografts due to abstention from immunosuppressive therapy, long distance from transplantation centers, and unreported episodes of acute rejection.[14]

VCA SOCIETIES AND MONITORING

The rapid growth of VCA has led to the formation of important international scientific societies. These societies include the annually held International Composite Tissue Allotransplantation Symposiums as well as the American Society for Reconstructive Transplant Surgery. Also, Web sites such as Handtransplant.com (Jewish Hospital Hand Care Center, Kleinert Kutz & Associates, and the University of Louisville) and Handregistry.com (International Registry on Hand and Composite Tissue Transplantation [IRHCTT]) have gone live. These sites provide a forum for public education, scientific- and media-related exchange, and an ongoing chronicle of transplants performed globally.

HAND TRANSPLANT PSYCHOLOGY

The history of modern hand transplantation has underscored the importance of a meticulous assessment of each patient's psychosocial support systems before surgery. A patient's psychological suitability for transplantation is as important as the surgeon's technical ability, the degree of HLA antigen matching, or the effectiveness of postoperative immunosuppression and antibiotic prophylaxis. Each candidate's willingness to partake in long-term physical therapy, endure potential side effects of immunosuppression, and weather the emotional challenges of organ transplantation should be evaluated.[19]

IMMUNOLOGY

Immunosuppression is an integral part of successful hand transplantation, with most, if not all, failures having stemmed from either noncompliance or lack of appropriate immunosuppression. Traditionally, patients are treated with initial induction agents followed by maintenance therapy. Most patients who have undergone hand transplant have received either polyclonal (antithymocyte globulins) or monoclonal (alemtuzumab, basiliximab) antibody preparations for induction.[14] Maintenance therapy consists of high-dose triple-drug combinations, including tacrolimus, MMF, and prednisone.[14]

Apart from the unique psychological burdens of hand and face transplantation, VCA differs from solid organ transplantation in 2 other important aspects. First, VCA uses allografts with highly immunogenic components such as skin and bone marrow, a problem that initially cast doubt on the biological feasibility of these transplants. Recent investigation has focused on the development of innovative new immunomodulating strategies to produce long-term survival and simultaneously decrease immunosuppressive requirements.[20] Unlike hidden solid organ transplants, acute rejection of skin-bearing allografts may actually be easier to detect and treat at an early stage. The skin, unlike a solid organ, is readily available for clinical examination, easy to biopsy, and amenable to different forms of immunosuppressive delivery such as topical ointments.

Second, the necessary functional recovery of the allograft is significantly different from that in solid organ transplantation. Unlike a heart or kidney, a hand must regain neurologic innervation to its muscles in order to function. Protective sensation, adequate 2-point discrimination, and motor innervation must be restored if the transplanted hand is to become useful. This restoration includes a period of neural regeneration and appropriate re innervations as the transplanted hand begins to respond to cortical signals. The beneficial effects of immunosuppressive therapy on neural regeneration as well as stem cell– and Schwann cell–based protocols are the focus of new research.[20–23] These efforts aim to decrease the immunosuppressive requirement while simultaneously promoting functional neural regeneration.

Immunosuppressive therapy in VCA has also focused on the induction of tolerance in recipients. Tolerance may be defined as a hyporesponsiveness to the donor without immunosuppression while maintaining adequate immune response to combat third-party antigens.[24] Chimerism and recipient conditioning are potential strategies of achieving tolerance. Chimerism is the presence of 2 pluripotent stem lines within one individual (donor and recipient). Chimerism of even 1% has been shown to significantly improve outcomes in VCA.[24,25] Newer approaches to tolerance have looked at the introduction of donor bone marrow in the recipient before transplantation as well as investigations in the roles of specialized T regulatory and facilitator cell subsets.[24]

IRHCTT

The IRHCTT reviewed hand transplants performed over an 11-year period (September 1998–July 2010) and reported on outcomes.[14] They accounted for 49 transplanted hands, 17 unilateral and 16 bilateral. Because of an inability to obtain complete patient information, a subset of transplants in China and a few other centers were not included. The authors believe the total number of hands transplanted to this date to be well over 65 worldwide.

In its most recent review, the IRHCTT reported 1 patient death (combined hand and face transplant) on day 65 from sepsis. Of transplants performed in patients in Western countries, 3 grafts have been lost. These grafts included a right hand of a bilateral transplant recipient as a result of bacterial infection, a single hand from noncompliance, and a single hand from intimal hyperplasia and possible chronic rejection.

The IRHCTT reported that all patients developed protective sensibility, 90% developed tactile sensation, and 82.3% had discriminative sensibility. Recovery of intrinsic and extrinsic motor function allowed patients to perform most activities of daily living. Moreover, 75% of recipients reported an improvement in quality of life, and many have returned to work. Side effects were related to immunosuppression and included opportunistic infections, metabolic disorders, and malignancies (1 case of posttransplant lymphoproliferative disease and a case of basal cell carcinoma of the nose).[14]

SUMMARY

Hand transplantation has proven itself to be a viable treatment option for upper extremity reconstruction. It has grown through advancements in several critical areas: microsurgery, transplant immunology, and psychiatry. The field has also benefited from a global effort with active transplant centers in 3 different continents. Continuing to build on this foundation, the future of hand transplantation may be advanced by new surgical techniques, further appreciation for psychosocial elements, and a continued effort to find innovative immunomodulation strategies.

REFERENCES

1. Kaufman CL, Blair B, Murphy E, et al. A new option for amputees: transplantation of the hand. J Rehabil Res Dev 2009;46(3):395–404.
2. Peacock EE. Homologous composite tissue grafts of the digital flexor mechanism in human beings. Transplant Bull 1960;7:418–21.
3. Peacock EE Jr, Madden JW. Human composite flexor tendon allografts. Ann Surg 1967;166:624–9.
4. Gilbert R. Transplant is successful with a cadaver forearm. Med Trib Med News 1964;5:20–3.
5. Benhaim P, Anthony JP, Ferreira L, et al. Use of combination of low-dose cyclosporine and RS-61443 in a rat hind limb model of composite tissue allotransplantation. Transplantation 1996;61:527.
6. Ustuner ET, Zdichavsky M, Ren X, et al. Long-term composite tissue allograft survival in a porcine model with cyclosporine/mycophenolate mofetil therapy. Transplantation 1998;66:1581–7.
7. Jones JW Jr, Ustuner ET, Zdichavsky M, et al. Long-term survival of an extremity composite tissue allograft with FK506-mycophenolate mofetil therapy. Surgery 1999;126:384–8.
8. Dubernard JM, Owen E, Herzberg G, et al. Human hand allograft: report on first 6 months. Lancet 1999;353:1315–20.
9. Jones JW, Gruber SA, Barker JH, et al. Successful hand transplantation. One-year follow-up. Louisville Hand Transplant Team. N Engl J Med 2000;343:468–73.
10. Kanitakis J, Jullien D, Petruzzo P, et al. Clinicopathologic features of graft rejection of the first human hand allograft. Transplantation 2003;76:688.
11. Composite tissue allotransplantation; history of hand transplantation. Available at: www.handtransplant.com. Accessed April 1, 2011.
12. Petruzzo P, Morelon E, Gazarian A, et al. Results of the first pilot study on bilateral hand allotransplantation. Transplantation 2010;90:166(S).
13. Petruzzo P, Badet L, Garzarian A, et al. Bilateral hand transplantation: six years after the first case. Transplantation 2006;6:1718–24.
14. Petruzzo P, Lanzetta M, Dubernard JM, et al. The international registry on hand and composite tissue transplantation. Transplantation 2010;90:1590–4.
15. Breidenbach WC, Gonzales R, Kaufman CL, et al. Outcomes of the first 2 American hand transplants at 8 and 6 years posttransplant. J Hand Surg 2008;33A:1039–47.
16. Carroll D. A quantitative test of upper extremity function. J Chronic Dis 1965;18:479–91.
17. Young V. Doctors perform first hand transplant in DOD. The Lackland Talespinner 2010;68(10):1–2 Newspaper article.
18. International Registry on Hand and Composite Tissue Transplantation. Available at: www.handregistry.com. Accessed April 1, 2011.
19. Klapheke M, Marcell C, Creamer B, et al. Psychiatric assessment of candidates for hand transplantation. Microsurgery 2000;20:453.
20. Brandacher G, Gorantla VS, Lee WP. Hand allotransplantation. Semin Plast Surg 2010;24:11–7.
21. Tanaka K, Fujita N, Higashi Y, et al. Neuro-protective and anti-oxidant properties of FKBP-binding immunophilin ligands are independent on the FKBP12 pathway in human cells. Neurosci Lett 2002;330:147–50.
22. Mosahebi A, Fuller P, Wiberg M, et al. Effect of allogeneic Schwann cell transplantation on peripheral nerve regeneration. Exp Neurol 2002;173:213–23.
23. Kuo YR, Goto S, Shih HS, et al. Mesenchymal stem cells prolong composite tissue allotransplant survival in a swine model. Transplantation 2009;87(12):1769–77.
24. Wu S, Xu H, Ravindra K, et al. Composite tissue allotransplantation: past, present and future-the history and expanding applications of CTA as a new frontier in transplantation. Transplant Proc 2009;41:463–5.
25. Ildstad ST, Sachs DH. Reconstitution with syngeneic plus allogeneic or xenogeneic bone marrow leads to specific acceptance of allografts or xenografts. Nature 1984;307:168–70.

World Experience After More Than a Decade of Clinical Hand Transplantation: Update on the French Program

Palmina Petruzzo, MD*, Jean Michel Dubernard, MD, PhD

KEYWORDS

- Hand allotransplantation
- Composite tissue allotransplantation • Immunosuppression
- Acute and chronic rejection • Functional recovery

Despite initial controversies and skepticism, hand transplantation has become the most common composite tissue allotransplantation (CTA) performed worldwide. The modern era of clinical CTA was initiated by the first hand transplantation performed in Lyon, France in 1998, despite the fact that several authors did not consider this type of transplant to be justified on an "ideal scientific basis." At that time only approximately 60 experimental rat and 2 primate limb transplants had shown sustained graft survival.[1] However, hand transplantation was rapidly and successfully replicated in the United States, China, Italy, Austria, and Belgium. Currently more than 60 upper extremities have been transplanted.[2] Moreover, other CTAs have been performed, such as larynx, face, abdominal wall, and knee.

The term *CTA* means grafting of skin, muscles, nerves, tendons, vessels, and bones as a unit, and provides ideal replacement of missing tissue after traumatic losses, tumor resections, or congenital absences using near-identical parts from a cadaveric donor, enabling reconstruction of "like-with-like." The goal of CTA, therefore, is not to save lives but rather to restore function and improve quality of life.

The first right hand[3] and bilateral hand transplantations[4] were performed in Lyon, France on September 23, 1998 and January 13, 2000, respectively. Four bilateral hand transplantations were subsequently performed at the authors' center. All transplants were funded by a national grant (PHRC) and approved by the Comité de Protection des Personnes Participants à la Recherche Biomédicale (CCPRB). This article reports on the functional results and complications.

CLINICAL CASES

The First Hand Allotransplantation

The recipient of the first single hand transplantation, a 48-year-old man from New Zealand, whose right arm was amputated in an accident in 1984, received the hand from a 41-year-old brain-dead donor on September 23, 1998. Donor and recipient had the same blood type but a complete 6/6 human leukocyte antigen (HLA) mismatch. The T-cell and B-cell crossmatch was negative. The immunosuppressive protocol included induction therapy with antithymocyte globulins and maintenance therapy involving prednisone, 5 mg/d; tacrolimus with blood levels between 5 and 10 ng/mL; and mycophenolate mofetil (MMF), 2 g/d.

During the first months the patient presented a well-vascularized hand graft with normal skin

Financial disclosure: The authors have nothing to disclose.
Department of Transplantation, Hopital Edouard Herriot, 5, Place d'Arsonval, 69437 Lyon, France
* Corresponding author.
E-mail address: palmina.petruzzo@chu-lyon.fr

Hand Clin 27 (2011) 411–416
doi:10.1016/j.hcl.2011.07.007

and rapid nerve regeneration, which resulted in protective and tactile sensation. He was able to perform most daily activities (eg, grasping a glass, writing) with his grafted right hand. In the first post-transplant month, he developed transient hyper-glycemia and a herpes virus infection as side effects of his immunosuppressive treatment. An acute rejection episode occurred 8 weeks post-transplant, which was characterized by erythema-tous maculopapular lesions disseminated on the skin of the transplanted hand. The lesions re-gressed after the oral dose of steroids was increased and topical immunosuppressants were used, such as tacrolimus and clobetasol creams.

In the first 6 months the patient adhered to his immunosuppressive treatment and physiotherapy protocol. Later, he adhered to the treatment only transiently before ultimately discontinuing it completely. During month 15 posttransplantation, signs of rejection appeared over the skin of the grafted hand and the lesions progressively wors-ened. The lesions were remarkably similar to those seen in chronic lichenoid cutaneous graft-versus-host disease. At the patient's request the hand graft was amputated in London on March 2, 2001 (29 months after his transplantation). After amputation, various tissue specimens were stu-died,[5] confirming that the more severe pathologic alterations (inflammatory infiltrate and necrosis) were mainly present in the skin component. The other tissues showed milder, if any, alterations. A lymphocytic infiltrate of moderate density forming loose perivascular aggregates was shown in the vicinity of muscles and tendons.

Although the results achieved in this first case showed the feasibility of hand allotransplantation, it also showed the great importance of patient compliance to immunosuppressive treatment and physiotherapy and patient motivation. Remarkably and somehow unexpectedly, the progression of this rejection process seemed slow although the long treatment-free period and the signs were mainly in the skin, and few in deeper tissue.

The Five Cases of Bilateral Hand Allotransplantation

Table 1 lists the donor and recipient characteris-tics of the five patients who underwent bilateral hand allotransplantation.

The immunosuppressive protocol in all patients included induction with antithymocyte globulins, and the 1-year maintenance treatment consisted of prednisone (5 mg/d), tacrolimus (blood level between 5 and 10 ng/mL), and MMF (2 g/d).

During the follow-up ranging from 1 to 10 years, the transplanted upper extremities looked grossly normal, based on color and texture of the skin, temperature, and hair and nail growth, except in patient 1 who showed nail alteration 5 years after transplantation.

Skin biopsies were performed periodically, and histologically the skin showed normal structure and contained all of its normal cell components (**Figs. 1** and **2**).

All patients experienced at least one episode of acute rejection (**Table 2**), characterized macro-scopically by erythematous macules over the graft skin. Acute rejection episodes were characterized mainly by the presence of a dermal perivascular lymphoid infiltrate consisting predominantly of CD3+/CD4+ T cells occasionally reaching and penetrating the epidermis.

These rejection episodes could be reversed through increasing the oral steroid dose in patients 1 and 2; patient 4 experienced only one reject-ion episode, which was successfully treated with

Table 1
Donor and recipient characteristics

	Patient 1	Patient 2	Patient 3	Patient 4	Patient 5
Transplantation date	13.01.2000	30.04.2003	19.02.2007	4.07.2008	11.07.2009
Sex	Male	Male	Female	Male	Male
Age at transplantation (y)	33	21	27	29	21
Amputation date	12.01.1996	14.09.2000	28.08.2004	13.04.2003	11.07.2004
Amputation cause	Explosion	Crush	Electrocution	Burn	Explosion
Amputation level	R: wrist L: wrist	R: mid-forearm L: distal forearm	R: mid-forearm L: distal forearm	R: palm L: wrist	R: distal forearm L: wrist
Donor age (y)	18	45	40	29	18
HLA mismatches	5	4	4	3	5

Abbreviations: L, left; R, right.

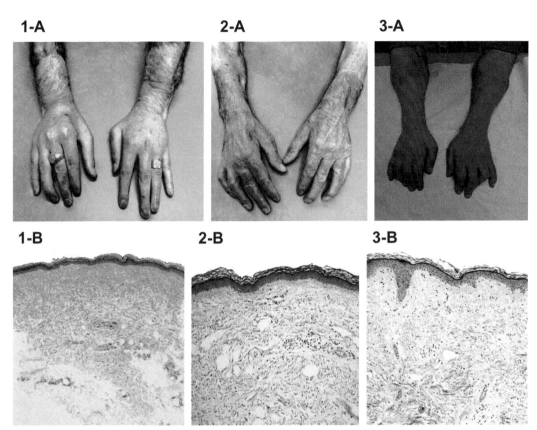

Fig. 1. Macroscopic aspect (*1-A, 2-A,* and *3-A*) and histology of skin biopsy (*1-B, 2-B,* and *3-B*) in patients 1, 2, and 3, respectively, at the last time point of the follow-up.

intravenous steroids, and in patient 5 the first rejection episode was treated with an intravenous steroid and the second through an increase in the oral steroid dose. In patient 3, the first two episodes were successfully treated with intravenous steroids, the third episode with antithymocyte globulins, and the fourth and fifth episodes with an increase in the oral steroid dose. In addition, after the last episode of rejection in November 2010, a low dose of sirolimus was added to the maintenance therapy for the patient. In all cases, topical immunosuppressants (clobetasol and tacrolimus ointments) were used with any rejection episode.

Anti-HLA antibodies were not detected, except in patient 2, who developed transiently anti-HLA class II antibodies in November 2009, which were not detectable 1 year later. None of the patients developed graft-versus-host disease or chimerism in the peripheral blood during follow-up.

At the most recent follow-up, histology, MRI, ultrasonography, and high-resolution peripheral quantitative CT scan of all tissue components of the grafted upper extremities detected no alteration that suggested a process of chronic rejection.[6]

Functional recovery is the final goal in upper extremity transplantation. This process is long and complex, and involves not only preservation of the viability of neural, muscular, and sensory end-organ components but also appropriate and timely reinnervation of neural targets and several degrees of cortical reorganization. The functional outcome that can be expected in limb transplantation is related to the level of amputation; this was confirmed by the authors' experience showing earlier functional recovery with amputation at the wrist level. However, late functional outcome seems very encouraging also at the forearm level, as shown by the results seen in the second and third recipient in the authors' series.

All of the recipients showed a relevant sensorimotor recovery, which was evaluated using the International Registry on Hand and Composite Tissue Allotransplantation[7] (IRHCTT) and the Disabilities of the Arm, Shoulder, and Hand (DASH) scores[8] (**Table 3**). The first two patients were graded as "excellent" based on both scores, whereas a discrepancy was seen in the evaluation of the other patients. The third patient and fifth

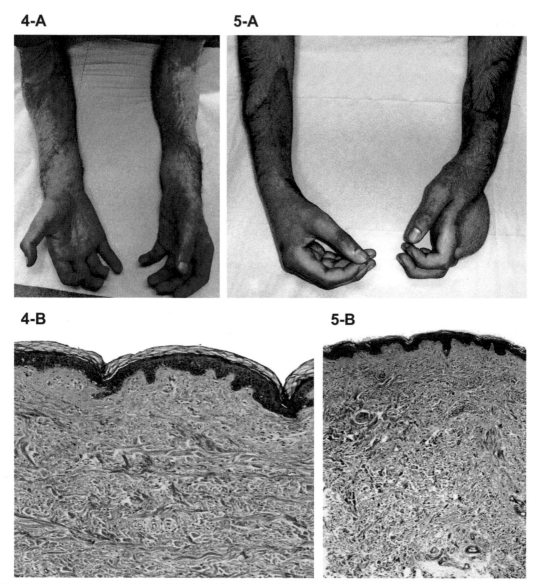

4-A

5-A

4-B

5-B

Fig. 2. Macroscopic aspect (*4-A* and *5-A*) and histology of skin biopsy (*4-B* and *5-B*) in patients 4 and 5, respectively, at the last time point of the follow-up.

patient self-evaluated as "excellent" with the DASH score, although they are "good" and "fair," respectively, based on the IRHCTT. The fourth patient presented a higher IRHCTT score compared with the DASH score, having ankylosis of right elbow (as a consequence of his burning accident) and being still unsatisfied of the achieved results, although they are considered encouraging.

Table 2
Acute rejection episodes

	Patient 1	Patient 2	Patient 3	Patient 4	Patient 5
Number of episodes	2	3	5	1	2
POD	53, 72	57, 86, 2759	16, 271, 635, 951, 1365	65	10, 350
Banff score	2, 2	2, 2, 2	2, 2, 3, 2, 3	2	2, 2

Abbreviation: POD, post-operative day.

Table 3
Functional recovery of the bilateral hand transplantations expressed by IRHCTT score and DASH score at the last time point of follow-up

	Patient 1		Patient 2		Patient 3		Patient 4		Patient 5	
Follow-up (y)	10		7		3		2		1	
IRHCTT score	R	L	R	L	R	L	R	L	R	L
	90.5	86	85.5	87	76.5	76	55.5	61	56	54
DASH score	4.84		6.25		4.31		31.45		12.10	

Abbreviations: L, left; R, right.

The IRHCTT is based on objective and subjective parameters, such as skin color and texture; hair and nail growth, which are important markers of hand vascularization and skin trophism; functional results (sensibility tests, measure of active range of motion, pinch and grip strength, intrinsic muscles activity); psychological outcome; social behavior; work status; subjective satisfaction; body image; and well-being. The well-known DASH score is based on patient self-evaluation of disability.

All of the recipients showed recovery of protective and tactile sensibility; in addition, a discriminative sensibility (S3+, based on Highet scale modified by Dellon and colleagues[9]) and a partial recovery of intrinsic muscles were shown in the first three patients 2 years after transplantation. Although the short follow-up period of the last two patients does not translate into a discriminative sensibility more than S3 and shows a limited recovery of intrinsic muscles, these patients are already able to perform most daily activities. In the authors' experience, recovery of intrinsic muscles started later, usually 6 months after transplantation, and evolved slowly compared with extrinsic muscles. However, extrinsic and intrinsic muscle recovery enabled all patients, from 1 to 10 years of follow-up, to perform most daily activities, including eating, driving, grasping objects, stringing a needle, riding a bicycle or a motorbike, shaving, using the telephone, and writing; they live a normal social life, and patients 1 and 5 were able to work again by 3 years and 15 months after transplantation, respectively. Despite the remarkable functional recovery, all patients had a limited range of motion of their joints because of fibrosis and adherences, a variable degree of muscular hypotrophy, and a diminished muscular power. Up to now, none of the recipients showed any decrease in sensorimotor recovery.

Cortical reorganization was assessed using functional MRI (fMRI) and transcranial magnetic stimulation. fMRI was performed before and after transplantation at different time points of the follow-up in the bilateral hand transplant recipients, and the results showed that hand transplantation resulted in global remodeling of the limb cortical map, reversing the functional reorganization induced by the amputation.[10] The spatial trajectory of these activations in time further indicates that the cortical rearrangement occurs in an orderly manner: the hand and arm representations tend to return to their original cortical area. Hence, brain plasticity seems to be accomplished with reference to a preamputation body representation. Thus, peripheral input can modify cortical hand organization in sensorimotor regions. Subsequent fMRI examinations performed at 12 and 18 months after transplantation showed no changes in the cortical map, suggesting that once hand neurons have reached their targets, brain plasticity processes in the motor areas become stable. Moreover, transcranial magnetic stimulation[11] showed the gradual reappearance of intrinsic hand-muscle representations in the motor cortex, with distinct time courses for right and left muscles and also an asymmetry between the two upper extremities. Although how the level of amputation and the quality of peripheral reconnection interacted with central factors in determining the degree and extent of functional recovery cannot yet be defined, the process of motor cortical plasticity clearly allows the recognition and integration of the transplanted muscles.

Risk versus benefit must always be considered carefully, because the main goal of hand transplantation is to improve patient quality of life. The recipients experienced some complications, which were fortunately reversible. Most complications were metabolic and infectious, such as hyperglycemia, which occurred in patients 1 and 5 in the first period after transplantation (first 30 and 10 postoperative days, respectively, and requiring insulin therapy). Currently both patients have normal values of glycemia and hemoglobin A1c. Osteitis of the left ulna was seen in patient 2 on day 152, which was successfully treated with antibiotics and removal of metallic materials; oral cellulitis from neutropenia was seen in patient 5 on day 81; and Epstein-Barr virus infection was seen in patient 3 on day 603. Patient 1 developed serum sickness on day 7.

Vascular complications also occurred in this series. Thrombosis of the left ulnar artery occurred in patient 2 on day 1, and thrombosis of the right radial artery and left ulnar artery occurred in patient 5 on day 12, which required a bypass between omeral and radial artery on the left side and an embolectomy on the other side. In addition, patient 5 was burned at the back of the left hand and underwent escharectomy with reconstructive surgery.

Despite these complications, and the necessity of taking daily immunosuppressive multidrug medication and following a rigorous program of rehabilitation, all of the recipients affirm that the bilateral hand transplantation improved their quality of life.

In conclusion, based on the experience and the results achieved in this first trial involving five cases of bilateral hand transplantation, patient compliance and careful recipient selection and evaluation during the follow-up are essential for the success of this type of transplantation.

SUMMARY

The Lyon team performed one single and five bilateral hand allotransplantations with a follow-up ranging from 1 to 10 years. The single hand transplantation was the first in the world, and the results showed the feasibility of the surgical technique, the efficacy of the immunosuppressive protocol, the limited adverse effects, and the importance of patient compliance and rehabilitation to ensure graft viability and functional recovery. Based on these findings and the positive results achieved in other single hand transplants performed around the world, the authors performed the first double hand transplantation, followed by four additional cases.

All recipients received the same immunosuppressive treatment, including tacrolimus, prednisone, MMF, and antithymocyte globulins for induction. Nevertheless, all patients showed episodes of acute rejection, which could be reversed after additional treatment. In addition, metabolic and infectious complications occurred during the follow-up.

All of the patients who had a bilateral hand transplant showed a relevant sensorimotor recovery, particularly of sensibility and activity of intrinsic muscles. They were able to perform most daily activities and to lead a normal social life. Results seen 12 years after the first hand transplantation are encouraging, because major adverse effects caused by surgery and the immunosuppressive regimen did not occur and the patients' quality of life improved considerably.

REFERENCES

1. Jones NF. Concerns about human hand transplantation in the 21st Century. J Hand Surg Am 2002;27(5): 771–87.
2. Petruzzo P, Lanzetta M, Dubernard JM, et al. The international registry on hand and composite tissue allotransplantation. Transplantation 2010;90(12):1590–4.
3. Dubernard JM, Owen E, Herzberg G, et al. Human hand allograft: report on first 6 months. Lancet 1999;353:1315–20.
4. Dubernard JM, Petruzzo P, Lanzetta M, et al. Functional results of the first human double-hand transplantation. Ann Surg 2003;238(1):128–36.
5. Kanitakis J, Jullien D, Petruzzo P, et al. Clinicopathologic features of graft rejection of the first human hand allograft. Transplantation 2003;76(4):688–93.
6. Petruzzo P, Kanitakis J, Badet L, et al. Long-term follow-up in composite tissue allotransplantation: in-depth study of five (hand and face) recipients. Am J Transplant 2011;11(4):808–16.
7. Petruzzo P, Lanzetta M, Dubernard JM, et al. The international registry on hand and composite tissue transplantation. Transplantation 2008;86(4):487–92.
8. Gummesson C, Ward M, Atroshi I. The shortened disability of the arm, shoulder and hand questionnaire (Quick DASH): validity and reliability based on responses within the full length DASH. BMC Musculoskelet Disord 2006;7:1–7.
9. Dellon AL, Curtis RM, Edgerton MT. Reeducation of sensation in the hand after nerve injury and repair. Plast Reconstr Surg 1974;53(3):297.
10. Giraux P, Sirigu A, Schneider F, et al. Functional cortical reorganization after transplantation of both hands as revealed by fMRI. Nat Neurosci 2001;4: 691–2.
11. Vargas CD, Aballéa A, Rodrigues EC, et al. Reemergence of hand-muscle representations in human motor cortex after hand allograft. Proc Natl Acad Sci U S A 2009;106(17):7197–202.

World Experience After More Than a Decade of Clinical Hand Transplantation: Update from the Louisville Hand Transplant Program

Christina L. Kaufman, PhD[a],*, Warren Breidenbach, MD[b,c]

KEYWORDS

- Hand transplantation • Bony union • Intimal hyperplasia
- Composite tissue allotransplantation

In the last 12 years, the Louisville CTA program has screened more than 600 interested hand transplant candidates and transplanted 6 patients with 7 hand allografts. The Louisville CTA program is a collaborative effort between the surgeons and staff of Kleinert, Kutz and Associates, Jewish Hospital and St. Mary's Healthcare, the Christine M. Kleinert Institute, and the University of Louisville. The functional outcome and long-term results of clinical hand transplantation have exceeded initial expectations both within the program, and within the community at large. This report summarizes the successes and challenges of the Louisville experience in composite tissue allotransplantation (CTA).

Follow-up time for the hand transplant recipients ranges from 6 months to 12 years. A summary of the patients is shown in **Table 1**. With the exception of a graft loss in Patient 4, very good to excellent results have been achieved. At this point our group believes that the graft loss in Patient 4 was due to graft vasculopathy. Function is good in all patients, and all patients have expressed satisfaction with their transplant. Even in the case of the graft loss, this patient continues to express interest in a second allograft.

The first patient received his transplant in January of 1999. He was 37 years at the time of transplant, and had a distal forearm amputation 13 years previously. Of note, he was diabetic at the time of transplant. This patient received basiliximab (Simulect) induction with standard triple-drug therapy of tacrolimus (Prograf), mycophenolate mofetil (MMF), and prednisone. He was weaned off steroids at 8 years after transplant and continues to do well, with good kidney function at 12 years after the transplant.

This work was supported in part by a grant from the Office of Navy Research (#N00014-06-1-0084) and the Office of Army Research (#W81XWH-07-1-0185). The US Army Medical Research Acquisition Activity, 820 Chandler Street, Fort Detrick MD 21702-5104 is the awarding and administering acquisition office. The content of the information does not necessarily reflect the position or the policy of the Government, and no official endorsement should be inferred.

Financial disclosure and Conflict of Interest obligations: The authors have nothing to disclose.

[a] Christine M. Kleinert Institute for Hand and Microsurgery, Kleinert Kutz Hand Care Center, Louisville, KY, USA
[b] Division of Plastic Surgery, University of Arizona School of Medicine, Tuscon, AZ, USA
[c] Division of Reconstructive and Plastic Surgery, Tuscon, AZ, USA
* Corresponding author.
E-mail address: ckaufman@cmki.org

Hand Clin 27 (2011) 417–421
doi:10.1016/j.hcl.2011.08.004

Table 1
Summary of Louisville CTA hand recipients

Patient	Time Post Transplant	Immunosuppression Regimen[a]	Severe Rejection Episodes	Complications	Two-Point Discrimination	Function
1	12 y	Simulect, Prograf, MMF, prednisone	3 (all in first year)	CMV	Yes 5–9 mm	Intrinsic muscle recovery, continues to improve
2	10 y	Simulect, Prograf, MMF, prednisone	7	Diabetes; osteonecrosis of hips	Can detect stimulus only	Good function; no intrinsics
3	4 y	Campath 1H (Prograf, MMF)	3	CMV, MZL	Can detect stimulus only	Good function, intrinsics lagging in thumb
4	9 mo[b]	Campath 1H (Prograf, MMF)	0	(chronic rejection at 9 mo)	No	Excellent for timeframe
5	2 y	Campath 1H (Prograf, MMF)	0	Weight gain, changes in kidney function	Can detect stimulus only	Good function, intrinsics returning
6	6 mo[c]	Campath 1H (Prograf, MMF, prednisone)	0	Wound closure issues and poor vascularity in right hand	Can detect stimulus only	Good early progress

Abbreviations: CMV, cytomegalovirus; IVIG, Intravenous immunoglobulin; MMF, mycophenolate mofetil; MZL, marginal zone lymphoma.

[a] Patient 1 and 2 were weaned off predinsone at 8 and 6 years post transplant.
[b] Patient 4 had graft amputated at 9 months due to ischemia secondary to end stage graft vasculopathy.
[c] This patient subsequently developed severe graft vasculopathy which responded to IVIG, plasmapheresis and a switch from MMF to Rapamycin.

The transplant itself was uneventful. This patient did have 3 episodes of rejection in the first year after the transplant, which were easily controlled with short courses of additional medication, most often with steroids. He has had minimal medical issues since the transplant. The patient developed cytomegalovirus (CMV) infection at 3 months that responded to medication. At 8 years after transplant he was weaned off prednisone without problems, and is currently maintained on MMF and tacrolimus. He has done an excellent job of managing his diabetes, and his hemoglobin A1c levels are within normal ranges.

Motor function improved from the end of the first year to 6 years, and has remained relatively stable. He does have functional abduction (4/5) of the thumb. He has 2-point discrimination that is near normal (5–9 mm). At 12 years after transplant this patient continues to experience sensory changes. His Carroll score at his 11-year annual evaluation was 69 out of a possible 99. He can feel hot and cold as well as rough and smooth textures. He is able to toss and catch a ball, turn the pages of the newspaper, unscrew the cap on a water bottle, pick up small objects, and independently complete all activities of daily living.

Our second patient was a 36-year-old Caucasian man who also had a distal forearm amputation from a blast injury, and successfully underwent hand transplantation in February 2001. This patient received a similar induction regimen to that of the first patient. However, within a few weeks of transplant he developed high blood sugars. As a means to allow targeting of lower tacrolimus levels, MMF was discontinued and he was switched to rapamycin. The patient still requires monitoring of his blood sugar, and takes medication to regulate levels. He does not require insulin treatment. Six years after transplant this patient was successfully weaned off prednisone. He had 5 episodes of acute rejection in the first year. One episode required antibody treatment with antithymocyte globulin to reverse rejection. In the fifth and seventh years after transplant he had another episode of rejection related to noncompliance with medications. The rejections responded to treatment, and compliance with his medication resumed. Because of an increasing donor-specific antibody (DSA) against class I donor antigens, he has recently been restarted on 7.5 mg/day prednisone, which has resulted in lowering of his DSA levels. Monitoring of the patient's DSA will continue. There are no obvious clinical sequelae from the DSA at this time. Skin biopsies are C4d negative.

The two major complications in this patient were the development of high blood sugars following transplant, that is, diabetes, and osteonecrosis of both hips (year 2 and year 6). Both of these complications are directly related to the prednisone and/or tacrolimus maintenance therapy. These side effects were part of the impetus for implementing alemtuzumab (Campath 1H) induction in the subsequent 4 patients. This steroid-free induction regimen is now routinely used in kidney transplantation.[1,2]

This patient achieved a level of fair function by 1 year. However, in contrast to Patient 1 he has not improved over the years with respect to intrinsic muscle function. His Carroll test was 59 at 9 years after transplant. Sensory return has been significantly less than that in Patient 1; however, he has not had a problem with ulcers on the transplanted hand, suggesting there is sufficient protective sensation as shown by monofilament testing. Touch localization (to tips of thumb, long, ring, and small finger) are poorly developed, but temperature and vibration sensation (256 cps) have returned. He does not have static or moving 2-point discrimination. He can detect the stimulus, but he cannot discriminate. He has a strong lateral pinch that allows him to pick up and grip objects. He is able to toss and catch a ball, turn the pages of the newspaper, unscrew the cap on a water bottle, pick up small objects, tie his shoes, and complete all activities of daily living, merely with a different technique than if using his right hand. He owns and operates a gutter installation business, and actively uses the hand in manual labor.

Our third patient is a Caucasian man, aged 54 years at the time of transplantation. He had

undergone a distal amputation of his dominant right hand 34 years prior in an industrial press accident. The transplant was performed in November 2006. He was the first subject in this series to receive Campath 1H induction, and was not started on methylprednisolone for maintenance immunosuppression. The transplant went well with no unexpected events. About 2 weeks after the transplant the patient developed a seroma on the ulnar forearm, which responded well to debridement and grafting with skin from the patient's thigh.

This patient has had 3 significant rejection episodes in the 2 years following his transplant. The first episode was a period of combined rejection and infection (CMV infection) at about 2 months after the transplant. The rejection resolved completely with treatment using topical agents (topical tacrolimus and topical steroids) only. He had a second episode of rash and swelling that occurred about 18 months after the transplant. His immunosuppression was transiently increased, and the swelling resolved in about 1 month. Of interest, function of the hand was not affected by the rash or swelling in the skin. Finally, the patient has had a severe episode of rejection in response to decreasing immunosuppression because of suspected posttransplant lymphoproliferative disorder (PTLD). This rejection resolved once immunosuppression was restored.

The other major complication noted in this patient was an unusual B-cell clone in the blood that was identified 23 months after transplant. At that time a monoclonal T-cell clone was also identified. These clones were identified in the course of doing routine blood work. The patient had no symptoms, positron emission tomography and computed tomography scans were negative, and marrow biopsy showed a small involvement of both clones. An initial diagnosis of PTLD was made, and the patient was sent home on reduced tacrolimus and discontinuation of MMF. The laboratory work was repeated and reviewed by several experts. No significant changes were seen in the absolute number of the clones following the reduction or resumption of immunosuppression. The World Health Organization classification histologically is of a marginal zone lymphoma (MZL). The group has monitored both of these clones by flow cytometry on a quarterly basis for more than 2 years, and have not seen any significant changes in their absolute number in the peripheral blood. The B-cell clone was also identified in pretransplant frozen peripheral blood leukocyte specimens, further suggesting that this is an MZL rather than PTLD.

At this patient's fourth annual checkup his function in the transplanted hand was measured as fair using the Carroll test (he scored 57 of a possible 99). The range of motion in metacarpophalangeal flexion and proximal interphalangeal hyperextension has increased over year 3. He does not have 2-point discrimination, but does have protective sensation on monofilament testing. He can feel cold and heat. Although by Carroll test he has not improved significantly over his prosthesis, this test does not take into account the ability to feel touch, heat, or cold. There are also several motor tasks he simply could not do with his prosthesis, such as turn a door knob, ride a snowmobile, or use power tools.

The fourth patient is a 32-year-old Caucasian man who had suffered an amputation of his dominant right hand following a firearm accident in 2002. He had a very distal forearm amputation. The transplant was performed in July 2008. Like the third patient, this patient received Campath 1H induction as part of his transplant. He was maintained on double therapy of tacrolimus and MMF.

This patient had a very quiet clinical course with respect to rejection. In the first 8 months he had 3 episodes of rash or slight swelling, all of which responded to topical tacrolimus and/or steroids. Unfortunately at 9 months he had unmanageable ischemia in the hand, resulting in amputation. Histologic analysis indicates that this was secondary to severe intimal hyperplasia primarily in the arteries of the allograft. No DSA was detected before or at the time of amputation. However, a blood sample taken 2 days after amputation, and 4 days after cessation of immunosuppression, did reveal significant class I and class II specific DSA, which has been maintained. C4d staining of various tissues of the amputated graft was nonspecific. Punch skin biopsies before and at the time of amputation were also negative for histologic rejection. Evidence of cellular infiltration was seen in deeper tissues, but the relation to humoral or cellular rejection versus a response to tissue damage as a result of ischemia is unclear. The severe intimal hyperplasia was confluent in all studied arteries of the amputated graft, and was restricted to donor vessels only, suggesting that this was an immunologic response. Based on the data reviewed, the loss of the graft may be attributable to aggressive chronic rejection.

The fifth patient received a hand transplant in late November 2008. This patient is a Caucasian man, 43 years old at the time of transplant, who lost his hand in a foundry accident in 2006. Again he had a distal forearm amputation. He also received Campath 1H induction, and was being maintained on tacrolimus and MMF. He had 4 episodes of grade II histologic rejection consisting of relatively localized rash in the first year after transplant, but no episodes of severe confluent rejection.

A surprising outcome in hand transplantation has been a lack of obvious chronic rejection in CTA patients who are several years post transplant. Early debate regarding hand transplantation predicted that chronic rejection would manifest as severe dermal fibrosis or dyskeratosis,[3,4] and it was even suggested that the early hand transplant recipients might eventually be remembered as a model of scleroderma.[5] The target organs were thought to be the skin and adnexal units, as has been seen in chronic graft-versus-host disease in recipients of stem cell transplantation.[6,7]

To date, the only report of severe changes resulting in pathology similar to chronic rejection were reported in the first French hand transplant recipient who independently stopped his immunosuppression, and who subsequently requested that the graft be removed.[8] In hindsight, these changes have been attributed to severe acute rejection as a result of noncompliance, rather than changes associated with chronic rejection. The Louisville CTA Program has transplanted 6 patients with follow-up of 12, 10, 4, and 2 years, and 9 and 6 months. Prior to the loss of the graft in Patient 4 at 9 months, no evidence of fibrosis, skin thinning, loss of adnexa, or atrophy in the skin had been documented; nor were any changes noted in vascular studies including annual brachial indices, magnetic resonance angiography, and duplex Doppler, which would indicate significant vascular disease.

The progam has performed extensive analysis of the graft and have also reevaluated 4 longer-term hand transplant recipients from their center. Although standard vascular studies did not show evidence of chronic rejection, review of deep tissue biopsies showed evidence of some intimal hyperplasia in all 4 patients. It was determined that the cause of graft loss in Patient 4 was severe obliterative intimal hyperplasia of the arterial tree, especially of the deep vessels, with relative sparing of the skin, muscle, nerves, and venous tissue. This analysis suggests a primary target of rejection in CTA recipients may not be the skin, but rather the arterial tree. Subsequent to this finding a research study was initiated using ultrasound biomicroscopy as a means to noninvasively monitor intimal hyperplasia. This technology, manufactured by Visual Sonics (Toronto, ON, Canada) is capable of noninvasively measuring the intima and medial layers of arteries from the brachial artery down to the digital arteries with a resolution of up to 30 μm.

In August 2010, the Louisville CTA Program transplanted their first bilateral hand recipient. This patient was unique because it was the first case of transplanting a patient who was not an amputee. He had his hands, though they were not functional secondary to a severe burn; this allowed maintenance of longer lengths and better quality of tendon and nerves than in a normal amputee. This patient did very well initially, and was able to form a partial fist on both sides at the first dressing change on day 3 post transplant. On the right side the patient developed a vascular occlusion of his arteries, which required a revision repair of the anastomosis. This procedure led to vascular compromise of the donor forearm tissue and eventually the distal thumb and small finger. Multiple debridements of the necrotic tissue and skin grafting of the forearm were necessary, followed by amputation of the thumb through the interphalangeal joint and the small finger through the distal interphalangeal joint.

During this period, the patient also had swelling of both hands and 2 biopsies with grade II histologic rejection. The second episode, which occurred on day 82 after transplant, was associated with significant swelling. Because of poor flow, this swelling contributed to the ischemia of the thumb and small finger, leading to the aforementioned distal amputation. The patient responded well to intravenous boluses of methylprednisolone (Solu-Medrol), with resolution of swelling and the rash. The patient was discharged to his home town on day 126, and is currently receiving therapy 3 times a week and is doing well.

Functionally this patient, who was severely disabled and required a 24-hour attendant at the time of surgery, is doing very well. He can now perform many activities of daily living, including eating, drinking from a water bottle, shaving, brushing his teeth, turning pages of a book, picking up a Kleenex and blowing his nose, opening doors (including a car door), pulling on his underwear and t-shirts, and turning lights on and off. His Carroll test score at the time of discharge was 59.

In summary, the functional outcomes and intermediate results of hand transplantation have far exceeded early expectations. Because of complications from immunosuppressive medications, our program has aggressively pursued immunosuppression minimization. The graft loss due to severe intimal hyperplasia may or may not be related to the reduced immunosuppression used in this patient. However, as a result of this event the program was motivated to pursue an experimental technology that should make future trials of immunosuppression reduction easier to monitor, and therefore safer. The Louisville CTA Program looks forward to working with colleagues at other CTA centers to achieve the ultimate goal of restoring function and quality of life to the thousands of patients living with devastating tissue loss.

ACKNOWLEDGMENTS

Any CTA program is a multidisciplinary effort between the surgeons, physicians, hand therapists, healthcare workers, scientists, institutions and the administration as well as our funding agencies. Specifically we would like to acknowledge the stellar surgeons who have donated their efforts including Drs Tsu-Min Tsai, Luis Scheker, Huey Tien, Tuna Ozyurekoglu, Rodrigo Moreno, Michelle Palazzo, Sunil Thirkannad and Rodrigo Banegas, as well as dozens of our hand surgery fellows who participated over the years. We would also like to thank the current Co-PIs of the study, Dr Joseph Kutz and Dr Michael Marvin, as well at the transplant groups at Jewish Hospital and St. Mary's Healthcare and the University of Louisville. Finally, we would like to acknowledge the dozens of colleagues and associates from around the world who have generously offered their support and guidance over the years.

REFERENCES

1. Magliocca JF, Knechtle SJ. The evolving role of alemtuzumab (Campath-1H) for immunosuppressive therapy in organ transplantation. Transpl Int 2006;19(9): 705–14.
2. Morris PJ, Russell NK. Alemtuzumab (Campath-1H): a systematic review in organ transplantation. Transplantation 2006;81(10):1361–7.
3. Brenner MJ, Tung TH, Jensen JN, et al. The spectrum of complications of immunosuppression: is the time right for hand transplantation? J Bone Joint Surg Am 2002;84(10):1861–70.
4. Jensen JN, Mackinnon SE. Composite tissue allotransplantation: a comprehensive review of the literature—part II. J Reconstr Microsurg 2000;16(2): 141–57.
5. Lineaweaver WC. Chronic rejection, hand transplantation, and the monkey's paw. Microsurgery 2006; 26(6):419–20.
6. Ferrara JL, Deeg HJ. Graft-versus-host disease. N Engl J Med 1991;324(10):667–74.
7. Ferrara JL, Levine JE, Reddy P, et al. Graft-versus-host disease. Lancet 2009;373(9674):1550–61.
8. Lanzetta M, Petruzzo P, Margreiter R, et al. The International Registry on Hand and Composite Tissue Transplantation. Transplantation 2005;79(9): 1210–4.

World Experience After More Than a Decade of Clinical Hand Transplantation: Update on the Innsbruck Program

Theresa Hautz, MD[a], Timm O. Engelhardt, MD[b],
Annemarie Weissenbacher, MD[a],
Martin Kumnig, PhD, MSc[c], Bettina Zelger, MD[d],
Michael Rieger, MD[e], Gerhard Rumpold, PhD, MSc[c],
Gerhard Pierer, MD[b], Marina Ninkovic, MD[f],
Markus Gabl, MD[g], Hildegunde Piza-Katzer, MD[b],
Johann Pratschke, MD[a], Raimund Margreiter, MD[a],
Gerald Brandacher, MD[h], Stefan Schneeberger, MD[i],*

KEYWORDS

- Hand transplantation • Composite tissue • Rejection
- Immunosuppression • Outcome • Psychological aspects

Composite tissue allotransplantation (CTA) is a valid therapeutic option for complex tissue defects in patients in whom conventional reconstructive surgery is insufficient to achieve satisfactory results.[1–10] Candidates for CTA are patients who have suffered massive or complex loss of tissue with prosthesis being either unavailable or insufficient to restore body integrity and function. In such cases, reconstructive transplantation holds the potential of restoring range of motion in

Funding support: TILAK Foundation, Innsbruck, Austria.

The authors have nothing to disclose.

[a] Department of Visceral, Transplant and Thoracic Surgery, Center of Operative Medicine, Innsbruck Medical University, Anichstrasse 35, A-6020 Innsbruck, Austria

[b] Department of Plastic, Reconstructive and Aesthetic Surgery, Center of Operative Medicine, Innsbruck Medical University, Anichstrasse 35, A-6020 Innsbruck, Austria

[c] Division of Medical Psychology, Department of Psychiatry and Psychotherapy, Innsbruck Medical University, Schöpfstraße 23a, A-6020 Innsbruck, Austria

[d] Department of Pathology, Innsbruck Medical University, Müllerstraße 44, A-6020 Innsbruck, Austria

[e] Department of Radiology, Innsbruck Medical University, Anichstrasse 35, A-6020 Innsbruck, Austria

[f] Unit of Physical Medicine and Rehabilitation, Department of Visceral, Transplant and Thoracic Surgery, Center of Operative Medicine, Innsbruck Medical University, Anichstraße 35, A-6020 Innsbruck, Austria

[g] Department of Trauma Surgery and Sports Medicine, Center of Operative Medicine, Innsbruck Medical University, Innsbruck, Austria

[h] Department of Plastic and Reconstructive Surgery, Johns Hopkins University School of Medicine, Ross Research Building 749D, 720 Rutland Avenue, Baltimore, MD 21205, USA

[i] Department of Plastic and Reconstructive Surgery, Johns Hopkins University School of Medicine, Baltimore, MD 21287, USA

* Corresponding author.

E-mail address: stefan.schneeberger@i-med.ac.at

doi:10.1016/j.hcl.2011.07.004

combination with sensation, resulting in independence and social integration in everyday life.

Between March 2000 and May 2006, 3 patients underwent bilateral hand or forearm transplantation at the Innsbruck Medical University Hospital. Because satisfactory functional outcomes were achieved in these cases and encouraging results with unilateral hand transplantation had been described by others,[7,11,12] unilateral hand amputation was accepted as an indication for transplantation and a first case was performed in July 2009. Widening the spectrum of indication was also influenced by the introduction of moderate-dose to low-dose immunosuppressive protocols. With a total of 7 hands/forearms transplanted, Innsbruck University Hospital represents one of the largest hand transplant centers.

This article reviews the clinical courses of the 3 bilateral hand transplant recipients at our institution, with emphasis on function, immunosuppression, rejection, complications, and graft vascular changes. Bilateral versus unilateral hand amputation as an indication for transplantation is discussed, as well as psychological aspects in hand transplantation.

THE INNSBRUCK HAND TRANSPLANT PROGRAM
Bilateral Cases

Between 2000 and 2006, 3 male patients (23–47 years old) underwent bilateral hand (n = 2) or forearm (n = 1) transplantation at the Innsbruck Medical University Hospital. Comprehensive descriptions of patients and donor selection were published earlier.[2,6,13–16] The first patient was a 47-year-old policeman who had lost his hands when he attempted to deactivate a bomb in 1994. He received a bilateral hand transplant at the level of the wrists in March 2000. In February 2003, the second patient, a 41-year-old electrical engineer, who lost his hands and two-thirds of his forearms in an electrical accident, received a bilateral forearm transplantation. The third bilateral case was performed at the level of the midforearm in a 23-year-old student from the Ukraine in May 2006. He had lost both hands in a bomb blast in 2000. The first 2 patients had been equipped with myoelectrical prothesis before transplantation, and the third patient refused prostheses.

During this period, only bilateral amputation was accepted as an indication for hand transplantation at our center. Restoration of hand function including sensitivity, allowing patients to regain independence in everyday live, was considered as the major goal.

Establishment of the Working Group Reconstructive Transplantation Innsbruck and Establishment of Unilateral Hand Transplantation

In unilateral hand transplantation, patient selection is more challenging because much of the functional deficit is compensated by the remaining hand and a prosthesis. However, the patients' functional needs and psychological impairment differ between individuals. To evaluate the necessity for unilateral hand transplantation in selected cases with significant psychological impairment caused by distal unilateral traumatic amputation, close interdisciplinary evaluation had been suggested.

To meet these aims, a working group called Reconstructive Transplantation Innsbruck (RTi) was founded by members of the Department of Visceral, Transplant and Thoracic Surgery, Department of Plastic Surgery, Department of Traumatology, and Department of Medical Psychology at the Innsbruck Medical University in November 2008. Guidelines for patient selection in bilateral and, in particular, unilateral transplantation have been developed based on surgical, immunologic, and psychological parameters. As a consequence, a 4-step candidate selection algorithm has been introduced and includes basic hand surgical, immunologic, psychological screening (step 1); advanced psychological evaluation (step 2); advanced hand surgical/immunologic diagnostics (step 3); helping to find an interdisciplinary consensus (step 4).

Recommendations have been developed for donor selection, surgical procedures, immunosuppression (IS) protocols, postoperative hand therapy, as well as psychological supportive therapy and detailed psychological follow-up testing including a preliminary suitability score for unilateral and bilateral transplantation.

Applying this novel selection algorithm, the first unilateral case was performed in July 2009 in a 54-year-old man, who lost his right hand in a woodworking accident in 2004. The unilateral hand transplantation was performed at the level of the very distal forearm. Inclusion criteria included significant psychological impairment following step 2 evaluation and loss of quality of life (manuscript in preparation).

PSYCHOLOGICAL ASPECTS IN HAND TRANSPLANT RECIPIENTS

One of the main psychological and psychosocial gains with hand transplantation is the improvement of quality of life, including the improvement of body image, after loss of 1 or both hands. A psychological assessment of potential hand transplant candidates includes evaluation of quality of life and describes psychological resources and coping strategies for the postoperative period.[17–20]

Motivation for Hand Transplantation

The motives driving patients to seek hand transplantation are diverse and depend on many factors such as functional impairment, lack of sensation, social integration, and the patients' overall physical or psychological status. In general, patients suffering from loss of 1 hand primarily report difficulties with coping and psychological burden, whereas patients with a bilateral loss particularly suffer from the functional impairment and loss of quality of life.

Body image has increasingly been functionalized and standardized by our society. Deviations from the ideal body image are often associated with self-esteem deficits. Body image is not only constituted by body shape, but it also depends on an individual's imagination of the body and the sum of body-related experiences and manifests itself mostly during puberty. Subsequently, body image is primarily influenced by social norms. Because body shape has gained increasing attention in the present, appearance-oriented society, it plays an important role in social integration and self-esteem.

As a consequence, it is increasingly difficult to live with physical deficits, to cope with the related psychological distress, and to compensate for the disadvantage in social integration. Reconstructive transplantation represents a novel method that allows for reconstitution of not only function but also body integrity. Therefore, the evaluation of emotional aspects represents an essential parameter in the psychological assessment of potential candidates for unilateral /bilateral hand transplantation.

Psychological Evaluation of Candidates for Reconstructive Hand Transplantation in Innsbruck

In the last decade, 4 candidates passed the clinical psychological assessment for bilateral or unilateral hand/forearm transplantation at our institution. All 4 candidates showed multiple, but minor, psychological irregularities as well as a reduced quality of life following hand/forearm amputation. Two candidates were declined because of psychiatric contraindications. Specifically, the required psychological resources and copying strategies were lacking.

Before transplantation, the strongest motivational aspect in the 3 bilateral hand or forearm transplant recipients was the expected improvement in function and quality of life. Concerns were primarily related to personal economic development. The primary motive in the patient suffering from unilateral hand amputation was his psychosocial well-being and the associated quality of life. Issues such as social withdrawal, embarrassment, reduced self-esteem, and a depressive coping style represented the essential elements in the psychological assessment of this patient.

To assess potential candidates for unilateral/bilateral reconstructive hand transplantation, a standardized Psychological Screening Program for Reconstructive Transplantation (iRT-PSP) was introduced recently. It consists of a detailed psychological interview that covers central issues related to reconstructive transplantation (eg, motivational aspects, coping skills, general compliance, concept of body and self, quality of life) and uses the following psychometric instruments for screening procedures and follow-up ratings: (1) Response Evaluation Measure (REM-71; a survey to evaluate an individual's defense mechanisms[21]), (2) Brief Symptom Inventory (BSI; a general evaluation of psychiatric symptoms[22,23]), (3) Essener Coping Questionnaire (a German questionnaire to measure disease-associated coping skills[24]), (4) Life Orientation Test-Revised (LOT-R; a test to assess individual differences in generalized optimism vs pessimism[25,26]), (5) Medication Experience Scale for Immunosuppressants (a German scale to evaluate compliance, focusing on immunosuppressants[27]), (6) Multidimensional Body-Self Relations Questionnaire (MBSRQ; a questionnaire to measure body image and organ fantasies[28,29]), (7) SF-36 Health Survey (a survey to measure quality of life[30,31]), and (8) the Transplant Effect Scale (TxEQ; a scale to measure potential post-transplant effects[32,33]) (**Table 1**).

We believe that pretransplant psychological assessment and posttransplant psychological counseling is essential for critical evaluation of the suitability of potential transplant candidates and may help to minimize the psychological morbidity of hand transplant recipients.[34–36]

Psychological Considerations and the Unilateral versus Bilateral Hand Transplantation Debate

Because restoration of function was considered to be the main goal, only bilateral amputees were accepted as candidates for hand or forearm

Table 1
Psychometric instruments of the Innsbruck Psychological Screening Program for Reconstructive Transplantation (iRT-PSP) and appendant constructs

REM-71 by Steiner et al[21]; German version Abwehrfragebogen by Schüßler et al (manuscript in preparation)	Survey to evaluate an individual's defense mechanisms
BSI by Derogatis et al[22]; German version by Franke[23]	General evaluation of psychiatric symptoms
Essener Coping Questionnaire (Essener Fragebogen zur Krankheitsverarbeitung) by Franke et al[24], (adapted for unilateral/bilateral hand transplantation)	German Questionnaire to measure disease-associated coping skills
LOT-R by Scheier et al[25]; German version by Glaesmern et al[26]	Test to assess individual differences in generalized optimism vs pessimism
Medication Experience Scale for Immunosuppressants (Medikamenten Skala für Immunsuppressiva) by Goetzmann et al[27]	German scale to evaluate compliance, focusing on immunosuppressants
MBSRQ by Brown[28]; German version by Mühlan and Schmidt[29] (additional items to evaluate potential organ fantasies [Kumnig et al, in preparation])	Questionnaire to measure body image and organ fantasies
SF-36 Health Survey by Ware et al[30]; German version by Bullinger and Kirchberger[31]	Survey to measure quality of life
TxEQ by Ziegelmann et al[32]; German version by Klaghofer et al[21,33]	Scale to measure potential posttransplant effects (eg, adherence, responsibility)

transplantation at our institute in the early stage of our program. For unilateral hand amputees, it was assumed that the remaining hand might suffice for most motoric, sensoric, and communicating functions. However, patients' functional needs and psychological impairment differ between individuals. Moreover, individual psychological distress may affect the benefit/risk ratio of the side effects caused by immunosuppression.

Therefore, the assessment of potential psychological assets and drawbacks of unilateral versus bilateral hand transplantation should include an evaluation of the patient's concept of body and self. Based on our clinical experience, the surgical restoration of a patient's damaged concept of body and self represents one of the central motivational aspects for surgery, especially in newly injured patients. In this regard, newly injured patients might be different from patients who have been living with the amputation for many years because they have learned to integrate the defect in their individual concepts of body and self and to cope with their imperfections. Some essential psychological differences between unilateral and bilateral amputees regarding motivational aspects, coping skills, compliance, concept of body and self, and quality of life should be assessed routinely by initial psychological assessment and continuous follow-up before and after hand transplantation. Particular

attention should be paid to differences between candidates for unilateral and bilateral hand transplantation. Ideally, a multicenter trial investigating psychological and psychosocial aspects in candidates for unilateral and bilateral hand transplantation should be pursued to obtain information on these important aspects and to serve as the basis for development of a standardized psychological screening protocol.

SURGERY

The surgical procedures were performed by teams comprising members of the Department of Plastic Surgery and Traumatology for all transplants. As described previously for cases 1 and 2, the recipient stumps and the donor forearms were prepared simultaneously.[2,6,13] Ulnar and radial artery, 1 palmar and 2 dorsal veins, the median and ulnar nerve, and the superficial branch of the radial nerve, as well as all extensor and flexor tendons, were identified proximally and distally and marked for musculoskeletal and microsurgical vascular/neural reconstruction.

In summary, following bone fixation, arterial and venous anastomoses were performed (radial and ulnar artery and a varying number of deep and superficial veins in the individual cases).[2,6,13,37] Subsequently, all hand and finger flexor and extensor tendons were attached. The ulnar and median nerve were coapted thereafter. Reconstruction of the radial nerve branches varied between patients. At the end of the procedure, skin flaps were approximated without tension. In patient 1, several muscles of the left forearm were insufficient or even missing, which required tendon repair en masse or by transpositioning.[2] Clinical observation and oxygen saturation monitoring confirmed patency of vessels and regular blood flow. Skin necrosis required skin grafts in all 3 bilateral hand transplant recipients. Long-term, patency of the vasculature was investigated using Doppler ultrasound.

To prevent ischemia/reperfusion injury (IRI), ischemia time was kept short in all cases. Time intervals between arteriovenous cross-clamping and reperfusion of the allograft were 150/170, 155/153, and 190/210 minutes in patients 1, 2, and 3, respectively. A short ischemia time was considered particularly important in the second case, in which a large quantity of skeletal muscle was transplanted. Allografts were flushed with cold Custodiol (HTK) or University of Wisconsin (UW) preservation solution.

Early Secondary Procedures

Split-thickness skin grafts were needed for defect coverage of the left forearm in patient 1.[2,14] Multiple arteriovenous fistulas required occlusion at 6 months after surgery. Skin grafting for wound closure was also necessary in case 2. In patient 3, 2 episodes of immediate postoperative soft tissue swelling caused by hematoma required surgical revision and defect coverage using split-thickness skin grafts at 1 week.

Late Secondary Procedures

Aesthetic scar excisions were performed in patient 2 in 2005.[14] In the third patient, surgical scar correction in the face and simultaneous scar and skin graft resection on both forearms was performed at 1 year. Two years after hand transplantation, insufficient palmar abduction and opposition of the thumb required an opponensplasty by transposing the superficial flexor tendon of the patient's ring finger.

Managing Neuromusculoskeletal Reconstruction in Forearm Transplantation

In forearm transplantation, detailed preoperative clinical, radiological, and neurologic examination is mandatory to evaluate the functional capacity of remaining neuromuscular units. Adequate length and intact innervation of the recipient's remaining musculature are critical for achieving normal functional capacity of the neuromuscular

units involved. Innervated short muscular remnants may need replacement by an entire neuromuscular unit of the donor with higher vulnerability to ischemia including motor nerve coaptation. Hence a longer time frame for neuromuscular regeneration in proximal forearm transplantation has to be expected when compared with hand transplantation at the wrist level.

In patient 2, missing and insufficient muscles required replacement by neuromuscular units of the donor.[6,15] Innervated remnants of forearm muscles were left untouched for possible use of a myoelectrical prosthesis in case of graft loss (lifeboat maneuver). Flexor muscles of the donor were attached to the medial epicondyle of the humerus, ulnar extensor carpi, and extensor digitorum communis to the periosteum of the ulna. Anterior and posterior interosseus nerve, as well as the motor branches of the median nerve for pronator teres, flexor carpi radialis, flexor digitorum superficialis, and palmaris longus, were coapted. Coaptation of the ulnar nerve was performed distal to the intact motor branches of the FCU.

GRAFT MONITORING

Grafts monitoring for rejection can be performed by visual inspection. Skin biopsies were regularly taken for histopathologic and immunohistochemical investigation (protocol biopsy) or whenever skin rejection was suspected (for cause biopsies). For evaluation of bone healing, radiographs and color Doppler sonography were performed regularly during the first year after transplantation. Graft vessels, nerves, muscles, and tendons were monitored by ultrasound. In addition, angiography and computed tomography angiography with three-dimensional reconstruction of graft vessels were performed once a year for assessment of chronic vascular changes.

No complications regarding bone regeneration were reported in any patient. As reported for patient 1, bone healing after hand transplantation was not influenced or altered by immunosuppression, compared with replantation.[37,38] Vascular invasion and callus formation appeared at week 3, calcified callus was observed at 4 months after transplantation, and bone union was completed after 11 months. In patient 2, the right forearm flexors revealed signs of fibrosis and ossification, resulting in dissection of this small compartment.[6] Vascular patency of graft vessels was documented in all cases, showing stable proportions and consistent perfusion of all tissue components.[14] No radiomorphologic signs of luminal narrowing as indicators for myointimal proliferation and chronic rejection were observed. In patient

1, kinking of the ulnar and radial arteries as a result of long vessels was observed.[2] In addition, an occlusion of the right radial artery was detected at 1 year in this patient, which was found to have recanalized at 4 years after transplantation.[4]

FUNCTIONAL OUTCOME
Rehabilitation Protocol and Functional Assessment

Principles of the rehabilitation program were published previously.[2,4] In brief, the rehabilitation program was based on an early protective motion program (EPM) in combination with cognitive exercise training after Perfetti, electrostimulation, and occupational therapy and adjusted to the type of transplant (hand vs forearm), the individual patient's needs, and the level of progress. The major goal of the rehabilitation protocol was to enable independence in basic activities of daily life and hence to increase the patient's quality of life and psychological well-being. Motor function and hand sensitivity, as well as electrophysiologic studies and somatosensory evoked potentials, were studied at close intervals during the first 5 years after surgery and annually thereafter. Hand function was evaluated and documented by a variety of tests and scoring systems, as described earlier.[6]

Function

For patient 1, updates on hand function were published at 1.5, 5, and 8 years, respectively.[2,4,13,14] The progress in functional and sensory recovery was outstanding in this patient. At 4 months, intrinsic muscle activity was observed for the first time. After the first year after transplantation, the patient was able to perform activities of daily life (except buttoning a shirt[2]), and was back to work at a police station by then. At 1 year, thermal discrimination, pressure sensation, sensitivity to pain, and 2-point discrimination sensation were present in hand and fingers of the right and left allograft. Hand function and sensitivity continuously improved until year 5 after transplantation and remained stable thereafter. The patient experienced a fracture of the left radius at month 56, which resulted in a transient decrease in active range of motion at 5 years. After 5 years, total active range of motion increased and decreased for some joints, but remained stable overall.

In the forearm transplant recipient, update on functioning was given at 3, 5, and 6 years' follow-up.[6,14,15] Compared with patient 1, motor function was inferior at all time points; however, a continuous improvement in hand function was observed during the first 3 years after surgery.

The patient described hand function as superior to the function he experienced with myoelectrical prostheses. Temperature discrimination was apparent for the first time at 6 months, although sensitivity overall remained poor. Dexterity was slightly inferior to that observed after hand transplantation.

In the third transplant recipient, rehabilitation was complicated by blindness. An update was provided at 2 years after transplantation.[14] At that time, the patient was still receiving intensive physiotherapy and rehabilitation. According to the Hand Transplantation Score System, functional outcome at 1 year after surgery was graded as 64 and 65.5 out of 100 for the left and the right hand, respectively.[39] Hand function improved during another year after transplantation and signs of intrinsic muscle recovery were detected by then.

Nerve conduction studies revealed that motor and also sensory action potentials not only increased by an early time point after transplantation but also after 4–5 years after transplantation.[14] These findings show that nerve regeneration can also be expected at later periods after hand transplantation.

IMMUNOSUPPRESSION AND IMMUNOLOGIC COMPLICATIONS
Immunosuppression

Induction therapy with antithymocyte globulin (ATG) was used in the first 2 patients and alemtuzumab (Campath-1H) in the third patient. Tacrolimus, prednisone, and mycophenolate mofetil (MMF) were used for maintenance. Tacrolimus trough levels of 15 ng/mL were targeted during the first month and reduced thereafter. Steroids were tapered in a stepwise fashion and withdrawn in patients 1 and 2 between year 3 and 5. In patient 1, sirolimus was started at 2 years and tacrolimus was eventually withdrawn at 5 years. In patients 2 and 3, everolimus was added to the maintenance IS and tacrolimus is currently being weaned.[4,6,14]

Rejection Episodes, Treatment and Current Immunosuppression

All patients experienced at least 1 acute rejection episode within the first year after transplantation. The onset of the first rejection episode was at postoperative day 55, 9, and 51 in patients 1, 2, and 3 respectively.[14] A total of 3, 6, and 4 rejection episodes were observed. The appearance of the skin lesions was mostly scattered, nonconfluent, and restricted to a defined region either on the forearm of dorsum of the hand. However, a characteristic pattern of rejection was observed for each patient.

Patient 1 experienced only 2 mild rejections[2,4] (grade 1–2). Treatment with topical tacrolimus and steroid ointments, intravenous (IV) steroids, and restart of tacrolimus treatment for 8 months (after tacrolimus had been withdrawn) were effective. The postoperative course of the forearm transplant recipient (patient 2) was challenged by increasingly severe rejections compared with patient 1. A comprehensive report on this topic is given elsewhere.[6,14,40] In brief, 2 mild rejection episodes occurred on days 9 and 46 followed by severe (grade IV and III) rejections on days 95 and 345 and 2 more mild (grade I) rejections on days 473 and 972. Therapy included IV steroids, topical steroids, basiliximab, ATG, and alemtuzumab. In patient 3, a first rejection was observed on day 51 (grade 2) followed by a rejection grade 3 that was restricted to the palm on day 60 and a rejection grade 2 on day 601.[14] Although the first rejection responded promptly to IV steroids, the second episode required administration of alemtuzumab. A detailed report of the second, atypical rejection episode was published earlier.[39] No donor cells were found in the blood of any recipient during the follow-up period, indicating that no chimerism is induced with hand or forearm transplantation and conventional immunosuppressive therapy.[14]

COMPLICATIONS AND SIDE EFFECTS

Aggressive immunosuppressive regimens have been used in hand transplantation and an intensified treatment is necessary on rejection. Infectious prophylaxis consisted of piperacillin/tazobactam (patient 1, 2) or amoxicillin/clavulanic acid (patient 3), fluconazole (patient 2), ganciclovir (patient 1) or ganciclovir/valganciclovir (patients 2 and 3) and trimetoprim/sulfametoxazole (given during the first year in all patients).

As published earlier,[41,42] cytomegalovirus (CMV)-associated disease was detected in all 3 double hand allograft recipients. The donor/recipient CMV combination was d+/r−, d+/r+, and d+/r+ for patients 1, 2, and 3 respectively. In the first 2 patients, CMV infection was resistant to valgancyclovir but controlled with anti-CMV hyperimmunoglobulin, foscarnet, and cidofovir. Because of foscarnet treatment, patient 1 experienced nausea and diarrhea, and patient 2 developed severe neutropenia triggered by valgancylovir around day 150. Cidofovir and anti-CMV hyperimmunoglobulin treatment resulted in edema of both transplanted hands in the second case. The third patient experienced repetitive, but mild, CMV infections, which were successfully treated with valgancyclovir. In the forearm recipient, an invasive fungal infection and human papilloma virus (HPV)–associated skin warts scattered over the thumbs of the allografts required treatment. Noninfectious side effects included hypertension (patient 2, 3) resulting in severe headaches in patient 2, a transient increase of creatinine levels (patient 1, 2, 3), non–insulin-dependent diabetes mellitus (patient 1), and hyperlipidemia (patient 2, 3). After repeated administration of alemtuzumab because of severe rejection episodes, patient 3 developed nausea, fever, headache, and edema requiring hospitalization and monitoring of hemodynamic parameters.

DISCUSSION

In summary, good functional results and a high degree of patient satisfaction have been achieved with bilateral hand transplantation in Innsbruck. Acute rejection episodes, especially during an early period, are common complications; this was also recorded in the latest update of The International Registry of Hand and Composite Tissue Transplantation.[43] The follow-up of approximately 80% of recipients was challenged by an acute rejection episode before year 1 after transplantation. Although immunosuppressive regimens were more aggressive during the early period, moderate-dose to low-dose IS protocols were successful in preventing additional rejections and graft loss in all 3 cases. Weaning from steroids, tapering IS trough levels, and conversion from calcineurin inhibitors to mammalian target of rapamycin (mTOR) inhibitors seems possible in all patients.

No radiomorphologic changes in graft bone, muscular texture, and nerve anastomoses were detected in any patient. Vascular changes were observed rarely and only 1 minor complication required further intervention. Monitoring for chronic vascular changes is of utmost importance. So far, no evidence of chronic vascular changes have been observed in any patient transplanted in Innsbruck.

Infections are common complications observed after reconstructive transplantation, especially on intensified IS. Early and accurate diagnosis, as well as specific treatment, is required in these cases. IS-sparing protocols might help to reduce complications and side effects.

REFERENCES

1. Dubernard JM, Henry P, Parmentier H, et al. First transplantation of two hands: results after 18 months. Ann Chir 2002;127(1):19–25 [in French].

2. Margreiter R, Brandacher G, Ninkovic M, et al. A double-hand transplant can be worth the effort! Transplantation 2002;74(1):85–90.

3. Petruzzo P, Badet L, Gazarian A, et al. Bilateral hand transplantation: six years after the first case. Am J Transplant 2006;6(7):1718–24.

4. Schneeberger S, Ninkovic M, Piza-Katzer H, et al. Status 5 years after bilateral hand transplantation. Am J Transplant 2006;6(4):834–41.

5. Schuind F, Van Holder C, Mouraux D, et al. The first Belgian hand transplantation–37 month term results. J Hand Surg Br 2006;31(4):371–6.

6. Schneeberger S, Ninkovic M, Gabl M, et al. First forearm transplantation: outcome at 3 years. Am J Transplant 2007;7(7):1753–62.

7. Breidenbach WC, Gonzales NR, Kaufman CL, et al. Outcomes of the first 2 American hand transplants at 8 and 6 years posttransplant. J Hand Surg Am 2008; 33(7):1039–47.

8. Petruzzo P, Lanzetta M, Dubernard JM, et al. The international registry on hand and composite tissue transplantation. Transplantation 2008;86(4):487–92.

9. Cavadas PC, Landin L, Ibanez J. Bilateral hand transplantation: result at 20 months. J Hand Surg Eur Vol 2009;34(4):434–43.

10. Jablecki J, Kaczmarzyk L, Domanasiewicz A, et al. Hand transplantation–Polish program. Transplant Proc 2010;42(8):3321–2.

11. Kaufman CL, Blair B, Murphy E, et al. A new option for amputees: transplantation of the hand. J Rehabil Res Dev 2009;46(3):395–404.

12. Jablecki J, Kaczmarzyk L, Domanasiewicz A, et al. Hand transplant - outcome after 6 months, preliminary report. Ortop Traumatol Rehabil 2010;12(1):90–9.

13. Piza-Katzer H, Ninkovic M, Pechlaner S, et al. Double hand transplantation: functional outcome after 18 months. J Hand Surg Br 2002;27(4):385–90.

14. Brandacher G, Ninkovic M, Piza-Katzer H, et al. The Innsbruck Hand Transplant Program: update at 8 years after the first transplant. Transplant Proc 2009;41(2):491–4.

15. Gabl M, Blauth M, Lutz M, et al. Musculoskeletal reconstruction in bilateral forearm transplantation. Handchir Mikrochir Plast Chir 2009;41(4):224–9 [in German].

16. Piza-Katzer H, Wechselberger G, Estermann D, et al. Ten years of hand transplantation experiment or routine? Handchir Mikrochir Plast Chir 2009; 41(4):210–6 [in German].

17. Klapheke MM, Marcell C, Taliaferro G, et al. Psychiatric assessment of candidates for hand transplantation. Microsurgery 2000;20(8):453–7.

18. Klapheke MM. The role of the psychiatrist in organ transplantation. Bull Menninger Clin 1999; 63(1):13–39.

19. Lees VC, McCabe SJ. The rationale for hand transplantation. Transplantation 2002;74(6):749–53.

20. Klapheke MM. Transplantation of the human hand: psychiatric considerations. Bull Menninger Clin 1999; 63(1):159–73.

21. Steiner H, Araujo KB, Koopman C. The response evaluation measure (REM-71): a new instrument for the measurement of defenses in adults and adolescents. Am J Psychiatry 2001;158(3):467–73.

22. Derogatis LR. Brief Symptom Inventory (BSI): administration, scoring, and procedures manual. 4th Edition. Minneapolis (MN): National Computer Services; 1993.

23. Franke GH. Brief Symptom Inventory von L.R. Derogatis (Kurzform der SCL-90-R). Deutsche Version. Göttingen: Beltz Test GmbH; 2000a.

24. Franke GH, Mähner N, Reimer J, et al. Erste Überprüfung des Essener Fragebogens zur Krankheitsbewältigung (EFK) an sehbeeinträchtigten Patienten. Z Diff Diag Psychol 2000;21:166–72 [in German].

25. Scheier MF, Carver CS, Bridges MW. Distinguishing optimism from neuroticism (and trait anxiety, self-mastery, and self-esteem): a reevaluation of the Life Orientation Test. J Pers Soc Psychol 1994; 67(6):1063–78.

26. Glaesmer H, Hoyer J, Klotsche J, et al. Deutsche Version des Life-Orientation-Tests (LOT-R) zum dispositionellen Optimismus und Pessimismus. Z Gesundheitspsychol 2008;16:26–31 [in German].

27. Goetzmann L, Klaghofer R, Spindler A, et al. The "Medication Experience Scale for Immunosuppressants" (MESI): initial results for a new screening instrument in transplant medicine. Psychother Psychosom Med Psychol 2006;56(2):49–55 [in German].

28. Brown TA, Cash TF, Mikulka PJ. Attitudinal body-image assessment: factor analysis of the Body-Self Relations Questionnaire. J Pers Assess 1990;55(1–2): 135–44.

29. Mühlan H, Schmidt S. Multidimensional Body-Self Relations Questionnaire - Deutsche version. In: Kupfer J, Schmidt S, Augustion M, editors. Diagnostische Testverfahren für die Dermatologie. Göttingen (Germany): Hogrefe; 2006. p. 152–6.

30. Ware JE, Snow KK, Kosinski M, et al. SF-36 Health Survey manual and interpretation guide. Boston, MA: New England Medical Center, The Health Institute; 1993.

31. Bullinger M, Kirchberger I. SF-26 Fragebogen zum Gesundheitszustand: Handanweisung. Göttingen: Hogrefe; 1998 [in German].

32. Ziegelmann JP, Griva K, Hankins M, et al. The Transplant Effects Questionnaire (TxEQ): the development of a questionnaire for assessing the multidimensional outcome of organ transplantation - example of end stage renal disease (ESRD). Br J Health Psychol 2002;7(Part 4):393–408.

33. Klaghofer R, Nera S, Schwegler K, et al. Questionnaire on emotional response after organ transplantation: German validation of the Transplant Effect

Questionnaire (TxEQ-D). Z Psychosom Med Psychother 2008;54:174–88.

34. Dew MA, Switzer GE, DiMartini AF, et al. Psychosocial assessments and outcomes in organ transplantation. Prog Transplant 2000;10(4):239–59 [quiz: 260–1].

35. Geller SE, Connolly T. The influence of psychosocial factors on heart transplantation decisions and outcomes. J Transpl Coord 1997;7(4):173–9.

36. Craven J, Rodin G. Psychiatric aspects of organ transplantation. Oxford: Oxford University Press; 1992.

37. Gabl M, Pechlaner S, Lutz M, et al. Bilateral hand transplantation: bone healing under immunosuppression with tacrolimus, mycophenolate mofetil, and prednisolone. J Hand Surg Am 2004;29(6): 1020–7.

38. Gabl M, Pechlaner S, Lutz M, et al. Bone healing in hand transplantation. In: Lanzetta M, Dubernard JM. Hand transplantation. New York: Springer-Verlag; 2007. p. 271–7.

39. Schneeberger S, Gorantla VS, van Riet RP, et al. Atypical acute rejection after hand transplantation. Am J Transplant 2008;8(3):688–96.

40. Schneeberger S, Kreczy A, Brandacher G, et al. Steroid- and ATG-resistant rejection after double forearm transplantation responds to Campath-1H. Am J Transplant 2004;4(8):1372–4.

41. Schneeberger S, Lucchina S, Lanzetta M, et al. Cytomegalovirus-related complications in human hand transplantation. Transplantation 2005;80(4): 441–7.

42. Bonatti H, Brandacher G, Margreiter R, et al. Infectious complications in three double hand recipients: experience from a single center. Transplant Proc 2009;41(2):517–20.

43. Petruzzo P, Lanzetta M, Dubernard JM, et al. The International Registry on Hand and Composite Tissue Transplantation. Transplantation 2010;90(12): 1590–4.

World Experience After More Than a Decade of Clinical Hand Transplantation: Update on the Polish Program

Jerzy Jabłecki, MD, PhD[a,b,*]

KEYWORDS

- Hand transplantation • Composite tissue allografts
- Cytomegalovirus infection • Bony union

Living with any type of deficit or deformity has become increasingly difficult in our modern societies, which value appearance that reflects on our emotional, physical, and social well-being. No doubt transplantation nowadays should be considered not only to prolong or to save lives but also to improve one's quality of life. It has been demonstrated over the past decade that the generally achieved functional outcomes of patients after hand transplantation (HTx) are better than those of equivalent replantations.[1,2] However, HTx should be performed in specialized centers with Institutional Review Board–approved transplantation programs. In Poland such requirements are fulfilled by The Subdepartment of Replantation of Limbs of St. Jadwiga Hospital in Trzebnica. The institutional strength of this subdepartment, which is the oldest of its kind in Europe (formed in 1973), lay in a large hand surgery program with a high number of extremity replants, and a strong multiorgan transplant division located nearby. The author's group declared its intention to proceed with HTx at this program through announcements in the lay press and professional journals as well as via public media. Along this line, a main emphasis of the subdepartment is to make the very involved process of donor recruitment, recipient screening, surgery, and postoperative treatment fully transparent. This article summarizes the experience of this center with HTx over the past 5 years.

This program adhered to the following inclusion criteria implemented by the groups of Lanzetta, Schneebherger, Brandacher[3–5] and others: recipient age between 18 and 55 years, traumatic amputation of dominant hand or bilateral upper limbs at any level below mid-humerus, patient tried and failed or refused different prosthetic alternatives, otherwise healthy and mentally stable, able to give informed consent, resident in the country, available for follow-up, and sufficient family support.

A total of 68 individuals were evaluated over a 5-year period. According to the selection process and inclusion criteria, 15 patients were considered to be potential candidates for HTx. These 15 patients then proceeded to a formal hospital admission after signing the detailed informed consent, to sustain a thorough evaluationincluding diagnostic tests (ie, blood tests, magnetic resonance imaging, psychological evaluation, muscle and sensory evaluation, ultrasound, human immunodeficiency virus and hepatitis C tests). The group invited for full screening consisted

The authors have nothing to disclose.
^a Subdepartment of Replantation of Limbs, St Jadwiga Hospital, 55-100 Trzebnica, ul Prusicka 53, Poland
^b State Higher Medical Professional School, 45–060 Opole, ul. Katowicka 68, Poland
* Subdepartment of Replantation of Limbs, St Jadwiga Hospital, 55-100 Trzebnica, ul Prusicka 53, Poland.
E-mail address: jerzy.jablecki@interia.pl

Hand Clin 27 (2011) 433–442
doi:10.1016/j.hcl.2011.08.003

hand.theclinics.com

of 13 male patients (aged 21–55 years) with single, dominant hand amputation and 2 women (age 18 and 23 years) with bilateral hand amputation. Several other patients are currently undergoing screening for HTx, and those selected for transplantation will be wait-listed in the near future.

In the process of donor acquisition, the team cooperated with the National Center for Tissue Transplantation "Poltransplant." However, only 7 hospitals provided the Subdepartment with donor notifications, with the great majority from one center (6 notifications, 3 of which eventually led to transplantation). In 13 cases donors identified for hand transplantation could not be called upon. Reasons for this consisted of donor family refusal in 4 cases, with the remainder attributable to blood-type incompatibility (5 cases), limb size discrepancy (3 cases), and donor neoplasm (chorionepithelioma) diagnosed prior to procurement (1 case).

A total of 7 HTx were performed at the author's center in 6 patients. These cases include 5 male recipients transplanted in the following years: 2006 (mid-forearm level), 2007 (mid-forearm level), 2008 (distal forearm level), 2009 (distal humerus level), and 2010 (bilateral HTx, wrist level); and one female recipient (mid-arm level).

The individual transplant procedures are summarized here.

PATIENT 1
History

The patient was a 32-year-old man who lost his dominant right hand in an accident with a grinder 14 years prior to HTx. He was a manual worker but did not try to work after the accident, and reluctantly used only a cosmetic prosthesis.

Indication for Transplantation

Mid-forearm level amputation, with sufficient proximal muscles remaining to power a hand transplant. The patient demonstrated a strong motivation confirmed by Rorshach-Catell test, did not accept his disability, which markedly affected his body image, and presented with a highly integrated personality and high intelligence quotient (IQ = 96). Since the accident he had been receiving support from family and friends. The hand transplant procedure was performed in April 2006.

Immunosuppression (IS) Regimen

Patient 1 and all other recipients in the center received the following regimen. Induction: basiliximab, tacrolimus (FK506) 5 mg by mouth, mycophenolate mofetil (MMF) 2 g by mouth, methylprednisolone 1 g intravenously. Day 1: tacrolimus 5 mg by mouth twice a day, MMF 1 g by mouth twice a day, methylprednisolone 500 mg intravenously; day 2: basiliximab intravenously tacrolimus 5 mg by mouth twice a day, MMF 1 g by mouth twice a day; days 3–7: tacrolimus (to serum level 20 ng/mL), MMF by mouth 2g daily, methylprednisolone 500 mg intravenously. Maintenance: tacrolimus (target trough level 10–15 ng/mL). At present, 56 months after transplantation, IS consists of tacrolimus (trough level 10 ng/mL), steroids (5 mg/d), and MMF (2 g/d).

Relevant Surgical Details

The limb was obtained from a 47-year-old male multiorgan donor. The limb was procured prior to solid organs by disarticulation at the level of the elbow joint. There were 3 out of 6 HLA mismatches between donor and recipient; the cross-match result was negative. The recipient operation was performed with repair of structures in the following order: bones (2 rush pins)-muscles-nerves (median and ulnar)-veins (3)-arteries (2)-remaining veins (2) (BMNVAV). The total ischemic time was 10.5 h. Except for prolonged wound healing requiring a skin graft, the posttransplant course was uneventful. No other surgical procedures were performed in this patient.

Rehabilitation

A program similar to that being used for replantation cases after amputation at the mid-forearm level was applied. Passive physiotherapy was started on the second postoperative day. During the postoperative hospitalization, the patient underwent 4 (1-hour) sessions of intensive hand therapy. After 2 weeks, a device for continuous passive motions (CPM), Artromot "F," was applied and the range of motion was successively increased. After 5 weeks, protected active motion was implemented. Three weeks later activities with light resistance were added, supplemented by global stretching technique. At that time a dynamic outrigger splint was introduced. Electrostimulation was started on day 70 and was carried out twice daily since then. Between therapy sessions, the limb was kept in a custom-made orthosis maintaining wrist extension, with the thumb in palmar abduction and the fingers in intrinsic plus position. To promote cortical reintegration a special program designed by Perfetti was applied. The patient was discharged from the ward on posttransplant day 64.

Rejection Episodes and Treatment

This patient had one single rejection episode (grade I) 20 months after HTx, which correlated with an attempt to decrease the IS dose of tacrolimus. This rejection episode was controlled with topical tacrolimus and increases in maintenance IS.[6]

Major Complications

No serious complications were observed. Both serum blood urea nitrogen (BUN) and creatinine levels remained within their baseline (30 mg/dL and 1.0 mg/dL, respectively). Previously increased serum glucose (up to 130 mg/dL and hemoglobin A1c 7.8%) normalized, which prompted cessation of oral hypoglycemic therapy (acarbose 50 mg/d).

Functional Outcome

All patients discussed in this article are seen at regular intervals as per protocol, and at least once a year for follow-up and functional evaluation.

In Patient 1, motor function continuously improved from the end of year 1 to year 3, and has remained relatively stable thereafter. Total active motion of fingers (TAM) equals 60% of fingers of unaffected hand (Video 1). Evaluation by the Short Form 36 Questionnaire (0–136 points) protocol revealed a score of 53; evaluation by the Disability of Arm, Shoulder, and Hand (DASH) questionnaire (30–150 points) gave a score of 92; Chen's score system commonly used for assessment of replantation cases rated the patient as II (good); and the Comprehensive Functional Score System (CFSS)[3] scored 84 points (rated as excellent). Cold intolerance is mild, and the patient can localize stimuli with his eyes shut but cannot discriminate between differently shaped objects. He can also distinguish between different thermal stimuli, and there is some discriminative sensation (2-point discrimination [2PD] = 15 mm). After 56 months, function of intrinsic muscles could be confirmed by electromyography, but it was weak. The patient cannot spread his fingers or oppose the thumb. The muscle strength is also weak, the 2- and 3-point pinch is immeasurable, and the grip strength is 3 kg. The patient has fully incorporated the transplanted limb into his body image and has also regained self-confidence in social relationships. In addition, he is able to write, drive a car, ride a bicycle, holds large and medium objects of any form and shape (see Video 1; Video 2), and has a full-time manual job.[7] All psychosocial evaluations find that the patient is experiencing great satisfaction and happiness with his transplant. Investigation of hand arteries revealed no signs of occlusion or stenosis.

PATIENT 2
History

This 42-year-old man lost his dominant left hand in a circular saw accident in 1999 (8 years prior to HTx). He had a cosmetic prosthesis but refused to wear it. He worked half-time as a telephone salesman in his house prior to HTx.

Indications for Transplant

Mid-forearm amputation. The patient was highly motivated and successfully underwent hand transplantation in January 2008.

Relevant Surgical Details

The limb was obtained from a brain-dead female multiorgan donor; there were 5 out of 6 HLA mismatches between donor and recipient. The limb was procured using standard procedures and by disarticulation at the elbow joint. The operative recipient technique/sequence was similar to the one described for Patient 1; 2 main arteries and 4 veins (including one large cephalic vein) were anastomosed. Some disturbances in blood circulation within the hand were encountered intraoperatively. As the arterial anastomoses seemed patent, 5000 units of unfractionated heparin were administered followed by a continuous infusion of 1500 units/h (total dose 12,000 units) resulting in temporary improvement of blood circulation in the hand (pulse oximetry reached 85%). Total ischemic time was 9 hours. However, 26 hours after completing the HTx the blood circulation worsened again, and a revision of the arterial anastomosis was performed. Intraoperatively, both arterial anastomoses were found to be patent. However, arterial collaterals in the hand were thrombosed. A large clot was extracted from the radial artery at the wrist level, distally to the site of prior arterial line catheter placement. Ultimately the transplanted limb could not be saved and had to be reamputated. The patient was discharged 14 days after reamputation without any additional complications.

PATIENT 3
History

This 29-year-old man lost his dominant right hand in an industrial accident 7 years prior to HTx . He was a manual worker part-time after the accident, and was reluctant to wear a hook prosthesis (**Fig. 1**).

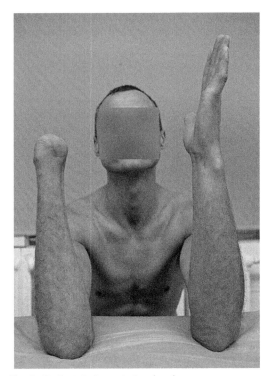

Fig. 1. Patient 3. Amputation level.

Indications for Transplant

Wrist-level amputation with intact wrist joint, with intact proximal row with some radiocarpal motion. The HTx was performed in September 2008.

Relevant Surgical Details

The limb was procured from a 52-year-old female multiorgan donor. The limb in this case was procured following solid organ harvest and was amputated at the mid-forearm level. There were 3 out of 6 HLA mismatches between donor and recipient. The recipient limb was shortened to enable HTx to be performed at a distal one-third forearm level. The recipient operation was performed in the following order: bones (2 rush pins)-tendons (separately sutured)-nerves (median, ulnar, superficial radial)-veins (2)-arteries (2)-remaining veins (1) (BTNVAV). The total ischemic time was 8 hours. The postoperative course was uneventful.

Rehabilitation

Physiotherapy protocol was similar to that for Patient 1. The patient was discharged from the hospital on posttransplant day 42. He continued his rehabilitation and hand therapy on an outpatient basis.

Rejection Episodes and Treatment

None. Neither donor-specific antibodies nor chimerism was detected.

Major Complications

Mild hyperglycemia requiring oral hypoglycemic therapy occurred. However, there were no post-transplant infections such as fungus, cytomegalovirus (CMV), human papilloma virus, or signs of malignancy.

Function of Transplanted Hand

Healing of bones was completed at 12 weeks. The hand's macroscopic appearance is very good, with proper matching of size and color with the contralateral hand. Texture and composition of the skin remained unchanged during the observation period. The pulse is distinctively palpable on both main arteries at the wrist. As luminal occlusion of graft vessels is considered to be an important sign of chronic rejection, special attention was paid to this component.[8] A high-resolution Doppler ultrasound device (Siemens THI/9.0 MHz) was applied to examine graft vessels. No luminal narrowing as an indirect sign of myointimal proliferation could be seen. Fingers' total active range of motion (AROM) is 210°, which equals 85% of active motion of the unaffected hand. Nerve regeneration progressed rapidly: 8 months after transplantation electromyographic signs of sensory reinnervation were observed in the tips of the ulnar fingers, and 4 weeks later in thumb and index finger as well. Cold intolerance was mild. After 36 months the sensibility was good, with some discriminative sensation (2PD = 10 mm).

The patient can distinguish between different thermal stimuli. Sweating is present; he can localize stimuli in each finger with his eyes shut, but cannot discriminate between differently shaped objects. The Semmes-Weinstein monofilament test gives positive results for both main hand nerves: ulnar nerve, blue (3.22–3.61 g) and median nerve, purple (3.84–4.31 g), which rates S3 and S3+, respectively. The function of intrinsic hand muscles is present. The patient can effectively spread his fingers and slightly oppose his thumb (**Fig. 2**). His grip strength is 4.5 kg, the DASH score is 65 (30–150 points), and the CFSS result is 92 (excellent). The patient has fully incorporated the transplanted limb into his body image and has also regained self-confidence in social relationships. In addition, he is able to write, drive a car, ride a bicycle, and hold small objects, and currently works (full-time manual job) as

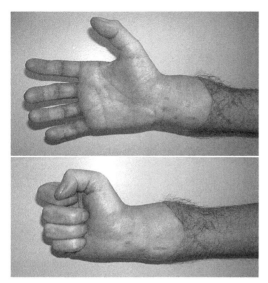

Fig. 2. Patient 3. Range of movement of fingers.

a cart-driver. He is also able to perform physical exercises (Video 3).

The patient's blood pressure is normal (130/90 mm Hg). His posttransplant diabetes has responded well to an oral hypoglycemic agent (metformin). At 2 years after transplant, urine glucose is normal and ketones are negative; serum creatinine and BUN levels are 1.2 and 49 mg/dL, respectively; and all other laboratory findings were within the normal range.

PATIENT 4
History

This 30-year-old man lost his dominant right upper limb as a child in a harvester accident 28 years prior to HTx. What is of particular importance is that this patient does not remember himself without the amputation. He worked as owner of a small computer firm and never wore any prosthesis (**Fig. 3**).

Indications for Transplant

Amputation at the elbow joint level. The patient was highly motivated, constantly trained his arm muscles, and was in a close contact with the group's prior HTx recipients (Patients 1 and 3). The HTx was performed in October 2009.

Relevant Surgical Details

The limb was procured from a 47-year-old female multiorgan donor. There were 5 out of 6 HLA mismatches between donor and recipient. Both donor and recipient were CMV negative. There

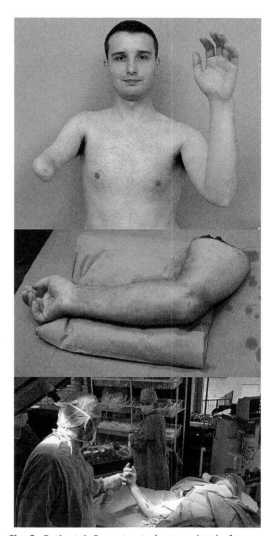

Fig. 3. Patient 4. From top to bottom: level of amputation, a procured limb, postoperative view.

was a size mismatch with regard to the diameter of recipient and donor humeral bones. Due to such an obstacle and prior period of cold ischemia, a bouquet osteosynthesis by means of a K-wire bundle was performed. The control radiograph revealed a 13-mm distension that could not be reduced. Surprisingly rapid progression of bony union was observed. After 6 months bone healing was complete (**Fig. 4**).

Similar difficulties were encountered on muscle anastomosis. There was a significant difference between the size of donor (strong, well developed) and recipient (small, atrophic) muscles, which in this situation had to be anastomosed and repaired in groups. The other anatomic structures (nerves, brachial artery, 3 veins) were reconstructed in a standard manner; total ischemia time was 9 hours.

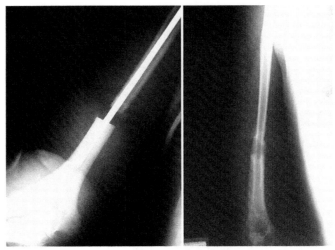

Fig. 4. Patient 4. (*Left*) postoperative radiograph, 13 mm distension; (*right*) complete consolidation achieved after 6 months.

Rehabilitation

Standard protocol for patients with arm replantation was used.

Rejection Episodes and Treatment

One acute episode of skin rejection (moderate, grade II) occurred 6 weeks after transplant, which correlated with the onset of CMV infection (treated with antiviral therapy and simultaneous tapering of IS). The rejection episode was successfully reversed with bolus steroids (Solu-Medrol 500 mg/d for 3 days) and topical tacrolimus.

Major Complications

The postoperative course was uneventful until posttransplant day 28 when the recipient's general condition worsened, with acute abdominal pain, fatigue, malaise, and a papular rash limited to the ribcage. An active CMV infection was confirmed with a polymerase chain reaction test. Once active viral replication was diagnosed, ganciclovir therapy was implemented, which resulted in a drop of CMV load from 500,000 to 34,000 copies/mL and significant improvement in the patient's general condition after 2 weeks of treatment. The therapy was continued with valganciclovir after discharge of the patient. Despite the aforementioned therapy, a viral load of 1500 copies/mL persisted. The patient is being thoroughly monitored for any new symptoms of infection.

Hand Function

After follow-up of 13 months the patient is able to flex his elbow joint 45° against gravity, and

effectively flex and extend his fingers (range of motion 110°) (**Fig. 5**). His protective sensation has reached the distal palmar crease. He is very satisfied with the result of the transplant at this stage.

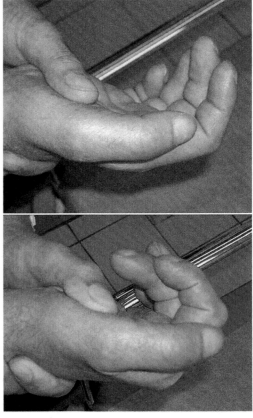

Fig. 5. Patient 4. Range of motion of fingers 12 months after operation.

PATIENT 5
History

This 33-year-old male soldier/ranger lost both of his hands during active duty as a result of a blast injury 2 years prior to HTx (**Fig. 6**).

Past Medical History

The patient suffered from a gunshot wound to his chest and abdomen that he also sustained in combat. In addition, his left eyesight is seriously impaired as a result of the same blast; several reconstructive procedures were unsuccessfully attempted on his right hand. The patient had a biomechanical prosthesis, which did not provide an adequate level of function for him.

Indications for Transplant

Short transradial amputation of the left hand and an extremely mutilated dominant right hand with its second and third ray spared. The remnant parts were deprived of any motor or sensitive function. The patient therefore opted for both of his hands to be transplanted. The HTx was performed in June 2010.

Relevant Surgical Details

The hands were procured from a 52-year-old female multiorgan donor. The left hand was transplanted at the distal forearm level close to the wrist and the right hand at the level of the radiocarpal joint. The sequence of reconstructive procedures was as follows (on both hands): bone-tendon (long tendon flexors)-nerve (2)-vein (2)-artery

(2)-vein (1). No circulatory/vascular problems were encountered on the right hand (ischemia 8 hours). However, on the left hand there were vascular problems encountered (ischemia 11 hours). This complication required a revision of the anastomosed vessels twice intraoperatively. A discovered arterial thrombosis was treated with bolused unfractionated heparin, 5000 units, followed by continuous infusion at 1500 units/h. The third revision was performed on the second postoperative day, resulting in thrombectomy of the superficial palmar arch. The fibrinolytic therapy was intensified using Plavix and Prostavasine. Ischemia resulted also in severe epidermolysis and necrosis of the distal phalanges, which ultimately had to be amputated on posttransplant day 13. Adequate blood flow was eventually achieved with fibrinolytic therapy, but excessive bleeding from both transplanted hands required transfusion of 65 units of blood over 12 days.

Rehabilitation

The physiotherapy protocol was similar to the one for Patient 3. The patient was discharged from the ward on posttransplant day 63 (**Figs. 7** and **8**). He then continued the rehabilitation and hand therapy on an outpatient basis.

Rejection Episodes and Treatment

Biopsies taken at 2-week intervals during the first 12 weeks showed persistent rejection (grade I/ grade II) which were not accompanied by any clinical signs such as rash, edema, and so forth. These findings were more severe (grade II) on the right hand (unaffected by thrombosis). Topical tacrolimus and increased doses of steroids were administered.

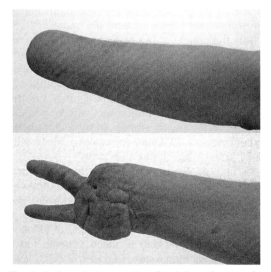

Fig. 6. Patient 5. Amputation level (see the text for details).

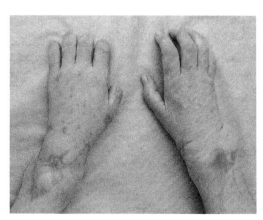

Fig. 7. Patient 5. Dorsal view of transplanted hands (6 months after operation).

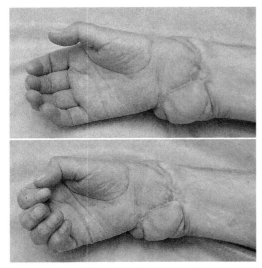

Fig. 8. Patient 5. Flexion of fingers of the right hand (6 months after operation).

Major Complications

During the first 10 postoperative days polyuria was observed (diuresis approximately 8–10 L/d). Surprisingly, during that time kidney function appeared normal by basic serum testing.

Hand Function

After 6 months of follow-up the patient can effectively use his right hand, performing most tasks of daily life (**Fig. 9**). The function of the left hand is still poor, with only very small finger movements being achieved.

PATIENT 6
History

Patient 6 was a 55-year-old housewife who lost her upper limb 2 years prior to HTx as a result of a car accident.

Indications for Transplant

Mid-arm amputation. The HTx was performed in September 2010.

Relevant Surgical Details

The limb was procured from a brain-dead 49-year-old female multiorgan donor. There were 4 out of 6 HLA mismatches between donor and recipient; The surgical technique applied as well as the rehabilitation protocol were very similar to those used for Patient 4. The postoperative course was uneventful, the wound healed properly, and the patient at this early stage post transplant is very satisfied with her new hand.

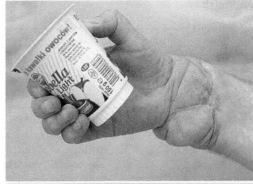
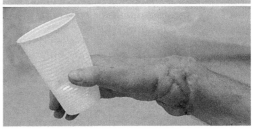
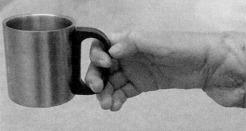

Fig. 9. Patient 5. Hand function of the right hand (6 months after operation).

DISCUSSION

The recipient age limit at the author's center (55 years), although significantly lower than that of several United States centers (65 years),[9,10] still meets the criteria of the majority of European reconstructive transplant programs.[3–5] It seems that age older than 55 years significantly increases the risk of both technical and metabolic complications. This aspect is particularly true for the Eastern-European population, where general health conditions, as expressed by a current life expectancy of 73 years for males, significantly differ from United States standards.

In the author's experience with screening patients for HTx in cases of unilateral amputations, the majority of patients encountered were so-called high/proximal amputations (proximal forearm or humerus). Apparently the loss of function and body integrity affects these patients much more severely than it does in cases of distal-level amputations. This factor obviously poses an important problem because the chances of restoring satisfactory hand/limb function through proximal forearm-level HTx are poor,[4] and in the case of shoulder disarticulation still remains questionable. However, as shown by the results from this center and the data collected from other transplant programs,[11] recipients of an HTx at a level distal to the midpoint of the humerus are able to regain good or even excellent limb function, exceeding the results obtained by patients after limb replantation (including all the limitations of this comparison).[1]

Two of the recipients experienced severe postoperative vascular complications within their grafts. For Patient 2 such a complication was probably attributable to late removal of a transducing arterial catheter placed in the radial artery and subsequent thrombus formation, which ultimately led to amputation of the graft on the first postoperative day. Such risk of arterial thrombosis due to invasive blood pressure monitoring has been estimated in some studies to be as high as 85%.[12] In this case, injury to the intima inflicted by the catheter was the cause of thrombi, which spread as far as the palmar arch. In Patient 5 thrombosis of both left hand arteries was observed despite numerous intraoperative attempts to revise their anastomoses. On postoperative day 2 the vascular anastomoses again required revision, and intensive fibrinolytic therapy was instituted at that time. The limb in this patient was saved; however, this recipient experienced massive blood loss during the multiple revision procedures. Ultimately, the distal phalanges of digits 1 to 5 required amputation. Despite these severe complications, the recipient is still satisfied with the overall outcome and motor function. Because HTx is not a life-saving procedure, the author's group continues to meticulously scrutinize these complications in this series. The available data regarding vascular complications in composite tissue allografts, however, show that these are extremely rare.[13]

The issue of bone healing in HTx patients has not drawn as much attention as certain other aspects of tissue regeneration such as soft tissue and wound healing, probably because very few complications have been observed with regard to bone union. Still, there is ongoing debate as to whether there is superior/expedited bony union after HTx in comparison with conventional bone osteosynthesis, and especially after replantation. The rapid bony union in the recipient after arm-level transplantation (Patient 4), despite an unstable osteosynthesis performed with a bundle of K-wires without osseous transplants and a postoperative bone gap of 13 mm, was somewhat surprising. The osteotomy site consolidated within 6 months. Gabl and colleagues[14] showed that the progress of bony union in limb transplants does not significantly differ from that observed after limb replantations. However, the pace of osteogenesis and bony union observed in Patient 4 in this series far exceeded that described in the author's patients with arm replantation.

Among all opportunistic infections complicating the postoperative course after limb transplantation, the most common is CMV, likely because of the high risk of transmitting latent forms of CMV with grafted leukocytes, and epithelial and hematopoietic bone marrow stem cells. Due to high numbers of cells potentially infected with the virus, strong IS and highly mismatched HLA, hand transplant recipients are probably as susceptible to CMV infection as are recipients of lung and small intestine transplants.[15] However, only one of the HTx recipients in this series demonstrated posttransplant CMV infection. Because CMV testing in this program has been performed as a screening test only since 2008/2009, one can only speculate as to whether this case of CMV infection was a "genuine" new infection or a reactivation.

In conclusion, hand transplantation, the most frequently performed type of composite tissue allotransplantation today, is capable of achieving very good results with regard to regaining motor and sensory function of the limb.[1,3,4,10,13] The author believes that the results obtained by his team in Trzebnica support this observation and encourage the continuation of this HTx program in the future.

SUPPLEMENTARY DATA

Supplementary data related to Patient 1 can be found online at doi:10.1016/j.hcl.2011.08.003.

SUPPLEMENTARY DATA

Supplementary data related to Patient 3 can be found online at doi:10.1016/j.hcl.2011.08.003.

REFERENCES

1. Schuind F, Abramowicz D, Schneeberger S. Hand transplantation: the state-of-the-art. J Hand Surg Eur Vol 2007;32(1):2–17.
2. Jablecki J, Kaczmarzyk L, Patrzalek D, et al. A detailed comparison of the functional outcome after midforearm replantations versus midforearm transplantation. Transplant Proc 2009;41:513–6.
3. Lanzetta M, Petruzzo P, Vitale G, et al. Human hand allotransplantation; what have we learned? Transplant Proc 2004;36:664.
4. Brandacher G, Ninkovic M, Piza-Katzer H, et al. The Innsbruck hand transplant program: update at 8

years after the first transplant. Transplant Proc 2009; 41:491–4.

5. Schneebherger S, Zelger B, Nincovic M, et al. Transplantation of the hand. Transplant Rev 2005;100: 107–11.

6. Jablecki J, Kaczmarzyk L, Patrzalek D, et al. Mild rejection episode evoked by modification of immunosuppressive protocol observed in a patient with forearm transplantation: case report. Transplant Proc 2009;41:557–9.

7. Jabłecki J, Kaczmarzyk L, Domanasiewicz A, et al. First Polish forearm transplantation—final report (outcome after 4 years). Ann Transplant 2010;15:61–7.

8. Breidenbach WC, Ravindra K, Blair B, et al. Transplant arteriopathy in clinical hand transplantation. Abstract Book of the 9th Meeting of the International Society of Hand and Composite Tissue Allotransplantation. Valencia (Spain), September 11–12, 2009.

9. Breidenbach WC, Gonzales NR, Kaufman LC, et al. Outcomes of the first American hand transplants at 8 and 6 years post transplant. J Hand Surg Am 2008;100:1039–47.

10. Kaufman CL, Blair B, Murphy E, et al. A new option for amputees: transplantation of the hand. J Rehabil Res Dev 2009;46:395–404.

11. Landin L, Cavadas PC, Nthumba P, et al. Preliminary results of bilateral arm transplantation. Transplantation 2009;88(5):749–51.

12. Martin C, Crama P, Courjaret P. Prolonged catheterization of the radial artery. Prospective evaluation of thrombotic risk. Ann Fr Anesth Reanim 1984;3:435–9 [in French].

13. Gazarian A, Abrahamian DO, Petruzzo P, et al. Hand allografts; experience from Lyon. Ann Chir Plast Esthet 2007;52:424–35 [in French].

14. Gabl M, Pechlaner S, Lutz M, et al. Bilateral hand transplantation: bone healing under immunosuppression with tacrolimus, mycofenolate mofetil and prednisone. J Hand Surg Am 2004;29(6): 1020–7.

15. Bonatti H, Brandacher G, Margreiter R, et al. Infections and complications in three double hand recipients in experience from a single centre. Transplant Proc 2009;41:517–20.

The Spanish Experience with Hand, Forearm, and Arm Transplantation

Pedro C. Cavadas, MD, PhD[a,b], Luis Landin, MD[a,b,*],
Alessandro Thione, MD, PhD[a,b],
Jose C. Rodríguez-Pérez, MD, PhD[c],
Miguel A. Garcia-Bello, MD[c], Javier Ibañez, MD[a,b],
Francisco Vera-Sempere, MD, PhD[d],
Pedro Garcia-Cosmes, MD, PhD[e], Luis Alfaro, MD[f],
Jose D. Rodrigo, MD[g], Federico Castro, MD[g]

KEYWORDS

- Hand transplant • Forearm transplant • Arm transplant
- Composite tissue allograft • DASH • Outcomes

Composite tissue allotransplantation (CTA) is increasingly being used as a reconstructive option for upper limb amputees. The procedure takes advantage of both previous experience of replantation and extensive knowledge of transplant immunology and immunotherapy. Hand allograft transplantation (HAT) has resulted in excellent success rates with respect to graft acceptance and survival.[1] However, outcomes after hand transplantation are reported frequently as single case reports, from different teams evaluating their results with different instruments.[2,3] To date, no report has specifically addressed changes in disability scores of the upper limb after HAT in a series of cases at a single institution.

Disclosure: There are no sources of support that require acknowledgment. The authors have no financial or personal relationships with other people or organizations that could influence (bias) this work inappropriately. The authors have no financial interest in any of the drugs mentioned in this work. Alemtuzumab, tacrolimus, sirolimus, and mycophenolate mofetil were used off-label to prevent and treat rejection of hand allografts. Authorship: Pedro C. Cavadas participated in the research design and writing of the paper. Luis Landin participated in the research design, data recovery and analysis, and writing of the paper. Alessandro Thione participated in the writing and reviewing of the paper. Javier Ibáñez participated in the writing and reviewing of the paper. Jose C. Rodríguez-Pérez participated in the data analysis. Miguel A. Garcia-Bello participated in the data analysis and reviewing of the paper. Francisco Vera-Sempere participated in the writing and reviewing of the paper. Luis Alfaro participated in the writing and reviewing of the paper. Pedro Garcia-Cosmes participated in the reviewing of the paper. Jose D. Rodrigo participated in the writing and reviewing of the paper. Federico Castro participated in the reviewing of the paper.

a University Hospital "La Fe," Avenida Campanar 21, 46009 Valencia, Spain
b Reconstructive Microsurgery, Clinica Cavadas, Paseo de Facultades 1, bajo 8, 46021 Valencia, Spain
c Nephrology Division, Dr Negrín University Hospital of Gran Canaria, Plaza Barranco De La Ballena S/N, 35012 Las Palmas De Gran Canaria, Spain
d Pathology Division, University Hospital "La Fe," Medical School, Valencia University, Avenida Campanar 21, 46009 Valencia, Spain
e Nephrology Division, University Hospital, Paseo San Vicente s/n, 37007 Salamanca, Spain
f Pathology Division, Hospital Virgen del Consuelo, C/Callosa de Ensarria n 7, 46007 Valencia, Spain
g Anesthesia Division, Clinica Cavadas, Paseo de Facultades 1, bajo 8, 46021 Valencia, Spain
* Corresponding author. Clinica Cavadas, Paseo de Facultades 1, bajo 8, 46021 Valencia, Spain.
E-mail address: landinsurgery@gmail.com

Hand Clin 27 (2011) 443–453
doi:10.1016/j.hcl.2011.08.002
0749-0712/11/$ – see front matter © 2011 Elsevier Inc. All rights reserved.

The Disabilities of the Arm, Shoulder and Hand (DASH) measure is a patient-reported outcome (PRO) measure that comprises a 30-item questionnaire, which is available free of charge. The questionnaire contains 21 items that assess physical function, 6 items on symptoms, and 3 social items that are related to the upper extremity.[4,5] It has been assessed with respect to its validity for face, content, convergent, and divergent constructs, and has been proved to be a consistent, reproducible, and responder-friendly tool. In general, the higher the DASH score the greater the disability that is indicated.[6] A decrease in DASH score of more than 15 points is the most accurate measure to discriminate between patients whose condition has improved and those who have not improved.[5] The advantages of the DASH measure include time efficiency, low administrative costs, and that it does not seem threatening or have any risks for the patients. This test does not focus on any particular condition but on the overall performance of the upper limb.[5]

This article is a retrospective review of a series of patients who underwent hand transplantation that summarizes their outcomes. We choose to use DASH because it can be used to evaluate disabilities of the upper limb before and after transplantation. In addition, details of the anesthesia, transplant procedure, secondary surgery, medical, psychological and immunologic status of the hand, forearm, and arm allograft recipients, and the medical complications observed are presented. The minimum follow-up period for every patient in this series was 2 years.

PATIENTS AND METHODS

A CTA program was approved at our institution by the Ethical and Institutional Review Boards. The candidates were recruited from consultations originated after reporting the approval of the transplant program in the media. Each candidate was evaluated surgically, psychologically, and medically. The exclusion criteria for our program included unilateral amputation, glenohumeral disarticulation, known psychiatric disorders, blindness, malignancy during the preceding 5 years, good functional and psychological adaptation, lack of economic support, congenital malformation, age greater than 50 years, and hepatitis B or C infection (**Box 1**). The selected candidates were examined on a case-by-case basis until consensus with the requirements for ethical and institutional approval was obtained. The recipients furthermore signed an informed consent form that included detailed information about the risks of malignancy, metabolic and infectious complications,

---

Box 1
Exclusion criteria

Unilateral amputation

Glenohumeral disarticulation

Known psychiatric disorders

Blindness

Malignancy during the last 5 years

Congenital malformation

Age older than 50 years

Hepatitis B or C infection

Lack of economic support

Good functional and psychological adaptation

---

and even death that might be associated with the procedure. Only 3 candidates fulfilled all the requirements during a screening period of 4 years.

Management of Anesthesia

Each case was planned in a similar manner to a solid organ transplant but with particular details that were related to microsurgery, namely maintenance of homeostasis, ensuring an optimum blood flow, avoidance of vasoconstriction, and favoring perfusion with a hyperdynamic state and decreased sanguineous viscosity.[7] The weight-bearing areas were protected, the operating room was maintained at a temperature of around 24°C, and the fluids that were administered were warmed. Standard cardiopulmonary parameters were monitored, including continuous and invasive measurement of hemodynamic parameters. Anesthesia was maintained by the inhalation of sevoflurane and oxygen/air; sevoflurane has advantages over propofol for this surgery in terms of diminishing interstitial edema[8] and avoiding ischemia-reperfusion injury.[9] Remifentanil was chosen as the analgesic, because it provides enhanced hemodynamic stability; the analgesic was perfused continuously. Cisatracurium was used for neuromuscular blockade. Appropriate fluid volume was maintained using crystalloids and colloids in a ratio of 3:1, with venous pressures increased sufficiently to ensure tissue perfusion. Blood was transfused in accordance with analytical results. The hematocrit and gasometric control of ions were checked every hour, and every 3 hours a complete hematology and biochemistry test was taken. Neither epinephrine nor norepinephrine was used, except in cases with severe hypotension that did not respond to fluid therapy. If hypotension occurred, a low dose of dobutamine was administered because, despite increasing metabolic demand and the frequency of heart contraction, it also increases intragraft blood flow.[10]

Surgical Technique

All the patients at our center underwent bilateral hand transplantation. The grafts were recovered from heart-beating brain-dead multiorgan donors who were matched with the recipient by gender and blood group but were not matched with respect to human leukocyte antigens.[11–16] All the allografts were obtained at a level above the elbow under tourniquet ischemia before cross-clamping for solid organ retrieval. Two teams were formed, each of which was composed of 2 surgeons and a nurse. One team prepared both recipient stumps whereas the other team moved to the donor operating room to harvest the allografts. Care was taken to evaluate the presence of any trauma to the upper extremities of the donor. The radial artery was checked for repeated gasometry punctures. Esmarch exsanguination was performed at the beginning of the procedure. The brachial artery was transected at the level of the upper arm, together with the median, ulnar, and radial nerves. The sensory nerves to the forearm were discarded. A transverse osteotomy was performed on each humerus using an oscillating saw. Afterwards, the brachial artery was cannulated and each allograft was perfused with 2 L of cold reconstituted Belzer solution until the superficial veins showed a clear effluent. Both limbs were recovered within 45 minutes, and cosmetic prostheses were subsequently fitted to avoid any donor disfigurement. The allografts were immersed in the perfusion solution and transported on ice. The recipient stumps were prepared using a fish-mouth skin incision and preservation of all neurotized muscle remnants. The bone stumps were osteotomized transversely for ease of repair. The vascular bundles at the forearm or the arm (depending on the individual case) and the median, ulnar, and radial nerves were identified as far distally as possible.

Bone fixation/synthesis was performed by the senior author (PCC). Transient reperfusion using whole blood from the recipient was performed in the first and second cases only.[15,17] An artery-last sequence of transplantation was performed to allow rapid repair of the nonvascular structures in all cases.[18] The transplant sequence was: bone, extensor tendons, flexor tendons, nerves, veins, and arteries. The allografts were trimmed to match the stumps of the recipient, with care being taken not to injure the posterior interosseous nerve. The bones were fixated using 3.5-mm and 4.5-mm locking compression plates (Synthes, Oberdorf,

Switzerland) for the forearm and the arm, respectively. Whenever possible, all the tendons were identified for primary repair using 4-strand Kessler and epitendinous techniques. Epineural neurorrhaphy was performed on the median, ulnar, and radial nerves.

The third recipient had suffered an electrical burn above the elbows and had undergone reconstruction of elbow flexion by means of transfer of a latissimus dorsi muscle 6 months before transplantation. In addition, this recipient required the preparation of long saphenous vein arteriovenous vascular loops from the brachial artery to the basilic vein at the proximal third of the arm for ease of vessel anastomosis to the allografts on the day of the transplantation.

The pretransplant cross-match, which was based on flow cytometry (LABScreen; One Lambda, Canoga Park, CA, USA), was negative in all cases. The induction protocol consisted of alemtuzumab (Mabcampath; Bayer Schering Pharma, Berlin, Germany; 30 mg administered before revascularization) and methylprednisolone (500 mg and 250 mg on the first and second postoperative days, respectively). Subsequently, patients were given tacrolimus (Prograf; Astellas Pharma, Berlin, Germany; initial trough level 15 ng/mL, reduced gradually to 10–12 ng/mL after 3 months) and mycophenolate mofetil (MMF; CellCept; Roche, Basel, Switzerland; 2 g/d). Different protocols for maintenance with steroid therapy were used (**Table 1**). All the patients required conversion to sirolimus (Rapamune; Wyeth, Madison, NJ, USA) with the aim of maintaining trough levels at 12 to 15 ng/mL. In 1 case, the switch was performed because of suspected neurotoxicity of tacrolimus,[12] whereas in the other 2 cases the switch was a result of increased serum creatinine (SCr) levels.[13] Laboratory test and drug trough levels were monitored weekly during the first month, biweekly until the sixth month, and monthly thereafter. Given that the relevant urine samples were not available for all time points, the Chronic Kidney Disease Epidemiology Collaboration formula was used to produce estimates of the glomerular filtration rate (GFR).

A total of 7 skin rejection episodes were clinically suspected and subsequently a 4-mm skin biopsy specimen was obtained from the severest clinical lesion (macula or erythema). Biopsies were graded according to the Banff consensus working classification after hematoxylin staining.[19]

Measurement of Function and Disability

Hand function before and after transplantation was measured using the Chen functional grade,[20]

Table 1
Steroid therapy protocols used in 3 hand allograft recipients

Patient	Methylprednisolone Induction (mg on day 1, mg on day 2, mg × consecutive days, …)	Maintenance with Prednisone (mg/d)	Steroid Boluses During Rejection (mg × d)
1	500, 250, 100 × 3, 60 × 5, 40 × 5, 20 × 20	2.5	1000 × 3 alternate days
2	500, 250, 100 × 3, 60 × 5, 40 × 5, 20 × 20	5	500 × 3 consecutive days
3	500, 250	5[a]	500 × 3 consecutive days

[a] Resumed on postoperative day 221.

whereas the disabilities of the upper limb were evaluated using the DASH score.[4] The Hand Transplant Score System (HTSS) was used to evaluate the functional abilities of the allografts after transplantation.[21] Functional magnetic resonance imaging (fMRI) could be performed only in the first and third recipients.

Rehabilitation

Passive mobilization of the forearm and arm allografts was started after 1 week and continued for 1 year. Active mobilization was initiated at 2 weeks after surgery, and exercises against resistance were allowed after 3 months. In the patient who received only hand allografts, active mobilization was delayed for 3 weeks to avoid tendon rupture because the patient had been given high doses of steroid. The tenorrhaphies were stretched progressively after 12 weeks. The hands were positioned strictly elevated for 4 weeks. Once the wounds had healed, splints were applied to maintain wrist extension at an angle of 45°. Physical therapy was performed for 2 hours daily for the following 15 months as an outpatient procedure.

All hand allograft recipients received clinical and functional follow-up similar to that for hand replantation. Secondary surgical procedures were indicated to improve limb function, including a total of 6 arthrodeses (**Table 2**). Cosmetic revision was performed on all the allografts.

The first patient presented with absent thenar function after 12 months. Bilateral trapeziometacarpal (TMC) arthrodeses using 1-mm Kirschner wires and intrinsic plasty of the long fingers by the Zancolli lasso procedure using FDS III (Flexor Digitorum Superficialis III) were performed. Arthrodesis of the metacarpophalangeal (MP) joint of the left thumb was performed using 1-mm Kirschner wires. Because of malunion, the right TMC joint was revised eventually using 2-mm plates and screws (Synthes, Oberdorf, Switzerland), and a volar arthrolysis was performed at the proximal interphalangeal joint of the fourth finger of the right hand. The concomitant administration of sirolimus did not impair bone healing in any of the cases.[22]

The second recipient presented with marked flexion contracture of the wrist. The long fingers could be extended only after forced flexion of the wrist. A double-bone shortening procedure and

Table 2
Secondary procedures on hand allografts

Patient	1	2	3
Indication	Lack of opposition Cosmesis	Contracture Cosmesis	Lack of grip Cosmesis
Postoperative day	375, 480, and 910	POM 5	POM 18
Surgical procedure	Bilateral TMC arthrodeses Left MP thumb arthrodesis TMC revision	Double-bone shortening	Bilateral wrist arthrodeses
Radiology	Consolidation	Consolidation	Consolidation

Abbreviations: POM, postoperative month; TMC, trapeziometacarpal.

fixation with 3.5-mm locking plates was performed to allow wrist and finger extension.[17]

The third recipient received bilateral arm allografts and presented with a lack of differential wrist and finger flexion. Bilateral arthrodeses of the wrist following the AO/ASIF (Association for the Study of Internal Fixation) technique were performed during postoperative month 18.[23]

Outcomes and Statistical Analysis

We hypothesized that disabilities related to the upper limb would be alleviated after hand transplantation. The null hypothesis was that there would be no differences in the disabilities of the upper limb after transplantation, when compared with the status before transplantation. The DASH instrument was used to evaluate disabilities of the upper limbs, whereas Chen and HTSS scores were used to evaluate the function of the allografts.

The 1-tailed paired t-test was used to evaluate the above hypothesis because ranking tests lack sensitivity to real treatment effects in studies that have few participants. The effect of the switch from a tacrolimus-based regimen to a sirolimus-based regimen was also evaluated. A linear mixed model was used with relative maximum likelihood estimation, as implemented in the lmer procedure of the lme4 library, which is a package that has been added to the open source statistical software R (R Development Core Team 2006, Vienna, Austria). The model included a main fixed effect model of the tacrolimus-sirolimus conversion and 2 random effect models, namely patient identification and residual error. The model could be expressed as $Y_{ij} = \mu + p_i + t_j + e_{ij}$, where $e_{ij} \sim N(0, \sigma^2)$ and $p_i \sim N(0, \sigma_p^2)$ are random effects, and t_j reflects the effect of the conversion. A P value of 0.05 or less was considered significant, without performing a Bonferroni correction.

RESULTS

The medical events that occurred in relation to the conversion to sirolimus are summarized in **Table 3**. In brief, a mean decrease in SCr of 0.21 mg/dL (95% confidence interval [CI], 0.26–0.427; P<.044) was observed.[13] There was a mean increase in the estimated GFR of 10.7 mL/min (95% CI, 1.6–18.4; P<.008) (**Fig. 1**). Other effects of sirolimus are summarized in **Table 4**. A mean decrease in the leukocyte count and absolute neutrophil count was observed, but only the mean percentage decrease in lymphocytes was statistically significant (P = .012). The mean increase in platelet count was 36×10^9/L (95% CI, −0.1–73.4; P = .05). The changes in other parameters, such

as an increase in cholesterol, decrease in triglycerides, and an increase in the level of glycated hemoglobin (HbA1c), were not statistically significant (P = .158, P = .90, and P = .34, respectively).

With regard to functional outcomes, the 3 patients had found that the functional benefits of their prostheses did not match their expectations, and they all presented with a pretransplant Chen grade of IV. The DASH score of the first patient, before transplantation, was 29.16. Four years after transplantation, the functional scores of this recipient were: Chen II (ability to resume some suitable work, range of motion that exceeded 40% of normal, nearly complete recovery of sensation, and muscle power grades 3 and 4), an HTSS of 74.5 (good), and a DASH score of 17.86 (Video 1; please go to http://www.hand.theclinics.com to view video.) The fMRI examination showed the cortical reintegration of the allografts. Two years after conversion from tacrolimus, the immunosuppressive (IS) regimen of this patient consists of sirolimus 2 mg/d, MMF 500 mg/12 h, and prednisone 2.5 mg/d.

Patient 2 presented a functional result that was limited to a Moberg-type key pinch on the left allograft, whereas the right allograft presented with excellent functional abilities (Video 2). The DASH score was 70.83 points before transplantation. Three years after transplantation, the patient presented with a Chen grade of II, the HTSS was 73.5 (good), and the DASH score had improved to 36.6 points. The patient had resumed the ability to work. His current IS regimen is sirolimus 4 mg/d, MMF 500 mg/12 h, and prednisone 5 mg/d.

Patient 3 was able to drive 2 years after the transplantation procedure, and fMRI showed cortical reintegration of the allografts. The patient presented with a Chen grade of II, an HTSS of 79.5 (good), and the DASH score had improved from 75 to 30.83 points (Video 3). His current IS regimen consists of sirolimus 4 mg/d, MMF 1 g/12 h, and prednisone 5 mg/d.

Among the 3 patients, there was a mean decrease of 29.9 ± 16.9 points in the DASH score after transplantation. This improvement in the disability of the upper limbs was statistically significant ($T_2 = 3.07$, P = .046) (**Table 5**). We observed 1 oncological incident (basal cell carcinoma of the nose)[11]; various minor infections, including 2 reactivations of herpes simplex virus and 6 reactivations of varicella zoster virus; and 1 case of cutaneous mycosis. Metabolic complications included new-onset diabetes mellitus in 1 case, increased levels of SCr in 2 cases, and hypertension in all cases.[13] However, all these side effects/complications were controlled successfully with appropriate medical treatment. A total

448

Table 3
Summary of data at baseline, before switch, and 6 months after conversion

	Baseline				Before Switch					After Conversion			
Patient	Age/Sex	IS Therapy	After Transplantation Day	Rationale	Tacrolimus Trough Levels (ng/mL)	Other Adverse Effects	Additional Drug Therapy	Infectious Complications	IS Therapy	SRL Trough Levels (ng/mL)	Rejection (Banff Grade)	Additional Drug Therapy	SRL Side Effects
1	43/Female	Tac + MMF + pred	190	Suspected visual acuity loss	10.1	Hypertension	Carvedilol Atorvastatin	VZV	SRL + MMF + pred	11.47	Yes (II)	Carvedilol Atorvastatin Gemfibrozil[a]	Mouth ulcers Hypertriglyceridemia
2	29/Male	Tac + MMF + pred	668	↑SCr	11.2	Hypertension	Carvedilol Nifedipine Atorvastatin	Mixed/fungal cutaneous infection	SRL + MMF + pred	19.25	No	Carvedilol Atorvastatin	Mouth ulcers
3	28/Male	Tac + MMF	332	↑SCr	11.6	Hypertension Anemia Hyperglycemia	Carvedilol Nifedipine Atorvastatin	—	SRL + MMF + pred Alemtuzumab Topical Tac + steroids	18.63	Yes (I)	Atenolol Lercanidipine Atorvastatin Gemfibrozil	Hypertriglyceridemia

Abbreviations: IS, immunosuppressive; pred, prednisone; SRL, sirolimus; Tac, tacrolimus; VZV, varicella zoster virus.
[a] for 6 months only.

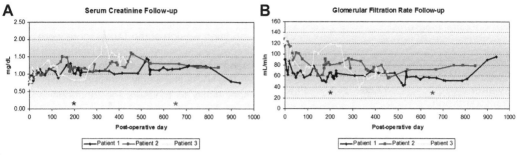

Fig. 1. (*A*) Follow-up of SCr levels of 3 recipients of bilateral hand allografts. (*B*) Follow-up of estimated GFR of 3 recipients of bilateral hand allografts. Asterisks mark the time point when the patients were switched from a tacrolimus-based to a sirolimus-based regimen.

of 7 episodes of acute skin rejection were diagnosed in these 3 patients. The severity of rejection showed Banff scores ranging from grade I to grade III. All episodes of rejection were controlled successfully using steroid boluses, adjustment of maintenance therapy, topical treatment, or rescue agents such as alemtuzumab.[11–16,19,24]

DISCUSSION

To consider hand transplantation there must be an acceptable trade-off between the restoration of function and complications that result from the required IS therapy. In this retrospective case series, a statistically significant alleviation in the disability scores of the upper limbs was observed in all patients after hand transplantation. Meanwhile, there were no life-threatening complications and the side effects of the IS therapy could be well controlled medically.

Although renal dysfunction after CTA is not common, it is a complication that is frequently seen in solid organ transplantation.[25] Minimizing the side effects of IS by reducing or switching the drugs that are administered might be a key factor in the preservation of the health status of

Table 4
Differences found after conversion to sirolimus

| Variable | Fixed Effects | | Random Effects (SD) | | | | |
	Intercept	Sirolimus Effect	Patient Identification	Residual Error	HPD$_{95}$	P Value (MCMC)
eGFR (mL/min)	59.3	10.7	7.2	8.4	1.6–18.4	0.008
SCr (mg/dL)	1.441	−0.213	0.188	0.202	−0.427; −0.026	0.044
Leukocytes ($\times 10^3$/mL)	4416	−587	1130	1517	−2028; 1000	0.454
Lymphocytes (%)	19.9	−7.556	6.8	5.12	−13.4; −2.2	0.012
Neutrophils ($\times 10^3$/μL)	0.75	−0.142	0.86	0.99	−1.1; 1.0	0.810
Platelets ($\times 10^9$/L)	217	36	65	28	−0.1; 73.4	0.05
Cholesterol (mg/dL)	198	28	13	40	−7; 69	0.158
Triglycerides (mg/dL)	179	−3.1	59	71	−77; 71	0.90
HbA1c (%)	5.7	0.14	0.56	0.22	−0.2; 0.5	0.34

Abbreviations: eGFR, estimated glomerular filtration rate; HPD$_{95}$, highest posterior density method; MCMC, Markov chain Monte Carlo method; SD, standard deviation. Patient identification represents the oscillation of mean value for the subjects; residual error represents the oscillation of each measure.

Table 5
DASH outcome measures

Patient	1	2	3
Pretransplantation	29.16	70.83	75
≥2 y after transplantation	17.86	36.6	30.83
Differences	11.3	34.23	44.17
Mean drop (± standard deviation)	29.9 ± 16.86 (T_2 = 3.07, P = .046)		

transplant recipients.[26] Sirolimus has been indicated in the prevention of solid organ graft rejection because it enhances kidney function and is associated with a low incidence of malignancy.[27] A recipient of a facial allograft was reported to suffer renal dysfunction that required conversion to sirolimus.[28] In this case series, we were able to show a statistically significant improvement in renal function after conversion from a tacrolimus-based to a sirolimus-based IS regimen. The use of sirolimus was not associated with a severe increase in cholesterol or triglycerides.

With respect to limb functionality, 2 types of measure may be used: clinician-based outcomes (CBOs) and PROs. CBOs measure mainly physiologic attributes that are believed to be associated with well-being and evaluate results from the perspective of the clinician.[29] CBOs have long been considered to be objective measures of the outcome of treatment, on the assumption that physiologic outcomes and patient well-being are highly correlated.[30] In contrast, PROs measure symptoms, function, and quality of life as they are perceived by the patient. In the past, PROs were considered to be subjective measures of the outcomes of treatment and were not considered to be a valid tool.[29,30] However, it is now recognized that the patient's subjective experience following a transplant is a critical factor in assessing the overall outcome. It is further recognized that the correlation between physiologic outcomes and patient well-being that is assumed by CBOs might not apply in all cases.[6,31]

At the time of writing this review, there was still no standardized definitive tool to evaluate the functional outcome of hand allografts. Therefore, in this study, both PROs and CBOs were used. Function was assessed using 3 measures: the HTSS, the Chen functional score, and the DASH score. The HTSS and Chen functional score use both CBOs and PROs. The DASH score represents an exclusive PRO. We chose to use all 3 measures and combine the results to provide

a more complete picture. The scoring systems of Tamai, Moberg, Jebsen, Smith, Carroll, and Ipsen's modified version of the Tamai score were not used because they have important limitations that have been discussed elsewhere in this journal.[32]

The HTSS is the only instrument that is designed specifically to measure the functional abilities of hand allografts. It contains 6 domains. The CBOs are appearance, sensibility, and movement. The PROs are psychological and social acceptance, daily activities and work status, and patient satisfaction and well-being. The face and content validity of the HTSS are being tested. The HTSS focuses on the functional aspects of the allografts and the recipient. However, it has the disadvantage that it is unable to detect differences in function before and after transplantation.

The Chen functional score classifies patients into 4 categories that identify only gross differences in function. It combines CBOs and PROs in simple designations (ie, excellent, good, fair, poor) that are used to summarize the status of the patient. Its advantages are that it is simple to calculate and can be used to evaluate the status of the patient before and after the transplant procedure.[20] However, it also has 2 major disadvantages. First, at any given time, patients might not fit well into any of the Chen grades because they present with characteristics from different grades. Specifically, return to work is not always correlated with the recovery of range of motion, sensitivity, and muscle power; this was true in the case of the first recipient in this study, who remains unemployed. Second, although this score has been accepted widely in replantation surgery, it has not been tested for validity, responsiveness, or reliability.

The DASH score quantifies symptoms and lack of function in patients suffering from disorders of the upper limb in a heterogeneous population, and covers a variety of conditions.[5] Its validity for measuring disability related to impairment of the upper limbs (construct validity) has been tested and confirmed.[33] It has been shown to measure change when observations are made before and after treatment and can verify patient's reports of significant improvements in their functionality and the presence of pain.[5,33] The DASH score was included in the evaluation of the functional status of the recipients because it can measure disabilities in the patient both before and after transplantation. Its precision lends it an advantage over the Chen functional score, whereas its range of applicability lends it an advantage over the HTSS. However, the DASH score was not specifically designed to evaluate the functional outcomes of hand allografts. Furthermore, as noted earlier, there is currently no definitive tool that can be used to evaluate the functional outcome of hand allografts, and hence no gold standard that can be used to determine the criteria that should be used to assess the validity of the DASH score for the evaluation of the functional outcome of hand allografts. In the present study the DASH score was used to evaluate the disability of the upper limb as a whole, rather than the function of the hand allograft, before and after transplantation, a purpose for which the DASH score has been shown to be a valid instrument.

There was a mean decrease of 29 ± 16 points in the DASH score, which was statistically significant ($P = .046$). This difference was almost double the number of points needed to discriminate between patients whose condition had improved and those who had not improved (15 points).[33] The minimum detectable change at the 95% CI (MDC_{95}) is the minimum change in score that must be observed before a clinician can be confident that a change in patient status has occurred. MDC_{95} is 12.7 points for the DASH. Our findings exceed the minimum change in score that can be interpreted as an improvement with a high degree of confidence.

Some limiting factors deserve comment. (1) Our 3 patients do not represent a random sample of the population who have received hand allografts. Thus, in the absence of a true control group, inferences should be discussed with caution. The limited number of patients represents a common weakness of reports on CTA transplants. However, short case series or even case reports in this field might be included in future systematic reviews and meta-analyses, and therefore are important. (2) Transient reperfusion might have exposed the allografts of the second recipient to further edema, which in turn might have impaired local microcirculation and caused ischemic contracture of the forearm muscles. Although transient reperfusion is a well-established technique in hand replantation,[18] its role in hand transplantation remains to be defined. (3) The use of alemtuzumab as a rescue treatment of rejection in the third recipient might have affected the analysis of the effect of sirolimus on some laboratory variables (ie, the leukocyte count). (4) The 1-tailed paired t-test suggested that the critical group size below which nonparametric tests were desirable was approximately 15 participants.[34] Because the ranking tests lack sensitivity to real treatment effects in studies with small numbers of participants, the results of the t-test need to be interpreted with caution. A sample size of 7 pairs with a correlation of 0.5 would have 80.7% power to detect a difference of 29.9 points between a mean difference for the null hypothesis of 0.0 and the mean difference of 29.9 at the 0.05 significance level (α) using a 2-sided Wilcoxon signed-rank test. These results were based on 10,000 Monte Carlo samples from the null distribution: normal (58.33–25.34) and the alternative distribution: normal (58.33–25.34) − normal (28.43–9.6).

This series of recipients showed good biologic and functional recovery, according to the Chen functional score. The subjective functional improvement was testified by the DASH score. In addition to good psychological and social acceptance, the use of the hands in activities of daily living and patient satisfaction were high, as shown by the HTSS score. Two patients were able to return to work, and all 3 patients acknowledged their ability to perform tasks of personal hygiene and the capacity for social exchange. In addition, none of the patients requested removal of the allografts because of side effects of the IS therapy. All side effects could be controlled surgically or medically and they have not posed a risk to the life of the recipients.

SUMMARY

Good functional outcomes after hand, forearm, and arm transplantation have been observed in our experience. The side effects of the IS therapy could be controlled successfully. The DASH questionnaire was selected to evaluate disabilities related to the upper limbs before and after transplantation. We found a statistically significant improvement with respect to disabilities of the upper limb in the posttransplantation period compared with pretransplant conditions. We therefore conclude that HAT had a positive risk/benefit ratio in this series of patients, although they might not represent a random selection of the patients who undergo hand transplantation.

SUPPLEMENTARY DATA

Supplementary data related to this article can be found online at doi:10.1016/j.hcl.2011.08.002.

REFERENCES

1. Petruzzo P, Lanzetta M, Dubernard JM, et al. The international registry on hand and composite tissue transplantation. Transplantation 2010;90(12): 1590–4.
2. Schneeberger S, Ninkovic M, Piza-Katzer H, et al. Status 5 years after bilateral hand transplantation. Am J Transplant 2006;6:834–41.

3. Petruzzo P, Badet L, Gazarian A, et al. Bilateral hand transplantation: six years after the first case. Am J Transplant 2006;6:1718–24.

4. Hudak PL, Amadio PC, Bombardier C. Development of an upper extremity outcome measure: the DASH (disabilities of the arm, shoulder and hand) [corrected]. The Upper Extremity Collaborative Group (UECG). Am J Ind Med 1996;29:602–8.

5. Solway S, Beaton DE, McConnell S, et al. The DASH outcome measure user's manual. Toronto: Institute for Work & Health; 2002.

6. Suk M, Hanson BP, Norvell DC, et al. Musculoskeletal outcomes measures and instruments, vol. 1. 2nd edition. Basel (Switzerland): AO Foundation; 2009.

7. Hagau N, Longrois D. Anesthesia for free vascularized tissue transfer. Microsurgery 2009;29:161–7.

8. Bruegger D, Bauer A, Finsterer U, et al. Microvascular changes during anesthesia: sevoflurane compared with propofol. Acta Anaesthesiol Scand 2002;46:481–7.

9. Lucchinetti E, Ambrosio S, Aguirre J, et al. Sevoflurane inhalation at sedative concentrations provides endothelial protection against ischemia-reperfusion injury in humans. Anesthesiology 2007;106:262–8.

10. Suominen S, Svartling N, Silvasti M, et al. The effect of intravenous dopamine and dobutamine on blood circulation during a microvascular TRAM flap operation. Ann Plast Surg 2004;53:425–31.

11. Landin L, Cavadas PC, Ibanez J, et al. Malignant skin tumor in a composite tissue (bilateral hand) allograft recipient. Plast Reconstr Surg 2010;125:20e–1e.

12. Landin L, Cavadas PC, Nthumba P, et al. Morphological and functional evaluation of visual disturbances in a bilateral hand allograft recipient. J Plast Reconstr Aesthet Surg 2010;63:700–4.

13. Landin L, Cavadas PC, Rodriguez-Perez JC, et al. Improvement in renal function after late conversion to sirolimus-based immunosuppression in composite tissue allotransplantation. Transplantation 2010;90:691–2.

14. Landin L, Cavadas PC, Nthumba P, et al. Preliminary results of bilateral arm transplantation. Transplantation 2009;88:749–51.

15. Cavadas PC, Landin L, Ibanez J. Bilateral hand transplantation: result at 20 months. J Hand Surg Eur Vol 2009;34:434–43.

16. Landin L, Cavadas PC, Ibanez J, et al. CD3+-mediated rejection and C4d deposition in two composite tissue (bilateral hand) allograft recipients after induction with alemtuzumab. Transplantation 2009;87:776–81.

17. Landin L, Cavadas PC, Garcia-Cosmes P, et al. Perioperative ischemic injury and fibrotic degeneration of muscle in a forearm allograft: functional follow-up at 32 months post transplantation. Ann Plast Surg 2011;66(2):202–9.

18. Cavadas PC, Landin L, Ibanez J. Temporary catheter perfusion and artery-last sequence of repair in macroreplantations. J Plast Reconstr Aesthet Surg 2009;62:1321–5.

19. Cendales LC, Kanitakis J, Schneeberger S, et al. The Banff 2007 working classification of skin-containing composite tissue allograft pathology. Am J Transplant 2008;8:1396–400.

20. Chen ZW, Yu HL. Current procedures in China on replantation of severed limbs and digits. Clin Orthop Relat Res 1987;(215):15–23.

21. Petruzzo P, Lanzetta M, Dubernard JM, et al. The international registry on hand and composite tissue transplantation. Transplantation 2008;86:487–92.

22. Cavadas PC, Hernan H, Landin L, et al. Bone healing after secondary surgery on hand allografts under sirolimus-based maintenance immunosuppression. Ann Plast Surg 2011;66(6):667–9.

23. Hastings H. Wrist arthrodesis (partial and complete). In: Green DP, Hotchkiss RN, Pederson WC, et al, editors. Green's operative hand surgery. 5th edition. Philadelphia: Elsevier Churchill Livingstone; 2005.

24. Schneeberger S, Landin L, Kaufmann C, et al. Alemtuzumab: key for minimization of maintenance immunosuppression in reconstructive transplantation? Transplant Proc 2009;41:499–502.

25. Christie JD, Edwards LB, Kucheryavaya AY, et al. The Registry of the International Society for Heart and Lung Transplantation: twenty-seventh official adult lung and heart-lung transplant report–2010. J Heart Lung Transplant 2010;29:1104–18.

26. Wilkinson A, Kasiske BL. Long-term post-transplant management and complications. In: Danovitch GM, editor. Handbook of kidney transplantation. 5th edition. Philadelphia: Lippincott Williams & Wilkins; 2010. p. 217–51.

27. Watson CJ, Gimson AE, Alexander GJ, et al. A randomized controlled trial of late conversion from calcineurin inhibitor (CNI)-based to sirolimus-based immunosuppression in liver transplant recipients with impaired renal function. Liver Transpl 2007;13:1694–702.

28. Devauchelle B, Badet L, Lengele B, et al. First human face allograft: early report. Lancet 2006;368:203–9.

29. Feinstein AR. Clinical biostatistics. XLI. Hard science, soft data, and the challenges of choosing clinical variables in research. Clin Pharmacol Ther 1977;22:485–98.

30. Deyo RA. Using outcomes to improve quality of research and quality of care. J Am Board Fam Pract 1998;11:465–73.

31. Bovens AM, van Baak MA, Vrencken JG, et al. Variability and reliability of joint measurements. Am J Sports Med 1990;18:58–63.

32. Herzberg G, Parmentier H, Erhard L. Assessment of functional outcome in hand transplantation patients. Hand Clinics 2003;19:505–9.

33. Beaton DE, Katz JN, Fossel AH, et al. Measuring the whole or the parts? Validity, reliability, and responsiveness of the Disabilities of the Arm, Shoulder and Hand outcome measure in different regions of the upper extremity. J Hand Ther 2001;14:128–46.

34. Bryman A, Cramer D. Quantitative data analysis for social scientists. London: Routledge; 1990.

Functional Outcome after Hand and Forearm Transplantation: What Can Be Achieved?

Marina Ninkovic, MD[a,*], Annemarie Weissenbacher, MD[b],
Markus Gabl, MD[c], Gerhard Pierer, MD[d],
Johann Pratschke, MD[b], Raimund Margreiter, MD[b],
Gerald Brandacher, MD[e], Stefan Schneeberger, MD[f]

KEYWORDS

- Hand transplantation • Rehabilitation
- Functional outcome • Assessment

The first successful hand transplant in the so-called modern era of reconstructive transplantation was performed in 1998.[1] Since then, more than 65 hand and upper limb transplantations have been performed around the globe, with encouraging results.[2]

The first bilateral hand transplantation in Austria was performed on March 7, 2000,[3] only 2 months after the worldwide first bilateral transplantation was performed in Lyon.[4] At that time, there had been a serious debate in the medical community as to whether hand transplantation was an appropriate therapeutic option. Because the procedure is considered life-enhancing as opposed to life-saving, ethical issues and balancing the risks and benefits were, and still are, a foremost consideration in hand transplantation. However, over the years, hand transplantation as a form of composite tissue allotransplantation has become an established means of limb reconstruction for patients with severe bilateral injuries to hands and forearms, as well as selected unilateral injuries.[5,6] The clinical outcome after hand transplantation is strongly dependent on, firstly, genetic matching and the chosen immunosuppressive regimen, to produce as few side effects as possible; secondly, precise and accurate surgery; and, thirdly, adequate rehabilitation and functional assessment. To prevent rejection of the transplant, various immunosuppressive strategies have been developed. Currently, several novel approaches of maintenance therapy are being tested to minimize the side effects of such medication.[7,8]

The reconstructive requirements of amputees, the mechanism and level of amputation, as well as soft tissue characteristics and the presence of

The authors have nothing to disclose.

[a] Unit of Physical Medicine and Rehabilitation, Department of Visceral, Transplant and Thoracic Surgery, Center of Operative Medicine, Innsbruck Medical University, Anichstraße 35, A-6020 Innsbruck, Austria

[b] Department of Visceral, Transplant and Thoracic Surgery, Center of Operative Medicine, Innsbruck Medical University, Innsbruck, Austria

[c] Department of Trauma Surgery and Sports Medicine, Center of Operative Medicine, Innsbruck Medical University, Innsbruck, Austria

[d] Department of Plastic, Reconstructive and Aesthetic Surgery, Center of Operative Medicine, Innsbruck Medical University, Innsbruck, Austria

[e] Department of Plastic and Reconstructive Surgery, Johns Hopkins University School of Medicine, Ross Research Building 749D, 720 Rutland Avenue, Baltimore, MD 21205, USA

[f] Department of Plastic and Reconstructive Surgery, Johns Hopkins University School of Medicine, Baltimore, MD 21287, USA

* Corresponding author.

E-mail address: marina.ninkovic@i-med.ac.at

Hand Clin 27 (2011) 455–465

doi:10.1016/j.hcl.2011.08.005

nerves and functioning muscle-tendon units of the recipient guide the planning of the surgical procedure and influence the subsequent functional outcome. The surgery involves accurate bone alignment, length, and fixation; revascularization of main arteries and veins; reconstruction of all functioning muscle-tendon units, achieving natural balance between extensors and flexors; nerve repair of all of the nerves of the recipient that are present; and adequate soft tissue coverage.[9] After the surgical intervention, nerve regeneration from the recipient nerve into the transplanted donor tissue is required to regain both sensation and motor function in the transplanted hand. Current experience suggests that a replantation at the wrist level achieves the best functional outcome, which is comparable with long-term outcomes after hand and upper limb transplantation.[10]

The main goal of upper limb transplantations is to enhance the patient's quality of life. The transplant must be successfully integrated into the patient's body and self-image and the recipient should be satisfied with the recovery of sensitivity and muscle function of the new limb.[11]

To achieve these goals, a proper and thorough design of the rehabilitation regimen is of critical importance.[12] In this regard, experiences with replantation procedures as well as their rehabilitation are helpful in choosing the right methods, protocols, and techniques.[13]

Hand transplantation is a logical extension of replantation surgery and functional outcome after transplantation is comparable with outcomes after replantation.[14] Such experience has also shown that the higher the level of amputation, the less successful the functional outcome after replantation.[15] The same might be expected for the recovery of sensibility and muscle function after hand transplantation.[16] However, special features of vascularized composite allotransplantation need to be considered.

PATIENTS

Since 2000, 4 patients have undergone hand (2 bilateral and 1 unilateral) and forearm (1 bilateral) transplantation at our center in Innsbruck, Austria.[17,18]

The demographic and surgical details have been described in detail previously (**Table 1**).[17,18]

REHABILITATION PROTOCOL

The goal for rehabilitation in this series was to achieve the best possible function concerning both nerve regeneration and motor unit recovery. The specific treatment was focused on the control of pain and swelling, prophylaxis of joint stiffness, prevention of soft tissue adhesion, maintenance of tendon glide, motor and sensory reeducation, and a significant regain of independence.

The rehabilitation program was therefore based on the well-established protocols used in hand replantation after distal forearm amputation: early protective joint motion (EPM)[19] combined with cognitive exercise training after Perfetti,[20] in combination with electrotherapy. Rehabilitation in our first recipient was started on the third postoperative day with passive EPM, sensory reeducation, and a protocol cortical reintegration. During the fourth postoperative week, active assisted exercises and electrical stimulation of thenar and hypothenar muscle groups for the right hand were added. One week later, the left hand was also included. The delay on this side was related to a different functional muscle reconstruction based on tendon transfer. Active finger movements and occupational therapy were started a week later. The patient was provided with thermoplastic splints[21] and was trained in all the basic and professional-related activities of daily life. From the ninth postoperative week, electromyogram (EMG) biofeedback training was introduced. The

Table 1 Patients' data				
	Patient 1	Patient 2	Patient 3	Patient 4
Age at transplantation (y)	46	41	24	54
Type of injury	Blast explosion	High-voltage burn accident	Blast explosion	Reprocessing unit
Level of amputation	Wrist, bilateral	Forearm, bilateral	Wrist, bilateral	Wrist, dominant hand
Myoelectrical prosthesis	Yes	Yes	No	Yes
Time between amputation and transplantation (y)	6	3	6	5
Follow-up (y)	11	8	5	2

whole rehabilitation program, especially the intensive cognitive exercise program, was performed for 12 months following surgery in our department. During the first 2 months, the patient received inpatient treatment with 3 to 4 hours of therapy 7 days a week, followed by outpatient treatment of another 10 months at our outpatient hospital facility: 6 hours daily, 5 times a week.

In our second patient, the rehabilitation program started on the second postoperative day. The patient was treated as an inpatient 4 hours a day for 10 months followed by outpatient treatment of a further 21 months, 5 times a week, 6 hours daily.

Our third patient received inpatient treatment on the first day after surgery and continued for 3.5 months with 3 hours of daily therapy, followed by outpatient treatment of another 2 years, 6 hours daily, 5 times a week. In this case, significant visual impairment and language barriers were a challenge to treatment.

The fourth patient received inpatient treatment 3 hours daily for 3 weeks, which was again initiated on the first postoperative day. Outpatient treatment then followed for a further 2.5 months; 3 hours daily, 5 times a week. This patient still receives outpatient treatment 2 hours daily, twice a week, in a designated rehabilitation center close to his home.

FUNCTIONAL OUTCOME

The standardized rehabilitation protocol used was the same in all 4 cases performed at our center.

Total active range of motion (TAROM) of wrist, metacarpal, and interphalangeal joints improved continuously for the first 2 years after unilateral and bilateral hand transplantation. This improvement was monitored in the first 5 years after the forearm transplantation. At 11 years after transplantation for patient #1, TAROM for the index finger was 192°, 200° for the middle finger, 199° for the ring finger, and 182° for the little finger on the right hand. On the left side, TAROM for the index finger was 186°, 179° for the middle finger, 192° for the ring finger, and 200° for the little finger, at the same time. The second patient showed TAROM of 138° for the index finger, 104° for the middle finger, 140° for the ring finger, and 147° for the little finger on the right side. On the left hand, TAROM for the index finger was 175°, 149° for the middle finger, 127° for the ring finger, and 130° for the little finger. Our third patient showed TAROM for the index finger of 176°, 206° for the middle finger, 200° for the ring finger, and 181° for the small finger on the right side, after 5 years. TAROM for the index finger was 151°, 130° for the middle finger, 179° for the ring finger, and 191° for the small finger on the left side. For patient #4, TAROM for the index finger was 212°, 222° for the middle finger, 233° for the ring finger, and 185° for the small finger, after 2 years. Abduction of thumb was reduced (19°).

The TAROM of the right thumb achieved in the unilateral and bilateral hand and forearm transplantation are shown in **Fig. 1**.

Kapandji score for thumb opposition improved until 2 years after transplantation in patient #1, in both hands. Updates at 5 years have revealed stable Kapandji scores: K5 on the right hand and K3 on the left side. Thumb opposition scored 6 on the right side and 4 on the left side, the maximum being achieved by 2 years after transplantation in our second patient. However,

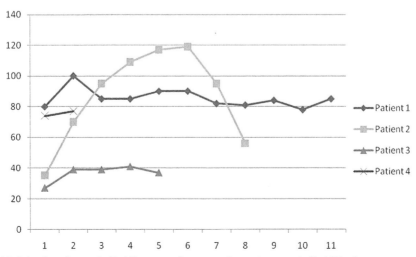

Fig. 1. TAROM right thumb. x axis (1–11): years after transplantation, y axis (0–140): degree.

subsequently the score decreased slightly until 7 years, but is currently showing an improved Kapandji score again. Thumb opposition on the left side could not be achieved during the first year in our third case. In contrast, the right side already showed Kapandji 3 at 6 months after transplantation. In patient #4, thumb opposition measured 5 after 2 years according to the Kapandji score.

In our first case, early signs of reinnervation of the abductor digiti minimi muscle on the left side were detected as early as 4 months after transplantation. At 9 months, electromyography confirmed the reinnervation process of the muscles innervated by the ulnar nerve on the left side and of the muscles innervated by the ulnar and median nerves on the right. Reinnervation of the muscles by the median nerve on the left side started at 1 year after transplantation. The amplitude of the detected action potentials increased significantly in the first 3 years after transplantation (**Fig. 2**).

After that, no changes in motor action potentials were found for about 1 year. Four years after transplantation, an improvement could again be observed, especially on the left side. In our second case, no clinical or electromyography signs of reinnervation of the intrinsic muscles were observed up to 18 months after the operation. Subsequently the functional recovery improved, but intrinsic function in this patient after forearm transplantation is still weak at 8 years. The abductor digiti minimi muscle on both sides showed the first signs of reinnervation at 6 months after transplantation in patient #3, both clinically and as assessed by electromyography. Intrinsic muscle strength was, on average, M3 at 5 years in this patient. The clinical signs of reinnervation of the abductor pollicis brevis muscle were present at 3 months in patient #4. At 2 years, the strength of this muscle was graded as M4. The first electromyography signs of reinnervation of the abductor digiti muscle were detected by 6 months.

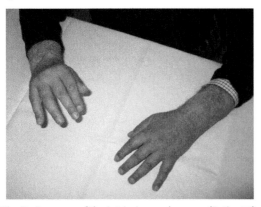

Fig. 2. Recovery of the intrinsic muscle group (Patient 1).

The Tinel sign was detected by 12 months on all fingertips bilaterally in patient #1. In the second case, Tinel sign was positive on the dorsal and volar side of both hands for all nerves except the radial nerve on the right side at 18 months. In our third case, Tinel sign for the ulnar and median nerve was detected on the fingertips on both sides by 12 months. In patient 4, Tinel sign was detected on fingertips at 2 years after transplantation.

Grip strength remained constant for the last 8 years in patient #1. Assessment by 1 year after transplantation showed a grip strength of 8.5 kg (third setting on a Jamar dynamometer) on the right side and 4.4 kg on the left. Until 5 years after transplantation, grip strength improved on both sides in our second patient. Thereafter, the grip strength showed a slight weakening on the right side. By 8 years, the strength was 6 kg on the right side and 6.6 kg on the left. Our third patient showed gradual improvement of grip strength, which was 4.6 kg at 5 years' follow-up. Grip strength increased constantly, beginning with the fourth month, and measured 7.5 kg (at the second setting on the Jamar dynamometer) by 2 years after transplantation in the fourth patient.

Results of the key pinch testing after the bilateral and unilateral hand and bilateral forearm transplantation are shown in **Fig. 3**.

Static 2-point discrimination (2-PD) returned to the normal range, bilaterally, in our first patient. However, dynamic 2-PD showed only fair results. Patient #1 is currently able to discriminate stimuli as well as shaped objects. Despite sensory recovery showing constant progression for 8 years after transplantation, it remains poor in patient #2. Sensory testing showed loss of protective sensation according to the monofilament test and protective sensibility according to the static 2-PD test at 8 years. Semmes-Weinstein monofilament test showed diminished protective sensation on both hands in patient #3. Static and moving 2-PD were already between 2 and 7 mm 2.5 years after transplantation in this patient. He is able to discriminate differently shaped objects. With our fourth patient, sensory recovery has improved slightly in the past 2 years. He is able to recognize a stimulus but still not able to localize it precisely, which is a stipulation of Semmes-Weinstein testing. According to this test, he showed loss of protective sensation (4.56). Two years after transplantation, static 2-PD was measurable with 14 to 15 mm for the first time. Moving 2-PD is still not detectable.

By 6 months, sensitivity to pain and thermal discrimination was present on both hands in all our cases except for patient #2. Cold discrimination was detected at the same time in our second case and hot discrimination 2 months later.

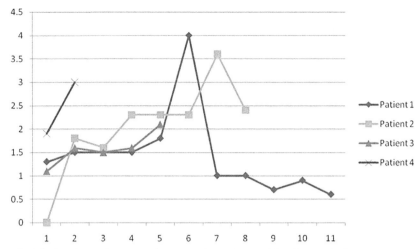

Fig. 3. Key pinch right hand. x axis: years after transplantation and for the y axis: kg.

Patient #4 has no cold intolerance, and the shape texture identification test is not possible at this stage after transplantation. Sweating is evident in the transplanted hand.

All of our patients can use their hands symmetrically. In daily living activities, only the fastening of a small button causes difficulties in patient #1. The second patient reports some problems in everyday life, such as picking up small objects, or diminished strength in both hands. The 2-PD test shows only protective quality. The third patient is nearly blind, which hindered therapy and impaired the functional outcome. Despite these obstacles, the patient shows encouraging clinical and EMG signs of recovery of the intrinsic muscles. Our fourth patient has no limitation in performing the activities of daily living. By 3 months after the transplantation, he was able to write, to grasp a glass, to ride a bicycle, to drive, to hold hands, and to pour water from a bottle (**Fig. 4**).

Patient 3 is extremely satisfied with his quality of life, and at 2 years after transplantation, his DASH (Disabilities of the Arm, Shoulder, and Hand questionnaire) score is 6.6. Changes in DASH scores for our patients are shown in **Fig. 5**.

The International Registry on Hand and Composite Tissue Transplantation (IRHCTT) was founded in 2002.[22] IRHCTT collects detailed information on every case of hand transplantation, and also data regarding functional outcomes according to the Hand Transplantation Score System (HTSS). HTSS evaluates 6 functional aspects with different weights for a total of 100 points. The score has good test-retest reliability and responsiveness. HTSS was also implemented at our center in Innsbruck. The collected data are presented in **Fig. 6**.

WORLD EXPERIENCE

The functional results achieved after unilateral and bilateral hand transplantation worldwide showed that all patients developed protective sensitivity, 90% of the recipients developed tactile sensitivity, and 84% also developed discriminative sensation.[23]

Motor recovery began with extrinsic muscle function, and the recovery of intrinsic muscles was observed only at a later stage, starting between 9 and 15 months after transplantation in most patients and correlated with the level of transplantation.

Because of sensorimotor recovery, the patients are able to perform most daily activities, such as eating, writing, dressing, and driving. The functional results achieved unilaterally and on the right side of the bilateral hand transplantation according to HTSS are shown in **Fig. 7**.

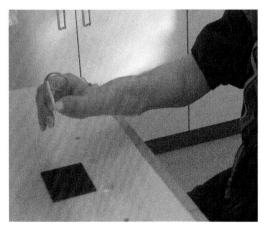

Fig. 4. Pinch grip while performing the Action Research Arm Test (Patient 4).

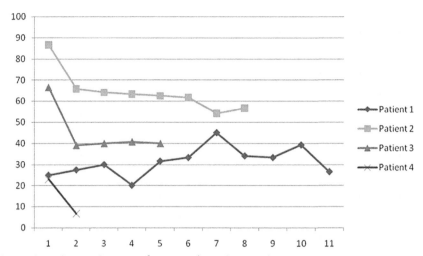

Fig. 5. DASH questionnaire. x axis: years after transplantation, y axis: score.

Patient quality of life improved in more than 75% of the recipients worldwide, and going back to work has been a consistent feature for most of them. DASH score improved as shown in **Fig. 8**.

Intrinsic muscle function was achieved earlier in the Innsbruck cases compared with other centers. However, the sensory recovery achieved is comparable with that of the IRHCTT cases. Furthermore, a faster progress was found in our 4 patients according to their DASH scores compared with the presented worldwide cases. The same observation was noted for HTSS functional outcome.

DISCUSSION

The rehabilitation of a patient after hand transplantation starts before surgery with the baseline examination by a multidisciplinary therapist team. From the beginning, we follow the principals of rehabilitation cycles, which entail a continuous cycle of assessment, assignment, intervention, and evaluation.[24] After finding/composing the right rehabilitation team, which has a significant influence on the functional outcome of the applied procedure, our attention is turned to the patient's compliance.

Components of a composite tissue transplant, such as bones, muscle-tendon units, nerves, vessels, and skin, do not only recover/regenerate

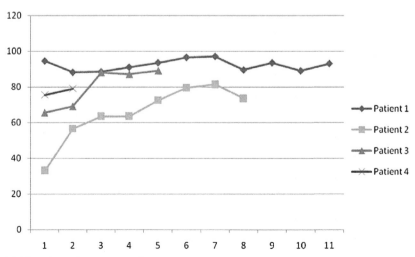

Fig. 6. HTSS right hand. x axis: years, y axis: score.

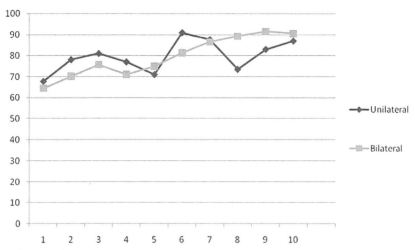

Fig. 7. HTSS results according to IRHCTT. x axis: years, y axis: score.

in different ways but also at a different pace, which requires the design of an individual and specialized rehabilitation protocol that focuses on the diverse regeneration times and different anatomic structures, always bearing in mind the main goal: a significant improvement of the function, quality of life, and self-esteem of the transplanted patient.

The aim of rehabilitation after hand transplantation is defined by the best outcome in motor and sensory function through the protection of the reconstructed structures during the healing process. This goal is applied to all levels of the ICF (International Classification of Functioning, Disability and Health) model.[25,26]

One challenge of the rehabilitation team is to identify the rehabilitation problems/limitations of each patient and to maintain the process of rehabilitation.

Physical therapy offers a wide range of treatment techniques that can be used successfully in the rehabilitation of hand transplant recipients.[27,28] In the planning stage of the rehabilitation program of our first patient, we applied the ICF model and related this to our experience with rehabilitation programs for patients who had undergone replantation of their hands after traumatic amputation.

Therefore, we introduced the early protective motion program at the beginning of the rehabilitation. These exercises maintain optimal length of ligament and joint capsular structure of the metacarpophalangeal joints, at the same time preventing swelling formation in finger joints and

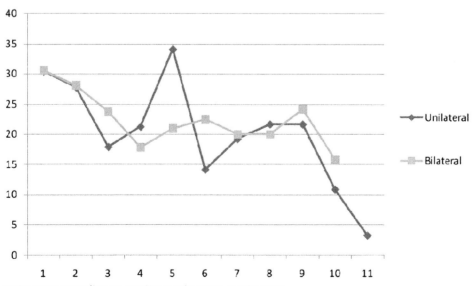

Fig. 8. DASH score according to IRHCTT. x axis: years, y axis: score.

balancing the tension between flexors and extensors.[29] We soon realized that our main attention had to be on sensory reeducation. Consequently, we added the specific cognitive exercise program, based on Perfetti,[20] to our rehabilitation program. This program is designed to induce a new mental concept-motor-imagery into the patients' programming of motor action and into their motor execution by using targeted, tailored tasks. Only such an individually tailored rehabilitation program secures a personalized protocol, flexible enough to be adapted to individual requirements, whenever needed. In the selection of applications of physiotherapy, particular attention has to be paid to including peripheral nerve stimulation to shape the organization of the sensorimotor cortex projection to the hand.[30,31]

Standardized tests and questionnaires were used at regular intervals to evaluate the patient's ability to use the transplanted hand properly.

There is a wide variety of published functional measures and questionnaires to assess upper extremity function and disability.[32–34] However, there is no specific method for patients having hand transplants that specifically documents the function and use of the transplanted hand in the patient's everyday life.

A prerequisite for the assessment of the patient's functional impairment and for evaluating the effects of rehabilitation is standardized measurement of the relevant parameters. The 3 broad categories of parameters[35] that can be measured are objective (eg, measurement of impairment of movement, strength, sensibility, and dexterity), subjective (eg, use of questionnaires to evaluate symptoms, disability, or handicap), and, if required, cost analysis (consideration of treatment costs). Measures for assessment and evaluation include both clinical measures and patient-orientated questionnaires. Clinical measures should include technical measures, such as imaging (functional magnetic resonance imaging), single clinical tests, or test batteries. Subjective assessment of treatment outcome can be obtained by questionnaires completed by patients at various stages in the rehabilitation process. Questionnaires reported by observers are especially significant for this type of rehabilitation. Outcome assessment is another essential tool for reporting, monitoring, and evaluating the results of interventions with patients, particularly because many different modalities of rehabilitation are used. However, it is important to assess patients' ability to use their hands.

One of the traditional single tests in our assessment protocol is active and passive range-of-motion measurement.[36] Published guidelines specify the starting position of the joint being evaluated and the correct placement of the goniometer in relation to the joint. The recurring measurements should be performed by the same examiner, because intratester reliability is higher than intertester reliability. This test can be performed manually with a goniometer, with biometrics, or with newer techniques such as optoelectronic, electromagnetic trackers, or kinematic devices.[37] However, there remains some doubt about the validity of this test system. The main concerns are twofold: first, is the measurement of the joint really passive, and, second, what are the normal values for the test concerning age, gender, and hand dominance?

Testing of muscle strength is one of the most frequently used means of hand assessment. Manual testing of muscle strength is reported on the Medical Research Council's scale from 0 to 5.[38,39] For more precise measurements, the dynamometer (isometric dynamometer, isokinetic dynamometer, pinch gauge) is used.[40] Normative data may vary with a participant's condition and the standard position is not always precisely defined. An instrumented keyboard and an instrumented mouselike device were also recommended for the individual evaluation of hand and finger force.[41]

When considering the appropriate tests for sensory assessment, the following facts should be taken into account: (1) restitution of functional sensibility correlates with specific central nervous system cognitive capacities.[42] (2) The new way that the hand communicates with the brain after hand transplantation cannot always be explained in an appropriate way. (3) The most commonly used tests that are assumed to measure sensibility actually measure pressure or vibration perception; others measure spatial discrimination, temperature sensation, or tactile gnosis. (4) Moving 2-PD and functional sensory testing such as the Moberg test may be influenced by the rehabilitation program, which is based on sensory retraining. Static 2-PD, which tests recovery of the slowly adapting fibers, is an objective reflection of the surgical team's performance.[43,44]

Dexterity has an impact on individual functional independence. Speed and precision are the criteria used to measure this skill. Finger dexterity and manual dexterity need to be determined. We are in favor of the Minnesota Manual Dexterity Test and the 9-hole peg test.

Self-reported questionnaires allow clinicians to understand a patient's experience. They are easy to perform and require no special equipment. One of these tests is the DASH. Its advantages are its sound development methodology and the normative data that are available.[42] Its drawbacks are that it was designed to measure disability and cannot measure impairment, handicap, or satisfaction.

Other important measures are objective, observer-reported questionnaires that assess the ability of the patient to perform the various tasks of daily life. One recent technique is the 400-points score.[45] The items are divided into 4 scales: hand mobility, prehensile strength, monomanual prehension, and bimanual function. This score provides an objective evaluation of hand function and adaptation to handicap. The test does not take pain or sensibility problems into account and evaluates dexterity incompletely. One of the well-known questionnaires is the Carroll test[46] and its successor the Action Research Arm Test (ARAT),[47] which we prefer and used in the assessment of our patients. The ARAT has been sufficiently proved for construct validity and is characterized by high correlation coefficients of its scores, with scores of validated impairment measures. The test also correlates with functional activities of daily living scales. We used this test for the first time for patients who had hand transplants and found that the test results strongly correlate with the results of the DASH questionnaire.

Until now, the only score that has been specifically developed for hand-transplanted patients is the HTSS, which evaluates 6 aspects with different weights for a total of 100 points: appearance, sensibility, movement, psychological and social acceptance, daily activities and work status, patient satisfaction, and general well-being.

With the currently available test systems mentioned earlier, the functional outcome of hand transplantation can be reported in a reproducible way.

In our experience, some critical points need to be emphasized to achieve optimal functional outcomes after hand transplantation. First, good teamwork is necessary to create an individually tailored rehabilitation program. Second, the rehabilitation activities should start as early as possible after surgery. Third, sensory reeducation must not be neglected. Fourth, the measurement instruments used should be valid, reliable, and feasible, and, fifth, standardized implementation of selected tests has to be reconsidered on a regular basis. In addition, the development of a specific ICF core set for hand transplantation patients should be advocated. Using a standardized method of describing a patient's condition and function, results can be followed and compared based on the same criteria. In addition, the rehabilitation protocol can be adapted and changed according to the functional development and achieved results.

The world experience with hand transplantation has shown some of our initial hypotheses to be correct; for example, the time between amputation and hand transplantation is not critical. It has been shown that an intensive rehabilitation program can improve function even several years after amputation and transplantation. The rehabilitation program tailored to the patient's particular needs should therefore start as early as possible, and should last for a period that is long enough to achieve a good functional outcome, superior to that with a prosthesis, combined with the additional advantage of regaining sensory function.

Although the list of factors that influence the outcome of hand transplantation is already long (eg, level and mechanism of amputation, surgical technique, ischemia time, immunosuppression therapy, rejection) there are other considerations in our personal experience.

First, the patients' compliance and understanding of their loss of body integrity are prerequisites for positive thinking and the development of the right motivation to undergo hand transplantation. These psychological indicators have to be tested and confirmed before surgery to obtain the optimal basis for a long-term alliance with the rehabilitation team and intensive rehabilitation program. If such factors are neglected, serious problems and difficulties in postoperative recovery may arise. The main goals of this high-technology procedure of hand transplantation are, and remain, to achieve complete independence in daily activities and successful integration of the transplanted limb into the patient's sense of self. Patients may not be interested in all assessment procedures, measurements, and data points. They need to have self-confidence according to achieved functional and sensory recovery. With a high level of identification and motivation, our expectations of the postsurgical outcome can be exceeded. It is possible to achieve intrinsic muscle recovery and precise hand movement with sensory recovery after distal forearm or hand transplantation, provided that the ischemia time is short and surgical nerve repair is successful. However, the patient's sensation of having complete body integrity and adequate function for daily life is more important than any other consideration. Therefore, our functional goals should be coordinated with the patient's requirements and wishes. Only a specialized, well-trained and well-organized interdisciplinary rehabilitation team should guide the patient safely through the complex and long-lasting postoperative period to achieve all the goals defined by CTA.

Today, more than a decade after the first hand transplantation, the initial mandate still holds true that graft survival alone, without restoration of an operational hand, lacks justification.

REFERENCES

1. Dubernard JM, Owen E, Herzberg G, et al. Human hand allograft: report on first 6 months. Lancet 1999;353:1315–20.
2. The International Registry on Hand and Composite Tissue Transplantation. Available at: http://www.handregistry.com/page.asp?page.4.
3. Margreiter R, Brandacher G, Ninkovic M, et al. A double-hand transplant can be worth the effort. Transplantation 2002;74:85–90.
4. Dubernard JM, Petruzzo P, Lanzetta M, et al. Functional results of the first human double-hand transplantation. Ann Surg 2003;238:128–36.
5. Brandacher G, Gorantla VS, Lee A. Hand allotransplantation. Semin Plast Surg 2010;24:11–7.
6. Tobin GR, Breidenbach WC, Ildstadt ST, et al. The history of human composite tissue allotransplantation. Transplant Proc 2009;41:466–71.
7. Sucher R, Hautz T, Brandacher G, et al. Immunosuppression in hand transplantation: state of art and future perspectives. Handchir Mikrochir Plast Chir 2009;41:217–23.
8. Schneeberger S, Gorantla VS, Hautz T, et al. Immunosuppression and rejection in human hand transplantation. Transplant Proc 2009;41(2):471–5.
9. Ninkovic M. Technical and surgical details of hand transplantation. In: Lanzetta M, Dubernard JM, editors. Hand transplantation. Milan (Italy): Springer; 2007. p. 197–205.
10. Meyer VE. Hand amputations proximal but close to the wrist joint: prime candidates for reattachment (long-term functional results). J Hand Surg Am 1985;10:989–91.
11. Ninkovic M. Rehabilitation and assessment of function after hand and forearm allotransplantation. In: Programs and abstracts of 1st ACRTS Conference. Philadelphia: ASRT; 2008. p. 54.
12. Schneeberger S, Ninkovic M, Margreiter R. Hand transplantation: the Innsbruck experience. In: Hewitt CW, Lee AW, editors. Transplantation of composite tissue allografts. New York: Springer; 2008. p. 234–50.
13. Buncke HJ, Jackson RL, Buncke GM, et al. The surgical and rehabilitative aspects of replantation and revascularization of the hand. In: Hunter JM, Mackin EJ, Callahan AD, editors. Rehabilitation of the hand: surgery and therapy. 4th edition. St Louis (MO): Mosby-Year Book; 1995. p. 1075–100.
14. Schuind F, Abramowicz D, Schneeberger S. Hand transplantation: the state-of-the-art. J Hand Surg Eur Vol 2007;32(1):2–17.
15. Chen ZW, Meyer VE, Kleinert HE, et al. Present indications and contraindications for replantation as reflected by long-term functional results. Orthop Clin North Am 1981;12:849–70.
16. Jablecki J, Syrko M, Arendarska-Maj A. Patient rehabilitation following hand transplantation at forearm distal third level. Ortop Traumatol Rehabil 2010;12:570–80.
17. Schneeberger S, Ninkovic M, Gabl M, et al. First forearm transplantation: outcome at 3 years. Am J Transplant 2007;7:1753–62.
18. Brandacher G, Ninkovic M, Piza-Katzer H, et al. The Innsbruck hand transplant program: update at 8 years after the first transplant. Transplant Proc 2009;41:491–4.
19. Silverman PM, Gordon L. Early motion after replantation. Hand Clin 1996;12:97–107.
20. Übungen. In: Perfetti C, editor. Der hemiplegische Patient- Kognitiv-therapeutische Übungen. München (Germany): Pflaum; 1997. p. 108–212.
21. Scheker LR, Hodges A. Brace and rehabilitation after replantation and revascularization. Hand Clin 2001;17:473–80.
22. Lanzetta M, Petruzzo M, Margreiter M, et al. The International Registry on Hand and Composite Tissue Transplantation. Transplantation 2005;79(9):1210–4.
23. Petruzzo P, Lanzetta M, Dubernard JM, et al. The International Registry on Hand and composite Tissue Transplantation. Transplantation 2010;90(12):1590–4.
24. Stucki G, Sangha O. Principles of rehabilitation. In: Klippel JH, Dieppe PA, editors. 2nd edition, Rheumatology, 11. London: Mosby; 1998. p. 1–11, 14.
25. International Classification of Functioning, Disability and Health (ICF). ICF full version. Geneva (Switzerland): World Health Organization; 2001.
26. Fitinghoff H, Lindqvist B, Nygard L, et al. The ICF and postsurgery occupational therapy after traumatic hand injury. Int J Rehabil Res 2011;34:79–88.
27. Schutt AH, Bengston KA. Hand rehabilitation. In: DeLisa JA, Gans BM, editors. Rehabilitation medicine: principles and practice. 3rd edition. Philadelphia: Lippincott; 1998. p. 1717–32.
28. Chan SW, LaStayo P. Hand therapy management following mutilating hand injuries. Hand Clin 2003;19:133–48.
29. Petengill KM, Van Strien G. Postoperative management of flexor tendon injuries. In: Hunter JM, Mackin EJ, Callahan AD, editors. Rehabilitation of the hand and upper extremity. 5th edition. St Louis (MO): Mosby; 2002. p. 431–57.
30. Delazer M, Domahs F, Bartha L, et al. Learning complex arithmetic – an fMRI study. Cogn Brain Res 2003;18:76–88.

31. Siemionow M, Mendiola A. Methods of assessment of cortical plasticity in patients following amputation, replantation, and composite tissue allograft transplantation. Ann Plast Surg 2010;65:344–8.

32. Amadio PC. Outcome assessment in hand surgery and hand therapy: an update. J Hand Ther 2001; 14(2):63–7.

33. Barbier O, Penta M, Thonnard JL. Outcome evaluation of the hand and wrist according to the International Classification of Functioning, Disability, and Health. Hand Clin 2003;19:371–8.

34. Thigpen C, Shanley E. Clinical assessment of upper extremity injury outcomes. J Sport Rehabil 2011;20: 61–73.

35. Bindra RR, Dias JJ, Heras-Palau C, et al. Assessing outcome after hand surgery: the current state. J Hand Surg Br 2003;28:289–94.

36. Cambridge-Keeling CA. Range-of-motion measurement of the hand. In: Hunter JM, Mackin EJ, Callahan AD, editors. Rehabilitation of the hand: surgery and therapy. 4th edition. St Louis (MO): Mosby-Year Book; 1995. p. 93–107.

37. Small CT, Bryant JT, Dwosh IL, et al. Validation of a 3D optoelectronic motion analysis system for the wrist joint. Clin Biomech 1996;11:481–3.

38. Medical Research Council. Aids to examination of the peripheral nervous system. Memorandum no. 45. London: Her Majesty's Stationary Office; 1976.

39. Paternostro-Sluga T, Grim-Stieger M, Posch M, et al. Reliability and validity of the Medical Research Council (MRC) scale and a modified scale for testing muscle strength in patients with radial palsy. J Rehabil Med 2008;40(8):665–71.

40. Mathiowetz V, Weber K, Volland G, et al. Reliability and validity of grip and pinch strength evaluations. J Hand Surg Am 1984;9(2):222–6.

41. Giansanti D, Morelli S, Maccioni G, et al. Health technology assessment of a homecare device for telemonitoring and telerehabilitation for patients after hand transplantation. Telemed J E Health 2008;14(1):69–75.

42. Lundborg G. Nerve injury and repair - a challenge to the plastic brain. J Peripher Nerv Syst 2003;8: 209–26.

43. Lundborg G, Rosen B. The two-point discrimination test-time for a re-appraisal? J Hand Surg Br 2004; 29:418–22.

44. Beaton DE, Katz JN, Fossel AH, et al. Measuring the whole or the parts? Validity, reliability, and responsiveness of the Disabilities of the Arm, Shoulder, and Hand outcome measure in different regions of the upper extremity. J Hand Ther 2001;14(2):128–46.

45. Schuind FA, Mouraux D, Robert C, et al. Functional and outcome evaluation of the hand and wrist. Hand Clin 2003;19:361–9.

46. Carroll D. A quantitative test of upper extremity function. J Chronic Dis 1965;18:479–91.

47. Lyle RC. A performance test for assessment of upper limb function in physical rehabilitation treatment and research. Int J Rehabil Res 1981;4(4): 483–92.

Immunosuppressive Protocols and Immunological Challenges Related to Hand Transplantation

Kadiyala V. Ravindra, MD[a], Suzanne T. Ildstad, MD[b],*

KEYWORDS

• Hand transplant • Immunosuppression • Immunology
• Vascularized composite allotransplantation

Transplantation of skin and composite tissues was thought to be impossible not long ago[1] and its full potential remains unfulfilled after nearly 6 decades of success in the field of solid organ transplantation. The first attempt at hand transplantation, in 1964 in Ecuador,[2] failed shortly after implantation owing to acute rejection. Immunosuppression was limited at that time to the only agents available: azathioprine and hydrocortisone. This experience reinforced prior experimental work and vascularized composite allotransplantation (VCA) had to wait until 1998[3] before interest was renewed. The landmark success of the first hand transplant in Lyon, France, has opened an entire new field. Over the last decade, VCA has made significant progress. It has emerged from the confines of basic research and it is well on its way to be considered standard of care as a therapeutic option.

Hand transplantation is the most widely performed and the most successful VCA procedure. Over 50 hand transplants have been performed worldwide, including bilateral and above-elbow transplants. In the United States, 12 patients have received hand transplants at three centers to date. There have been four bilateral procedures. The worldwide experience[4] currently includes over a dozen hand recipients who have had grafts in place for more than 5 years, providing confirmation of the long-term success of the procedure.

IMMUNOLOGY OF TRANSPLANTATION

The human immune system is intricate and it has evolved to eliminate foreign antigens, usually in the form of infectious agents. This is possible because the cells of our immune system are able to recognize self from nonself antigens; ignoring the former while attacking the latter. Unfortunately, a transplanted allograft is subject to similar scrutiny by a competent immune system. Transplantation, as treatment for end-stage disease or for reconstruction of an amputated limb, was never part of the evolution of the immune system.

To prevent rejection, immunosuppressive drugs must be given to transplant recipients immediately before receiving the allograft and continued

---

This work was supported in part by The Department of the Army, Office of Army Research. (Any opinions, findings, and conclusions or recommendations expressed in this material are those of the authors and do not necessarily reflect the views of the Office of Army Research.) This publication was made possible by Awards No. W81X WH07-1-0185, W81XWH-09-2-0124, and W81X WH10-1-0688 from the Office of Army Research); the Commonwealth of Kentucky Research Challenge Trust Fund; the W. M. Keck Foundation; and The Jewish Hospital Foundation.

[a] Department of Surgery, Duke University, Durham, NC 27710, USA
[b] Institute for Cellular Therapeutics, University of Louisville, 570 South Preston Street, Suite 404, Louisville, KY 40202, USA
* Corresponding author.
E-mail address: stilds01@louisville.edu

Hand Clin 27 (2011) 467–479
doi:10.1016/j.hcl.2011.07.001

indefinitely as maintenance therapy afterwards, to prevent the body from mounting an immune response towards the allograft resulting in rejection. Curbing the immune system's ability to effectively mount an immune response against the graft is the goal of transplant surgery. As the various components of the immune response are defined and their mechanisms of action delineated, more specific immunosuppressive agents have been developed.

However, the long-term use of these drugs comes at a price. Many of these drugs, particularly the calcineurin inhibitors (CNIs), which are the most commonly used agents, are nephrotoxic.[5] Furthermore, because they nonspecifically suppress a normal immune response, these agents increase the susceptibility to infection and, in the long term, cancer. Maintenance immunosuppression involves a delicate art of balancing the prevention of graft rejection (under-immunosuppression) while avoiding the risks of sepsis, end-organ damage, and neoplasia (over-immunosuppression). The traditional approach to immunosuppressive therapy involved a one-size-fits-all triple-drug regimen. More recently, induction immunosuppression at the time of transplant with lymphodepleting agents, such as thymoglobulin[6–8] and alemtuzumab,[9,10] has allowed steroid elimination and, sometimes, even monotherapy. Despite these advances, an unequivocal improvement in long-term results has yet to be demonstrated.[11] A clear understanding of the immunology of transplantation provides insight into novel approaches to minimize immunosuppression and maximize outcomes.

Basics of Transplantation Immunology

There are two categories of immune responses: innate immunity and adaptive immunity. The innate immune responses are present from birth and generate immediate nonspecific killing of foreign antigens. When the epithelial lining of the skin, gastrointestinal tract, and respiratory tract serving as a protective barrier from the external world is violated, for example by surgical incision, the injury can result in the introduction of microbes into the body that are capable of causing infection. The dominant players of innate immunity include macrophages, neutrophils, and natural killer cells. These cells migrate to the sites of infection, ingest, and kill microbes, such as bacteria and virus, generating the first line of attack against foreign antigens. They do not require priming and the action is rapid. This process can involve the complement system. The response is nonspecific and neither attenuates nor amplifies, even after multiple exposures to the same antigen. Cells of the innate immune system, such as macrophages and dendritic cells, also play a major role in presenting alloantigen to lymphocytes and are called antigen-presenting cells (APC). They ingest and process microbes and display the packaged alloantigens bound to self-major histocompatibility complex (MHC) molecules on the cell surface. Some of these antigen-presenting cells then migrate to the lymph nodes and spleen and present themselves to lymphocytes, the key players of adaptive immunity. An important property of T cell antigen recognition is self-MHC restriction. This term relates to the ability of T cells to recognize alloantigen only when it is presented by the APC attached to self-MHC molecules. However, the direct pathway of transplant alloantigen presentation, in which the APCs of the donor present their own antigens, is an exception to this rule.

In contrast to the nonspecific and nonincremental innate immune response, adaptive immunity is very specific and retains memory, resulting in an amplified and rapid response at second exposure. Lymphocytes play the primary role in adaptive immunity, the largest components of which are B lymphocytes (B cells) and T lymphocytes (T cells). On average, the human body contains 1×10^{12} lymphocytes, which are 20% to 40% of all leukocytes. These lymphocytes reside in the bone marrow, thymus, lymph nodes, spleen, and can be found in the periphery. B cells are derived primarily in the bone marrow. Interaction between T cells and a specific antigen processed and presented by APCs results in activation of B cells and antibody production against that antigen (**Fig. 1**).

Immature T cells are produced in the bone marrow and migrate to the thymus as precursor T cells. Of these precursor T cells, 98% will be eliminated in the early period of development by positive selection and negative selection (**Fig. 2**). In positive selection, T cells are selected that recognize only self-MHC. Of this population, T cells that recognize self-MHC with too high affinity are deleted to avoid autoimmunity. T cells are the forerunners of the cell-mediated immune response. There are two classes of T cells: the CD4[+] helper T cell and the CD8[+] cytotoxic T cell. CD4[+] T cells help B lymphocytes produce antibodies and phagocytes to destroy ingested microbes. CD8[+] T cells lyse cells harboring intracellular microbes. Activation of T cells is a complex process that requires the binding of the T cell receptor (TCR) to antigens processed by APCs in the context of MHC proteins.

The MHC proteins are present on the surface of cells and give unique identity. In humans, the MHC is the human leukocyte antigen (HLA) system. The MHC are encoded by genes on chromosome 6 and

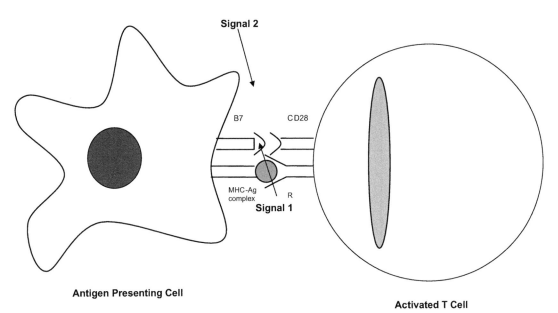

Fig. 1. APC present antigen to T cells via signal 1 (T cell receptor). T cell-activation requires signal 2 costimulatory molecule stabilization to proceed.

play a major role in adaptive immunity. The MHC is the most important determinant of acceptance or rejection of tissues exchanged between individuals—identity of the MHC genes (inbred animals and identical twins) promotes acceptance, whereas disparity is associated with a rejection response. HLA genes are divided into three classes: class I, class II, and class III. The most widely recognized are A, B, and C (class I) and DP, DQ, and DR (class II). These genes exhibit great polymorphism, making MHC identity among unrelated individuals a rarity. HLA proteins encoded by HLA genes are expressed on the cell surface and play a crucial role in transplant immunology. Class I proteins are expressed on all nucleated cells, whereas class II are expressed mainly on the surface of APC. Exposure to nonself-HLA antigens (through blood transfusion, pregnancy, or previous organ or tissue transplant) leads to the development of antibodies against these antigens. These antibodies can cause immediate rejection (hyperacute rejection) of a graft from a donor bearing the same nonself-HLA specificity. The routine practice of cross-match testing before kidney transplantation helps to identify the presence of preformed donor specific antibodies in the recipient. CD4$^+$ T cells recognize antigens bound to class II MHC, whereas CD8$^+$ T cells recognize antigens bound to class I MHC.

Activation of T Cells: Signals 1, 2, and 3

After transplantation, the protein products of the donor (alloantigen) are recognized by the recipient's lymphocytes. The donor HLA antigens expressed by the donor's APC may be directly recognized by the recipient's lymphocytes (direct pathway) or the donor HLA antigens may be processed by the recipient's APC and presented along with self-MHC to the host's lymphocytes (indirect pathway). The direct pathway of presentation of donor antigen is unique to the immune response to transplants. How do recipient T cells recognize donor alloantigen and initiate the immune response? The TCR that is present on the surface of the host T lymphocytes recognizes the appropriate antigen-MHC complex, thereby initiating the cell-mediated immune response. This binding of TCR on the T lymphocyte to the alloantigen-MHC complex on the APC is described as the first signal. However, the first signal by itself is insufficient to initiate activation of the intracellular pathway that leads to a full-blown immune response. Simultaneously, there must be binding of accessory molecules such as B7 on the APC to the CD28 molecule on the surface of T cells. This crucial process is called costimulation and is the second signal necessary to start the intracellular cascade, which results in T cell activation. When signals 1 and 2 occur concurrently, the immune response proceeds and there is activation of phosphatases in the cytoplasm that then lead to activation of the nuclear factor of activated T cells (NFAT). NFAT activation results in the transcription of genes that lead to production of important cytokines that lead to a runaway immune response. Various cytokines, such as IL (interleukin)-2, IL-4, and IL-5, are produced

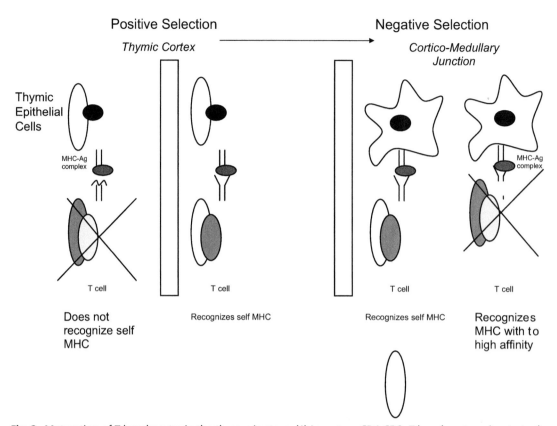

Fig. 2. Maturation of T lymphocytes in the thymus in steps. (1) Immature CD4-CD8- T lymphocytes migrate to the thymus from the bone marrow. (2) Positive selection: T lymphocytes begin to express T cell receptors, CD4, and CD8 on their surface. Those T cells that interact with a cortical epithelial cell presenting MHC class I go on to become CD8+ T cells. Those T cells that interact with a cortical cell presenting MHC class II go on to become CD4+ T cells. Those T cells that possess T cell receptors that are unable to interact with either MHC class I or II undergo apoptosis. (3) Negative selection: the still maturing T cells migrate towards the thymic medulla. There they interact with specialized dendritic cells presenting self antigens. Those T cells that interact with self antigen undergo apoptosis, whereas those that do not interact migrate to the periphery.

and the result is proliferation of an antigen-specific T cell population and differentiation of T cells into effector T cells capable of destroying foreign antigens (**Fig. 3**).[12] The binding of IL-2 to receptors on the surface of the activated T cells triggers the mammalian target of rapamycin (mTOR) to induce T cell proliferation and further cytokine production. This step is referred to as signal 3. If signal 2 is blocked while signal 1 is activated (costimulatory blockade), activation does not result. This observation has resulted in a new generation of immunosuppressive agents currently under clinical evaluation. Approaches to induce anergy through costimulatory molecule blockade are being tested clinically as a novel form of immunosuppression.[13–15]

Immunological Challenges of Composite Tissue

Why have skin-containing structures defied transplantation for so long? Studies in the 1960s documented the challenges of transplanting composite tissues. Murray[1] reported that skin was the most antigenic of all tissues tested. The immunogenicity of skin may be related to skin-specific antigens in the epidermis and the presence of a large number of APCs that could quickly be involved in direct presentation of alloantigens.[16] When Lee and colleagues[17] compared individual vascularized limb tissues (skin, subcutaneous tissue, muscle, bone, and blood vessels) and a whole limb with respect to the intensity of cell-mediated and humoral immune responses, they reported that no single tissue predominated in the elicited immune response and that, surprisingly, the whole limb allograft generated a less potent immune response than the individual components. The general perception that the skin component would mirror the immunological activity in the VCA graft has recently been questioned. In the first human hand allograft removed because of rejection

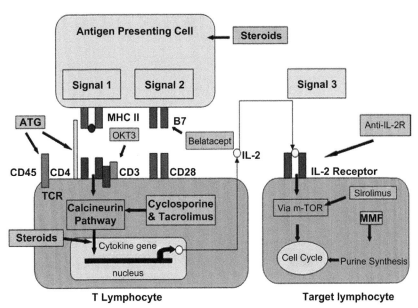

Fig. 3. 3 Signal model of T cell activation and sites of action of different drugs. The signal 3 pathway is essential for the immunological response following transplantation. Signal 1 is the binding of the between the nonself protein and CD3 receptor. Signal 2 that occurs almost simultaneously is the essential costimulation with the binding of B7 and CD28. The events that follow the generation of IL-2 constitute signal 3. (*Reprinted from Arias M, Campistol JM, Vincenti F. Evolving trends in induction therapy. Transplantation Rev 2009;23(2):94–102; with permission.*)

secondary to noncompliance, the histological changes were most intense in the skin.[18] Contrasting findings were reported from China by Wang and colleagues.[19] A recent report from Louisville describing the loss of a hand transplant at 9 months pointed out that blood vessels may be the dominant target of rejection.[4]

MECHANISM OF ACTION OF IMMUNOSUPPRESSIVE AGENTS

The various immunosuppressive agents used clinically may be grouped as follows:

1. Induction agents
2. CNIs
3. Antimetabolites
4. mTOR inhibitors
5. Costimulatory molecule blockers.

The exact site of action of each category of these agents in the immune response cascade is depicted in **Fig. 4**. Broadly, the lymphodepleting agents act at signal 1 by destroying lymphocytes and preventing activation. CNIs and IL-2 blocking agents act at signal 1 and 3, respectively, by inhibiting cytokine production and IL-2 mediated activation of mTOR. Antiproliferating agents, azathioprine and mycophenolate mofetil (MMF) and mTOR inhibitors sirolimus and everolimus act downstream from signal 3, causing inhibition of T lymphocyte proliferation. Many newer agents are being evaluated to target other sites of the immunological activation pathway. The most promising is belatacept (binds CD80 and CD86), which acts at signal 2 by inhibiting binding to the costimulation receptor.

Induction Agents

By convention, the word induction has been largely used to describe the use of biological agents or monoclonal antibodies that deplete T or B cells, or modulate the cellular or antibody responses at the time of antigen presentation, with the goal of preventing early acute rejection. These agents are given at the time of transplantation and the aim is sudden and large-scale suppression of the immune response. The use of biologic induction agents has steadily increased during the past decade. Most renal and pancreas transplant patients undergo induction therapy. The sole exception is liver transplantation where only 20% of patients receive induction therapy.[20] Antibody therapy has been used with a variety of aims: (1) to delay the initiation of CNI in the immediate posttransplant period, (2) to treat highly sensitized individuals, (3) to foster steroid avoidance and withdrawal, (4) to lower dose of CNI, and (5) as a means of achieving prope tolerance. During the past decade, there has been a dramatic shift from the use of OK-T3 and

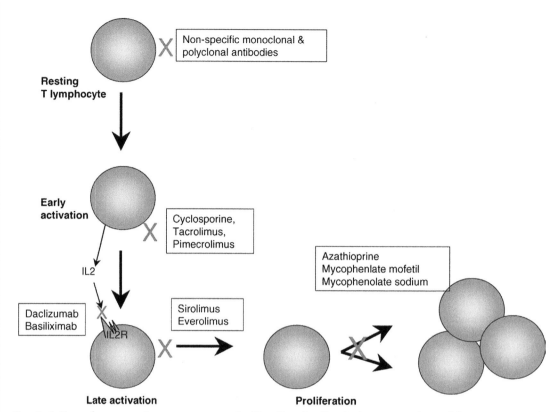

Fig. 4. Action of common immunosuppressants. The site of action is the commonly used immunosuppressive agents. Lymphodepleting agents act on the resting lymphocytes to prevent initiation of the rejection cascade, CNIs act in the early phase following activation, IL-2 blocking monoclonal antibodies block activated lymphocytes, sirolimus acts during late activation, and MMF prevents active proliferation of lymphocytes. (*Reprinted from* Taylor AL, Watson CJ, Bradley JA. Immunosuppressive agents in solid organ transplantation: mechanisms of action and therapeutic efficacy. Crit Rev Oncol Hematol 2005;56(1):23–46; with permission).

equine-derived polyclonal antithymocyte antibody to the better tolerated rabbit-derived antithymocyte antibody (thymoglobulin) and anti–IL-2 monoclonal antibodies basiliximab and daclizumab.[20] Of late, many centers have initiated the use of alemtuzumab (Campath-1H), an anti–CD-52 monoclonal antibody that depletes T cells, B cells, and NK cells, for induction therapy.[10,21]

Maintenance Agents

These agents include CNIs, prednisone, MMF, and sirolimus. Tacrolimus and cyclosporine A, both CNIs, act by blocking downstream propagation of signal 1 and are the most potent agents we currently use. Tacrolimus has been the backbone of most immunosuppression protocols in hand transplantation. The therapeutic levels used in hand transplantation have been higher (10–15 ng/ml) than those used in liver and kidney transplantation. The drawback is the long-term side effects, including nephrotoxicity, diabetes, hypertension, posttransplant lymphoproliferative disorder, and

infection. Tacrolimus, however, has been demonstrated to enhance nerve regeneration[22] and may be beneficial in hand transplantation.

MMF has been used extensively in hand transplantation and is the second most commonly used agent. Its active component, mycophenolic acid, inhibits the synthesis of guanosine nucleotides required for the proliferation of activated lymphocytes. Thus, it is cytostatic and prevents amplification of the immune response. It is part of most current immunosuppressive regimes. Major drawbacks include gastrointestinal side effects and bone marrow suppression.

Sirolimus blocks the mTOR step in signal 3 and, thus, the multiplication of lymphocytes. It is being used as a renal protective agent to eliminate or reduce the dose of CNI. The major side effects include poor wound healing, anemia, and elevated lipids.

IMMUNOSUPPRESSION PROTOCOLS

The combination and sequence of agents used varies widely from organ to organ and center to center. Triple-drug immunosuppression with a CNI, an antiproliferative agent, and prednisone was the most widely used regimen at most of the centers for solid organ transplantation until the past decade. Marked changes have been documented in this practice in the past decade.

The CNI used predominantly is tacrolimus. The use of cyclosporine A has diminished, although it continues to be the agent to be compared against when new agents are being tested. The chronic use of corticosteroids has been challenged by the use of lymphodepleting agents. The increased interest in steroid-free immunosuppression has been fuelled by the recognition that nearly half the transplant loss is related to patient death from cardiovascular disease and infectious complications. Long-term steroid use is blamed for the elevated cardiovascular morbidity. Many studies during the past decade have clearly demonstrated that steroids can be eliminated without an increase in short-term or intermediate-term detriment to the graft or patient. There has also been some evidence that factors that contribute to cardiovascular morbidity, such as hypertension and diabetes, may be favorably altered with steroid avoidance. However, the use of these agents with the idea that prope tolerance would be achieved has not been realized. The long-term outcomes with these strategies have not shown improvements compared with the older triple-drug combination regimens.

Thymoglobulin and alemtuzumab are the most commonly used agents in the steroid avoidance protocols. These drugs are given in the perioperative period as induction agents and patients are then maintained long-term on tacrolimus and MMF.

Challenges of Immunosuppression in Hand Transplantation

The single most important obstacle that currently prevents clinical application of limb transplantation is the risk associated with immunosuppressive therapy.[3] There has been controversy about whether it is ethical to potentially shorten the life of recipients owing to the cardiovascular, infectious, and neoplastic complications that will surely follow. The debate continues; however, the long-term success of the procedure, along with the improved quality of life of the recipients, has helped convince many skeptics that the procedure has a role.

There is a delicate balance between administering sufficient immunosuppression to prevent rejection and avoiding over-immunosuppression to reduce the associated complications. The incidence of acute rejection in hand transplant recipients is 85% in the first year.[23] This is higher than that currently seen in solid organ transplantation. For example, the incidence of acute rejection with the use of lymphodepletion in kidney transplantation is less than 10% in the first year.[10] The vastly different incidence of acute rejection is largely due to the easy visibility of the hand graft, which enables prompt and safe biopsy based on even minor changes in appearance.

SUMMARY OF IMMUNOSUPPRESSION DATA IN HAND TRANSPLANTATION

There is no standard immunosuppression protocol. The first successful hand transplant recipient (performed in Lyon, France) received induction with thymoglobulin (8 mg/kg for 10 days) and was maintained on tacrolimus, MMF, and prednisone.[3] The level of tacrolimus was adjusted to 10 to 15 ng/ml during the first month and 5 to 10 ng/ml thereafter. Prednisone dose was rapidly tapered to 20 mg/day in the immediate postoperative period and further lowered to 15 mg/day by 6 months. In addition, the patient received anti–CD-25 monoclonal antibody on days 26 and 100. Complications included diabetes and herpes infection. The patient lost the graft 29 months after transplantation following noncompliance with medication after 15 months.[18] Subsequent patients at Lyon have received similar immunosuppression and have satisfactory results.[24]

Most of the hand transplant patients have received induction agents.[4] Thymoglobulin has been the most widely used agent and was administered to 50% of patients. Basiliximab has been the second most commonly used agent, reported as used in 25% of patients. Alemtuzumab has

Table 1 Long-term complications related to immunosuppression reported in hand transplant recipients[4]	
Complications	**N**
Infections	29
Cytomegalovirus	10
Bacterial	9
Skin Mycosis	5
Herpes	3
Clostridium difficile	2
Metabolic Problems	23
Renal Dysfunction	6
Need for Hemodialysis	1

N, Number.

Table 2
Summary of the individual reports from different centers highlighting the immunosuppression and reported complications

Center/Year	Age	Induction	Maintenance	Rejection Treatment	Metabolic Problems	Infections	Cancers
Lyon 1998	48	Thymoglobulin × 10 days CD25 agent × 2 (d 6 and 100)	FK, MMF, and prednisone	Oral steroids, Topical agents	Diabetes	Herpes	—
Louisville 1999	37	Basiliximab × 2 doses	FK, MMF, and prednisone, prednisone stopped at 8 y	IV Solu-Medrol, topical agents	—	CMV tinea (skin)	—
Guangzhou 1999	39	Thymoglobulin × 7 d	FK, MMF, and prednisone	—	—	Tinea (skin)	—
Guangzhou 1999	27	Thymoglobulin × 7 d	FK, MMF, and prednisone	—	—	—	—
Lyon 2000 (Bilateral)	33	Thymoglobulin × 10 d CD25 agent × 2 (d 12 and 20)	FK, MMF, and prednisone	Oral steroids, topical agents	Transient hyperglycemia	—	—
Innsbruck 2000 (Bilateral)	47	Thymoglobulin	FK, MMF, and prednisone; weaned to sirolimus and MMF	Steroids	Diabetes, hyperlipidemia	CMV	—
Louisville 2001	36	Basiliximab × 2 doses	FK, sirolimus and prednisone	IV Solu-Medrol topical	Diabetes, hyperlipidemia, osteonecrosis hips	Pneumonia	—
Milano 2002	33	—	FK, MMF, and prednisone	Thymoglobulin	—	CMV	—
Belgium 2002	22	Thymoglobulin	FK, MMF, and prednisone	—	—	—	—

Center (year)	Patients	Induction	Maintenance	Rejection treatment (Oral steroids / Topical agents)	Metabolic complications	Infectious complications	Other (Osteomyelitis / malignancy)
Lyon 2003 (Bilateral)	21	Thymoglobulin × 4 d	FK, MMF, and prednisone	Oral steroids Topical agents	Hypertension	Osteomyelitis	—
Innsbruck 2003 (Bilateral)	41	Thymoglobulin	FK, MMF, and prednisone; weaned to everolimus and MMF	Steroids, basiliximab alemtuzumab	—	1. CMV 2. Invasive fungal (*Alternaria*) 3. Papilloma warts	—
Lanzetta 2004 (French 3 and Italian 3)	43, 33, 35 32, 33, 22	Thymoglobulin 3 Basiliximab 3	FK, MMF, and prednisone	Systemic steroids and topical drug	Transient hyperglycemia and hypertension	Clostridium infection	—
Louisville 2006	54	Alemtuzumab × 1 dose	FK, MMF	Topical	Hyperlipidemia	CMV	Mantle zone lymphoma
Innsbruck 2006 (Bilateral)	23	Alemtuzumab	FK, prednisone	Steroids, IV alemtuzumab	—	CMV	—
Poland 2006	32	Basiliximab	FK, MMF, and prednisone	Oral steroids, topical FK	Diabetes	Candida (wound)	—
Valencia 2006 (Bilateral)	47	Alemtuzumab	FK, MMF, and prednisone; FK replaced with sirolimus	IV Solu-Medrol	1. Diabetes 2. Hypertension 3. Hypertriglyceridemia	1. Varicella zoster 2. Fungal—skin	—
Poland 2008 (Bilateral)	29	Basiliximab	FK, MMF, prednisone	—	—	—	—
Valencia 2008 (Bilateral arm)	29	Alemtuzumab	FK, MMF	—	—	—	1. Basal cell carcinoma
Innsbruck 2009	47, 41, 23	ATG 2 Alemtuzumab 1	FK, prednisone in all MMF in 2	IV steroids, basiliximab, alemtuzumab, topical	Diabetes, hyperlipidemia Hypertension	CMV in all Tissue invasive fungus (*Alternaria*), papilloma warts	—

Abbreviations: ATG, anti-thymocyte; CMV, cytomegalovirus; FK, tacrolimus; IV, intravenous.

been used in about 14% of patients—as part of the steroid-sparing protocol at Louisville[25] and Valencia, and with steroid use at Innsbruck.[26]

Triple-drug therapy, resembling what is currently the most widely used in solid organ transplantation, has been the mainstay at most centers performing hand transplantation. The only exception has been the third hand transplant recipient (Louisville) who was on a steroid-free protocol for nearly 2 years. Long-term maintenance therapy has varied: 21.7% of patients received only steroids and tacrolimus; 8.7% were switched to sirolimus; 8.7% were on low-dose tacrolimus, steroids, and everolimus; 4.3% were on sirolimus and MMF; and 13% were completely weaned off steroids.[23] The reasons for switching to sirolimus included renal protection,[27] lowering of tacrolimus that was responsible for poor glycemic control,[25] and avoidance of chronic rejection and neurotoxicity.[27]

Topical tacrolimus and steroids ointment were used as part of the immunosuppression protocol in the two recipients who did not receive induction.[28] They were also primarily used in two patients who were only on two-drug maintenance therapy. However, most centers have utilized the topical agents only during episodes of acute rejection.[24,25,29] There has been paucity of data on the schedule and duration of use of these agents.

The University of Pittsburg has recently presented data on their initial experience with the use of donor bone marrow infusion in hand transplant recipients. The goal is induction of chimerism with the intent to promote tolerance and minimize immunosuppression. The patients received alemtuzumab induction and maintenance immunosuppression in the form of tacrolimus monotherapy. This study is currently ongoing and long-term results are pending.

The Louisville experience highlights the dilemma surrounding minimization of immunosuppression in hand transplantation. Although it would be ideal to give enough immunosuppression to prevent rejection, there are risks associated with the approach. The first two Louisville patients received basiliximab induction and triple-drug immunosuppression with tacrolimus or sirolimus, MMF, and prednisone.[25] These two patients have functioning grafts at 11 and 9 years respectively—one of them has been completely weaned off steroids 8 years after transplant. The third patient received alemtuzumab induction and maintenance with tacrolimus and MMF, which worked well for 18 months. However, due to the detection of mantle zone lymphoma (later proven to have been present before the hand transplant), the immunosuppression was withdrawn for 6 weeks, leading to acute rejection. This led to reinstitution of triple-drug

therapy. The fourth patient was managed with a similar protocol to the third but was further weaned to half the dose of MMF at 9 months. The graft developed features consistent with severe arteriosclerosis, thought to be due to chronic rejection versus humoral rejection, and was lost.

The overwhelming message seems to be that conventional immunosuppression, similar to that used in renal transplantation, works well in hand transplantation. Attempts to withdraw medications based on the assumption that visible changes will help detect and prevent a runaway rejection episode may have to be reconsidered. As of now, induction with a CD-25 antibody or a lymphocyte-depleting agent followed by maintenance with at least two drugs at optimum dose is recommended.

Side-Effect Profile in Hand Transplantation

The risks associated with the use of long-term immunosuppression remain the chief concern in this unique set of patients. Most of them are in good health, few have preexisting medical conditions, and have been through rigorous screening required by the individual institution's review board protocols. The trough level of tacrolimus has been high in most protocols, particularly in the first few months posttransplantation. The trough levels of 15 ng/ml are higher than that used in most solid organ transplant recipients. As expected, this has been associated with a significant number of posttransplant complications—infectious and metabolic. These are highlighted in the most recent report from the International Hand Transplant Registry (**Table 1**).[4] Some of the individually reported complications have been tabulated in **Table 2**.

Cardiovascular disease is a leading cause of mortality in solid organ transplantation. In data collected by the US Renal Data System, any immunosuppressive agent was identified as a risk factor for cardiovascular disease.[30] However, traditional risk factors such as hypertension and diabetes are preexistent in most renal recipients. In contrast, most hand transplant recipients are in good health and data on the prevalence of risk factors is not available.

Posttransplant hypertension and diabetes are commonly seen in solid organ transplant recipients. New-onset diabetes after transplantation occurs in 5% to 20% of transplant recipients within the first year posttransplant.[31] Tacrolimus and sirolimus have been reported to be diabetogenic.[32,33] Hyperglycemia has been reported in 9 out of 33 patients in the recent publication from the International Registry on Hand and Composite Tissue Allotransplantation.[4] Hypertension was reported in 5 out of 33 patients. The data on hyperlipidemia is lacking.

Infections have been reported in nearly two-thirds of recipients; cytomegalovirus (CMV) infection has been common.[34] It has caused serious problems in some patients, often forcing centers to avoid the use of CMV-positive organs into naïve recipients.[35] The high incidence of CMV infection in hand transplant recipients is probably related to the higher levels of immunosuppression agents used (widespread use of lymphodepletion, high tacrolimus levels). It may be worthwhile considering other options, such as a longer duration of CMV prophylaxis and/or closer monitoring of CMV antigenemia, after the prophylaxis ends.

Data on osteoporosis in hand transplant recipients is lacking. One patient required bilateral hip replacement following steroid-related avascular necrosis of femoral head.[25]

Following the transplantation of a nonrenal organ, chronic renal failure believed to be secondary to the CNIs has been reported in 16.5% of recipients during 36 months follow-up.[5] Some hand transplant recipients have been reported to have elevated serum creatinine levels and one patient has end-stage renal disease.[4] So far, none has received a renal transplant.

Since the first report of de novo cancer occurring in renal transplant recipients, data from registries have confirmed that malignancies are a common complication after transplantation.[36,37] The incidence is threefold to fivefold greater in transplant recipients compared with the general population and increases with the duration of follow-up. The most frequent types of malignancies are nonmelanoma skin cancer, lymphoma, and other viral-related cancers.[38] These data have important implications for the follow-up of hand transplant recipients. Most recipients have been followed for fewer than 5 years—the true risks to hand recipients remains unknown.

The Valencia Hand Transplant Unit has recently reported the first case of skin malignancy following hand transplantation.[39] The patient was a 48-year-old woman who received induction with alemtuzumab and maintenance with tacrolimus, MMF, and prednisone. Two episodes of acute rejection during months 4 and 8 were treated with intravenous methylprednisolone. She developed a 3 mm basal cell carcinoma on the right nasal ala that was successfully resected.

This report underscores the importance of close long-term surveillance in hand transplantation. If a hand recipient develops a life threatening neoplasm such as a lymphoma, the treatment options might have to include complete cessation of immunosuppression with removal of the graft. The risks of neoplasm and the strategy to be adopted in the event of tumor development must be discussed during the consenting process.

In summary, complications related to immunosuppression in hand transplant recipients are similar to incidences among solid organ recipients. With longer follow-up, the increased cardiovascular risk factors or the development of a neoplasm will likely translate into causes of mortality. Standardizing immunosuppression in hand transplantation with the long-term goal of minimization is critically needed.

SUMMARY

Few new immunosuppressive agents have been introduced into clinical practice in organ transplantation during the last decade. Transplant centers' continuous scrutiny of short-term (1 and 3 year) organ and patient survivals might hinder willingness to test new agents and strategies. The result is inadequate emphasis on long-term (>10 years) results following organ transplantation. Hand transplantation is ideally suited to address this issue. Most recipients are healthy and the goal should be long-term success of the graft without significant morbidity to the patient.

The induction of donor-specific tolerance has been the ultimate goal in organ transplantation. Different strategies have been successfully used in experimental animal models. These include the use of total lymphoid irradiation, costimulatory blockade, depletion of recipient T cells, infusion of regulatory cells, and donor bone marrow infusion. The only success in clinical transplantation has been with the use of donor bone marrow infusion. Kawai and colleagues[40] at Massachusetts General Hospital, Scandling and colleagues[41] at Stanford, and Leventhal and colleagues[42] at Northwestern reported success with donor bone marrow infusion in living donor renal transplant recipients using different nonmyeloablative conditioning regimens. There has been much enthusiasm about this approach recently. The key is to minimize the toxicity of the conditioning and demonstrate durable tolerance. This exciting approach has tremendous potential in hand transplantation because it would reduce the long-term risks of immunosuppression that are currently hindering widespread application.

ACKNOWLEDGMENTS

The authors thank Dr Olayemi Ikusika for preparation of **Figs. 1** and **2**, Carolyn DeLautre for manuscript preparation; and the staff of the animal facility for outstanding animal care.

REFERENCES

1. Murray JE. Organ transplantation (skin, kidney, heart) and the plastic surgeon. Plast Reconstr Surg 1971;47:425–31.

2. Barker JH, Francois CG, Frank JM, et al. Composite tissue allotransplantation. Transplantation 2002;73: 832–5.

3. Dubernard JM, Owen E, Herzberg G, et al. Human hand allograft: report on first 6 months [see comments]. Lancet 1999;353:1315–20.

4. Petruzzo P, Lanzetta M, Dubernard JM, et al. The international registry on hand and composite tissue transplantation. Transplantation 2010;90(12):1590–4.

5. Ojo AO, Held PJ, Port FK, et al. Chronic renal failure after transplantation of a nonrenal organ. N Engl J Med 2003;349:931–40.

6. Patlolla V, Zhong X, Reed GW, et al. Efficacy of anti-IL-2 receptor antibodies compared to no induction and to antilymphocyte antibodies in renal transplantation. Am J Transplant 2007;7:1832–42.

7. Jindal RM, Das NP, Neff RT, et al. Outcomes in African-Americans vs. Caucasians using thymoglobulin or interleukin-2 receptor inhibitor induction: analysis of USRDS database. Am J Nephrol 2009; 29:501–8.

8. Willoughby LM, Schnitzler MA, Brennan DC, et al. Early outcomes of thymoglobulin and basiliximab induction in kidney transplantation: application of statistical approaches to reduce bias in observational comparisons. Transplantation 2009;87: 1520–9.

9. Shapiro R, Basu A, Tan H, et al. Kidney transplantation under minimal immunosuppression after pretransplant lymphoid depletion with thymoglobulin or campath. J Am Coll Surg 2005;200:505–15.

10. Kaufman DB, Leventhal JR, Axelrod D, et al. Alemtuzumab induction and prednisone-free maintenance immunotherapy in kidney transplantation: comparison with basiliximab induction–long-term results. Am J Transplant 2005;5:2539–48.

11. Ciancio G, Burke GW III. Alemtuzumab (Campath-1H) in kidney transplantation. Am J Transplant 2008;8:15–20.

12. Arias M, Campistol JM, Vincenti F. Evolving trends in induction therapy. Transplant Rev (Orlando) 2009; 23:94–102.

13. Vincenti F, Larsen C, Durrbach A, et al. Costimulation blockade with belatacept in renal transplantation. N Engl J Med 2005;353:770–81.

14. Vincenti F, Charpentier B, Vanrenterghem Y, et al. A phase III study of belatacept-based immunosuppression regimens versus cyclosporine in renal transplant recipients (BENEFIT study). Am J Transplant 2010;10:535–46.

15. Ferguson R, Grinyo J, Vincenti F, et al. Immunosuppression with belatacept-based, corticosteroid-avoiding regimens in de novo kidney transplant recipients. Am J Transplant 2010;11:66–76.

16. Siemionow M, Nasir S. Immunologic responses in vascularized and nonvascularized skin allografts. J Reconstr Microsurg 2008;24:497–505.

17. Lee WP, Yaremchuk MJ, Pan YC, et al. Relative antigenicity of components of a vascularized limb allograft. Plast Reconstr Surg 1991;87:401–11.

18. Kanitakis J, Jullien D, Petruzzo P, et al. Clinicopathologic features of graft rejection of the first human hand allograft. Transplantation 2003;76:688–93.

19. Wang HJ, Ding YQ, Pei GX, et al. A preliminary pathological study on human allotransplantation. Chin J Traumatol 2003;6:284–7.

20. Kaufman DB, Shapiro R, Lucey MR, et al. Immunosuppression: practice and trends. Am J Transplant 2004;4(Suppl 9):38–53.

21. Schneeberger S, Landin L, Kaufmann C, et al. Alemtuzumab: key for minimization of maintenance immunosuppression in reconstructive transplantation? Transplant Proc 2009;41:499–502.

22. Kuffler DP. Chapter 18: enhancement of nerve regeneration and recovery by immunosuppressive agents. Int Rev Neurobiol 2009;87:347–62.

23. Petruzzo P, Lanzetta M, Dubernard JM, et al. The International Registry on Hand and Composite Tissue Transplantation. Transplantation 2008;86: 487–92.

24. Gazarian A, Abrahamyan DO, Petruzzo P, et al. Hand allografts: experience from Lyon team. Ann Chir Plast Esthet 2007;52:424–35 [in French].

25. Ravindra KV, Buell JF, Kaufman CL, et al. Hand transplantation in the United States: experience with 3 patients. Surgery 2008;144:638–43.

26. Brandacher G, Ninkovic M, Piza-Katzer H, et al. The Innsbruck hand transplant program: update at 8 years after the first transplant. Transplant Proc 2009;41:491–4.

27. Landin L, Cavadas PC, Rodriguez-Perez JC, et al. Improvement in renal function after late conversion to sirolimus-based immunosuppression in composite tissue allotransplantation. Transplantation 2010;90: 691–2.

28. Lanzetta M, Petruzzo P, Dubernard JM, et al. Second report (1998-2006) of the International Registry of Hand and Composite Tissue Transplantation. Transpl Immunol 2007;18:1–6.

29. Dubernard JM, Burloux G, Giraux P, et al. Three lessons learned from the first double hand transplantation. Bull Acad Natl Med 2002;186:1051–62 [in French].

30. Lentine KL, Brennan DC, Schnitzler MA. Incidence and predictors of myocardial infarction after kidney transplantation. J Am Soc Nephrol 2005;16:496–506.

31. Weir MR, Fink JC. Risk for post transplant diabetes mellitus with current immunosuppressive medications. Am J Kidney Dis 1999;34:1–13.

32. Vincenti F, Friman S, Scheuermann E, et al. Results of an international, randomized trial comparing glucose metabolism disorders and outcome with cyclosporine versus tacrolimus. Am J Transplant 2007;7:1506–14.

33. Johnston O, Rose CL, Webster AC, et al. Sirolimus is associated with new-onset diabetes in kidney transplant recipients. J Am Soc Nephrol 2008;19:1411–8.

34. Schneeberger S, Lucchina S, Lanzetta M, et al. Cytomegalovirus-related complications in human hand transplantation. Transplantation 2005;80:441–7.

35. Bonatti H, Brandacher G, Margreiter R, et al. Infectious complications in three double hand recipients: experience from a single center. Transplant Proc 2009;41:517–20.

36. Murray JE, Gleason R, Bartholomay A. Third report of the human kidney transplant registry. Transplantation 1965;3:294–302.

37. Vajdic CM, McDonald SP, McCredie MR, et al. Cancer incidence before and after kidney transplantation. JAMA 2006;296:2823–31.

38. Kauffman HM. Malignancies in organ transplant recipients. J Surg Oncol 2006;94:431–3.

39. Landin L, Cavadas PC, Ibanez J, et al. Malignant skin tumor in a composite tissue (bilateral hand) allograft recipient. Plast Reconstr Surg 2010;125:20e–1e.

40. Kawai T, Cosimi AB, Spitzer TR, et al. HLA-mismatched renal transplantation without maintenance immunosuppression. N Engl J Med 2008;358:353–61.

41. Scandling JD, Busque S, jbakhsh-Jones S, et al. Tolerance and chimerism after renal and hematopoietic-cell transplantation. N Engl J Med 2008;358:362–8.

42. Leventhal JR, Gallon L, Miller J, et al. Facilitating cell enriched stem cell infusion results in durable chimerism, donor specific tolerance, and allows for immunosuppressive drug withdrawal in recipients of HLA disparate living donor kidney allografts [abstract]. Vancouver (Canada): XXIII International Congress of The Transplantation Society; 2010.

Acute and Chronic Rejection in Upper Extremity Transplantation: What Have We Learned?

Vijay S. Gorantla, MD, PhD[a], Anthony J. Demetris, MD[b],*

KEYWORDS

- Hand/upper extremity transplantation
- Composite tissue allograft • Acute rejection
- Chronic rejection

Vascularized composite tissue allografts (CTA), such as forearm transplants, differ from solid organ transplants (SOT) in several important aspects.[1] First, CTAs are comprised of tissues derived from multiple germ lines such as ectoderm, endoderm, and mesoderm, such as skin, muscle, blood vessels, nerve, fat, cartilage, bone, and bone marrow. Second, the functional allograft is easily and grossly visible for inspection by the patient and clinical management team. Third, for the most part, CTAs are not strictly life sustaining.

Transplantation of multiple tissue constructs such as CTAs is associated with a quantitatively graded recipient immune response to individual graft components. Traditionally, skin has been considered the most immunologically difficult allograft tissue to transplant. This impression has been verified experimentally. Skin, subcutaneous tissue, muscle, bone, nerve, and blood vessels have been evaluated for their intrinsic and relative antigenicities.[2] Skin is the most immunogenic component and it usually triggers and is the primary target of acute rejection (AR).[3] After skin, it is muscle, bone, cartilage, and nerve that predictably induce a relatively lower immune response, in that order.

Skin is the largest organ in the body and is both a physical and immunologic barrier.[4,5] Owing to its exposure to the environment, the skin, like the small bowel and lung, has a robust and effective local immune system, called the skin immune system, which contributes to its heightened antigenicity.[6,7] Langerhans cells (LC) are immature dendritic cells (DC) that are the primary dermal antigen presenting cells. They are extremely efficient at initiating innate responses to trigger sensitization and priming of naïve host T cells to attack the graft.[8] LCs make up 2% to 4% of epidermal cells. Keratinocytes make up 90% of epidermal cells and play an accessory role in initiating or supporting cell-mediated immune responses.[9] Apart from LCs, skin also has other types of DCs such as dermal DCs. These DCs, because of their migratory capability, can carry antigenic information from skin to secondary lymphoid organs and present to lymphocytes for priming and stimulation.[10] Human skin also has tissue-specific minor antigens that may contribute to its antigenicity.[11] These are similar to antigens such as skin antigen (Skn) and embryonic prealbumin 1 (EPA-1), which are potent contributors to skin antigenicity in murine models and swine models.[12,13]

[a] Pittsburgh Reconstructive Transplantation Program, Division of Plastic Surgery, Department of Surgery, 3550 Terrace Street, Pittsburgh, PA 15261, USA
[b] Department of Pathology, Division of Transplantation, University of Pittsburgh Medical Center, Pittsburgh, PA 15213, USA
* Corresponding author.
E-mail address: demetrisaj@upmc.edu

Hand Clin 27 (2011) 481–493
doi:10.1016/j.hcl.2011.08.006
0749-0712/11/$ – see front matter © 2011 Published by Elsevier Inc.

Skin antigenicity correlates with clinical findings in hand transplants. It initially shows the first signs of rejection and is associated with maximal cellular infiltrate in established rejection.[14,15] Experimentally, it has been possible to induce tolerance toward all tissues of a CTA except the skin (split tolerance).[16] More powerful conventional or standard immunosuppression regimens have successfully treated skin rejection and prolong CTA-graft survival, but, like other allografts, in most cases standard baseline immunosuppression is still unable to prevent long-term skin rejection or deterioration. Although other tissues are less antigenic, rejection of even one component of a CTA could result in graft dysfunction or compromise.

The gross visibility and accessibility of CTAs, such as hand transplants, enables direct visual inspection with comparison to nonallograft tissues for routine clinical evaluation, directed biopsy, and topical therapy. This potentially enables more localized therapy and, possibly, reduced systemic exposure to standard immunosuppressive medications, which lessens side effects for recipients who, for the most part, are healthy.[17]

WORLD EXPERIENCE IN HAND TRANSPLANTATION

Early attempts at hand transplantation in 1964 failed owing to inadequate immunosuppression. The advent of modern, high efficacy combination therapies including calcineurin inhibitors, such as tacrolimus, changed the landscape of SOT in the 1980s and 1990s, enabling successful transplantation of other "immunologically difficult" organs, such as small intestine, multivisceral, and CTA allografts.[18,19] Consequently, reconstructive transplantation has emerged as a new field over the past 2 decades, with hand transplants being performed around the world at multiple centers.[20] The overall world experience counts 78 hands transplanted in 55 recipients. Good functional results have been achieved with excellent patient satisfaction, acceptably low morbidity, and no mortality.[21]

The first United States' patient has the longest surviving hand transplant 13 years after surgery.[22] There have been exceptions to this encouraging record. These include the first French patient[14] and the discouraging Chinese experience.[23] Bilateral hand transplants performed in conjunction with face transplants were lost to complications in two cases in Amiens, France, and Boston, MA, USA. One patient in Louisville, KY, USA, lost his graft to chronic allograft rejection (CR).[24] In some of the above cases, transplanted hands were amputated more than 2 years after transplantation. These cases have shown that the operation is fully reversible. More importantly, reamputation provided an opportunity to observe the evolution of untreated acute rejection in the event of noncompliance and treatment withdrawal, and early chronic rejection.

REJECTION IN HAND TRANSPLANTATION
Acute Cellular Rejection

Almost all patients receiving hand transplants experience AR. Of all patients, 85% had at least one episode of acute skin rejection within the first year; multiple rejections were seen in 56%.[21] Noncutaneous tissues seem to be affected to a lesser extent. Review of these AR episodes leads the authors to believe that AR in hand transplants are similar to AR in SOTs. As in SOTs, AR in hand transplants is a predominantly lymphocytic response normally reversible with an increase in systemic immunosuppression or with bolus steroid or antibody treatment.

Macroscopically, "classic" AR in hand transplants manifests as an erythematous (**Fig. 1**) or maculopapular rash (**Fig. 2**) that is either localized or diffuse in distribution over the allograft. Clinical signs may also include edema (**Fig. 3**), vesiculation, desquamation, ulceration, and/or necrosis. Recently, "atypical" AR in a cohort of hand transplant recipients was described.[25] All patients were young and exposed to repetitive and persistent mechanical stress of the palm. This pattern is unlike the classical pattern of rejection and is novel in involving the palmar skin (**Fig. 4**) and the nails. Hallmarks of this atypical AR included a desquamative rash associated with dry skin, red papules, and palmar thickening or lichenification. Skin lesions were associated with nail dystrophy, pitting, degeneration, deformation, or loss. Such lesions may appear similar to leuconychia or dermatophytotic lesions.

Histopathology remains the gold standard methodology for diagnosing AR in CTAs, as in SOTs. It not only facilitates the diagnosis and management of AR but also plays a critical role in elucidation of pathophysiology. The routine preparation of biopsies involves hematoxylin and eosin (H & E). As needed, periodic acid-Schiff (PAS) staining can be used to delineate fungal infection and immunohistochemical staining can be performed for identification of specific cell subsets or types bearing markers such as CD3, CD4, CD8, CD19, CD20, CD68, HLA-DR, and Fox-P3. Masson trichrome or elastin stains can be used to delineate fibrogenic or vascular processes that may be associated with chronic graft changes. The objective utility of detecting complement deposition through C4d staining is

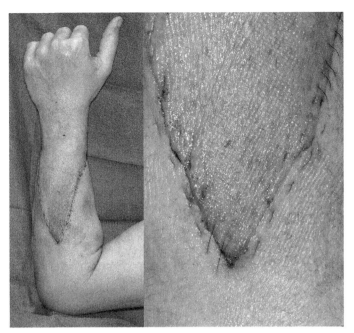

Fig. 1. Grade 3 AR. Diffuse erythematous rash that is limited to the donor skin flap.

debated in hand transplantation, but the authors have used it routinely for monitoring along with simultaneous measurement of circulating donor-specific antibodies (DSA).

AR in CTAs such as hand transplants is associated with characteristic changes. However, there are no changes that are the sine qua non for AR in hand transplants. These changes are neither specific to these grafts in terms of appearance nor in cellular composition, localization, or distribution. Given the emerging nature of this field, the manifestations of AR in hand transplants are just beginning to be understood. They can pose diagnostic challenges for the novice pathologist or be potentially missed without attention to detail.

Recently, an international consensus conference on CTA pathology held in La Coruna, Spain, on June 26, 2007, proposed the Banff Working Classification for CTAs such as hand transplants.[26] It represents the first internationally accepted, standardized grading scheme for scoring, diagnosis, and reporting of AR in CTA, and is based on four previously published scoring systems.[15,27–30] Because it is a tiered, working classification for interpretation of AR, it is open to modification with continued insights into clinical CTA rejection.

The primary histologic feature of classic AR is a variable lymphohistiocytic and eosinophilic infiltrate that first appears in cuffing small venules and capillaries in the superficial reticular dermis and periadnexal areas. As with other solid organ allografts, in our experience AR can present with predominantly eosinophilic inflammation. However, eosinophils have not been not yet recognized

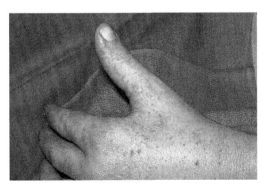

Fig. 2. Grade 2 AR. Maculopapular rash that is localized in distribution to the radial dorsum of the hand.

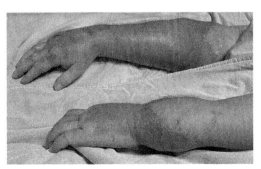

Fig. 3. Grade 2–3 AR. Diffuse erythema and edema with rash delimited to the suture line.

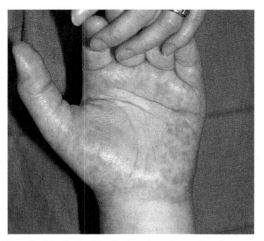

Fig. 4. Atypical AR. Isolated palmar involvement (Grade 2–3 AR).

as rejection-related by the Banff CTA Working Group.[26]

With progression of AR, the infiltrate spreads to the interface zone between dermis and epidermis and/or adnexal structures. An intraepidermal infiltrate is typical for moderate rejection. Without reversal of AR with treatment at this stage, it progresses to loss of single keratinocytes or adnexal epithelial cell apoptosis or necrosis associated with focal dermal-epidermal separation. With further worsening, AR ultimately results in necrosis and loss of the epidermis and/or adnexal structures—a stage that is often irreversible and results in permanent graft damage. Varying degrees of dermal edema and spongiosis may be seen in AR of hand transplants. This often results from dermal microvascular injury with fluid transudation.

In a recent study, 174 skin biopsies from five human hand transplant recipients were examined for AR.[31] The predominant cells in the infiltrates of AR in hand transplant recipients have been shown to be CD3+ T lymphocytes with most being CD4+ with lower numbers of CD8+ cells. Perivascular infiltrates, however, had a reversal of this pattern: CD8+ greater than CD4+ cells. Fewer than 5% were CD20+ and CD79a+ B-lymphocytes. Immunohistochemical analysis of infiltrates revealed that the preponderance of T-cells were CD5+, with only a few CD7+ cells indicating that most T cells were mature.[32–34] During ongoing AR (grade II and III), 10% to 50% of the infiltrating cells were CD68+ (histiocytic or macrophage lineage) that were localized to the epidermis. This percentage increased with worsening (grade IV) AR, as in other organs. Most (88.14%) samples with moderate AR were remarkable for HLA-DR+ cells mostly in the perivascular zones of the papillary dermis. With severe AR, similar cells were seen in the epidermis. Immunohistochemical analysis for adhesion and other markers in samples from rejecting patients revealed staining for the cell and vascular adhesion markers lymphocyte function-associated antigen-1 (LFA-1), intercellular adhesion molecule-1 (ICAM-1), E-selectin, and P-selectin. Psoriasin (S100A7), a protein expressed in psoriasis patients was detected in some biopsies. In this and other studies, few cells in skin biopsies from hand recipients were found to express FoxP3+, which can be seen on T regulatory cells (Treg). However, characterization beyond FoxP3 is needed to link T cells with regulatory properties and, even so, a conclusive role for Treg in promoting graft survival is still unclear. Without exception, T cells were also noted to be of recipient origin (as evidenced by the expression of recipient's specific HLA-class I antigens). In some cases of AR, there may be an admixture or predominance of cells of histiocytic, macrophage, eosinophilic, or mast cell lineage. Tissue biopsies from the amputated graft of the first French patient reveal that in severe AR the infiltrates are more dense and appear as a subepidermal "lichenoid" streak localized with less marked involvement of the epidermis per se. Varying degrees of lymphocytic exocytosis, keratinocyte vacuolization or necrosis, formation of colloid or cytoid bodies in the deeper epidermis, and (rarely) hyperkeratosis and lichenification can be seen. Lymphocytic inflammation of adnexal structures is also frequently seen in AR and is associated with adnexal epithelial cell apoptosis/necrosis.

Histopathologic changes of classic AR in hand transplants, albeit characteristic, lack absolute diagnostic specificity as they are observed in a wide variety of dermatoses (inflammatory, infectious, autoimmune or rarely neoplastic). The differential diagnosis of classic AR from these phenomena has been described.[35] Histology of the skin and nail bed in atypical AR was also mostly comparable to the previously described classic type or rejection with predominance of T cells and a small numbers of B cells. Regardless, when an inflammatory disorder preferentially, or exclusively, involves the allograft, rejection must be placed at the top of the diagnosis list. Therefore, close clinicopathologic correlation is even more helpful in skin allograft pathology than in other SOTs.

Hand transplants are unique as they contain a skin component that serves as a visual monitor for AR and allows ready access for directed biopsy of clinically suspicious areas. Additionally, hand transplants enable topical intervention with immunosuppressive medications, potentially minimizing the need for augmenting systemic therapy. Recent evidence from hand transplants suggests that the skin may not be a true "sentinel" of graft immune activity.[26,36] As with other organs, histologic evidence of AR in the skin can occur without gross clinical signs. An additional concern, however, is that skin may be histopathologically quiescent while smoldering rejection is occurring in underlying tissues, such as deep dermis or muscle. The sensitivity and specificity of clinical signs of AR in the skin as true reflectors of rejection remain to be validated. Similarly, there is lack of consensus on the endpoints for treatment intervention of AR (eg, is it resolution of cellular infiltrates from repeat biopsy or resolution of clinical rash?). The heterogeneity of manifestations of AR in CTA, such as hand transplants, and the possibility of unrelated immune or nonimmune phenomena, that can mimic AR, make clinicopathologic correlation important in diagnosis, monitoring, and management of AR in limb transplant recipients. It also underlines the importance of individualized interpretation and correlation of clinicopathologic findings with results of other immune monitoring assessments (eg, antibody assays and immune profiling tests).

All of the preceding discussion on AR is based on experience with skin biopsies. Hand transplant teams around the world have been limited to routine punch biopsies of skin evaluated using routine methods (**Fig. 5**). Hand transplant biopsies usually contain representation from several tissue types, including adnexa, adipose tissue, small blood vessels, collagen, and epidermis. However, as for other organs, the issue of "sampling problems" is raised in hand transplants with respect to deeper tissues such as muscle, larger nerves, blood vessels, and bone or marrow. Access to

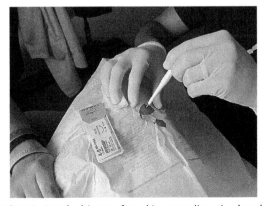

Fig. 5. Punch biopsy for skin sampling in hand transplantation.

these tissues has been limited because of concern for morbidity or inadvertent damage to vital structures. Thus, very limited information is available on the involvement of other tissue components by AR. In select cases (eg, where reamputation was necessitated), it has been possible to sample deeper tissues such as bone, vessels, nerves, or muscles. In some patients, repeat reconstructive procedures (eg, removal or refixation of hardware or tendon imbrication) have provided the opportunity for teams to obtain deep biopsies. Reports indicate that components other than the skin may also be affected at a lesser extent with or without ongoing evidence of cellular infiltrates or clinical signs of AR in the skin.[32,37]

Antibody-Mediated Rejection

Although cellular AR remains the most commonly recognized form of rejection after CTA, the possibility of combined cell and antibody-mediated rejection (AMR), or AMR alone, must not be ignored. Recent evidence from SOT strongly suggests that AMR also contributes to CR.[38] In renal transplants, AMR occurs in 20% to 30% of AR cases, has a poorer prognosis than isolated cellular rejection, is refractory to conventional immunosuppressive, and (importantly) contributes to allograft loss. In general, AMR manifests as microvascular injury classically characterized by endothelial cell activation, leukocyte margination, microvasculature injury, and eventual destruction that contributes to progressive fibrosis associated with CR and eventual allograft failure.

There is insufficient evidence to clearly delineate the contribution of AMR to overall rejection and transplantation outcomes, which is likely related to relative inexperience. Generic diagnostic criteria for AMR, as derived from SOT,[39,40] includes (1) presence of C4d deposition in vasculature as confirmed by immunohistochemistry, (2) evidence of graft injury or dysfunction (eg, endothelial cell hypertrophy, leukocyte margination, congestion/hemorrhage), and (3) presence of circulating DSA that are anti–HLA-specific or otherwise.

C4d is the degradation product of the activated complement factor C4, a component of the classical complement cascade, which is typically initiated by binding of antibodies to specific target molecules. Following activation and degradation of the C4 molecule, its product C4d binds to endothelial cell surfaces and extracellular matrix components of vascular basement membranes near the sites of C4 activation. C4d is also found in intracytoplasmic vacuoles of endothelial cells. Covalent binding renders C4d a stable molecule that can easily be detected by immunohistochemistry.

C4d deposition is regarded as an indirect "fingerprint" of the antibody response[41–44] and it has proven to be a marker of AMR in SOTs, including kidney, heart, pancreas, and lung.[45–50] However, it should be noted that, apart from the classical antibody-mediated route of complement activation, C4 could also be activated via an alternative, antibody-independent mechanism.[51]

Indeed, although C4d remains a specific marker of a humoral response, recent evidence in renal transplants indicates that a considerable fraction of biopsies showing AMR are C4d-negative, even by immunofluorescence.[52] Two separate studies by the Innsbruck, Austria, and Valencia, Spain, teams showed that C4d expression was present but did not correlate with cellular skin rejection.[31,53] In contrast, the Lyon, France, group studied a total of 60 samples from four patients receiving CTA (three hands, one face) obtained as early as 7 days to as late as 7 years after surgery but did not detect any C4d deposits.[54] Further, none of these patients was positive for circulating DSA during the study period. These clinical studies in SOT and CTA support the existence of C4d-negative AMR. It is yet to be seen if this entity, if untreated, may lead to the development of scarring within the graft and even graft loss. Alternatively, some have suggested that in ABO-incompatible renal transplants, biopsies that are positive for C4d in the absence of significant histologic abnormalities may indicate stable graft "accommodation."[55] Therefore, detection or absence of C4d in a graft biopsy ideally should be supplemented by correlative clinical information as well as by DSA levels. In our experience interpretation of C4d stains can be problematic in CTA due to high background in dermal collagen. This problem can be avoided somewhat by restricting C4d stain interpretation to endothelial cells lining interstitial capillaries feeding adnexal structures and adipose tissue.

The contribution of anti-HLA antibodies to AMR in CTAs is in the early stage of evolution. CTA recipients are mostly young, otherwise healthy, and less likely to be sensitized, as manifested by low panel reactive antibodies (PRAs) for eligibility. Some investigators suggest that this might lower the risk of developing posttransplant DSA. Conceptually, it seems likely, as in SOTs, that both preexisting long-lived plasma cells and the conversion of B memory cells to new plasma cells play a role in the increased DSA production.[56,57] Some hand transplant teams have relied on the use of depletional induction regimens such as alemtuzumab, which has been associated with production of memory cells after transplantation. Such therapy, therefore, might increase the propensity for long-term development of DSAs in some patients.[58] Also, reliance on systemic DSA levels alone, as a marker for presence or absence of antibodies, can be falsely reassuring in CTA recipients. The United States' fourth hand transplant recipient, who was amputated because of ischemic complications secondary to chronic rejection, had normal DSA levels as measured by single antigen bead assays. Following amputation, however, the patients' DSA levels surged, indicating that the graft may have served as a "sump" for the DSA,[24] (Dr Warren Breidenbach, personal communication), as seen in SOT.[59] Thus, anti-HLA antibodies can contribute to chronic allograft injury and vasculopathy in an occult and insidious fashion with gradual graft dysfunction.

Chronic Rejection

Unlike AR, we are still unclear regarding the magnitude or risk for CR or how it manifests in CTA, but there is enough experience with animal models and other SOT that manifestations can be reasonably and accurately predicted. What is unknown, however, are (1) the realized side effects of prolonged immunosuppression (renal, infective, metabolic or neoplastic)[18] and their impact on the incidence of CR; and (2) the mitigating effect, if any, of cotransplantation of donor bone marrow and consequent hematopoietic microchimerism on susceptibility to CR.

At 5 years, the incidence of CR is about 40% in cardiac transplants,[60] 80% in lung transplants,[61] and 5% in liver transplants[62]; the net incidence of CR is reduced to 10% to 20% in combined heart-lung transplantation.[63] This reduction in incidence of CR is even more significant when other organs are combined with liver transplantation, which is widely recognized as a tolerogenic organ. It is possible, therefore, that transplantation of multiple tissues[2] or organs[64] attenuates or modifies their antigenic character. The effect of imperfect HLA matching on the incidence or pathogenesis of CR is controversial. Some studies indicate that any degree of mismatching results in progressive loss of graft function due to CR,[65] whereas others conclude that this effect is less than would be expected.[66]

In SOTs, both immunologic and nonimmunologic factors play a role in CR pathogenesis (**Box 1**).[67] Immunologic risk factors are, by far, the most important for all allografts. Included are the frequency, severity, and temporal onset of AR; greater HLA mismatch; PRA status of recipient; racial mismatch between donor-recipient

> **Box 1**
> **Immunologic and nonimmunologic factors implicated in CR in SOT that could be important or relevant to CTA**
>
> *Immunologic*
>
> Timing of AR (late vs early)
>
> Severe, repetitive, humoral AR
>
> Greater HLA mismatch
>
> Higher PRA of recipient
>
> CMV+ Donor to CMV− Recipient
>
> Steroid resistant AR
>
> Antidonor antibodies + C4D
>
> *Nonimmunologic*
>
> Older donor
>
> Donor atherosclerosis
>
> Cadaver donor
>
> Prolonged cold ischemia
>
> Hypertension, DM, obesity, high cholesterol
>
> Unstable donor
>
> Noncompliance

(eg, white donor into non–white recipient); sex mismatching (female donor into male recipient and vice versa); and cytomegalovirus (CMV) seromismatch (CMV+ donor into CMV− recipient), listed largely in order of influence. Data from almost every form of solid organ transplantation have indicated decreased graft survival in the face of CMV infection.[68] CMV infection has a far greater effect on the allograft than on native organs, increasing the risk of both AR and CR.[69] This is engendered by cytokines, chemokines, and growth factors.

CR may begin weeks to months after transplantation, especially if there are many high-grade AR episodes. In kidney transplants, late, severe, or persistent AR episodes occurring more than 1 year after transplantation are particularly strong and consistent predictors of CR.[70] The AR may be predominantly cellular or antibody-mediated. AMR rejection has a considerably worse prognosis than acute cellular rejection.[71] Thus, in kidney transplants, severe, late-onset AR with a significant humoral component may be more predictive of CR. However, such a correlation may not be totally valid in other organ transplants. For example, in liver transplants, early, mild AR and late episodes of AR are usually not associated with later CR.[72]

Late-onset AR may be seen in inadequately immunosuppressed or noncompliant patients.[73] Medication noncompliance accounts for one-third of late-graft losses and is an important factor contributing to CR. Though the exact determinants are unclear, some factors associated with noncompliance include improper physician-patient relationship, long-duration after transplant surgery, multiple immunosuppressive medications, nontolerance of medications, missed clinic visits, and poor transplant outcomes.[74]

Common histopathologic features of chronic rejection in SOT include (1) patchy organized (lymphoid neogenesis) interstitial inflammation; (2) patchy interstitial fibrosis and associated parenchymal atrophy (atrophy of adnexal structures and thinning of the epidermis); (3) graft vascular disease (GVD), which primarily manifests as concentric fibrointimal hyperplasia of arteries; (4) destruction of epithelial-lined conduits; and (5) destruction and atrophy of organ-associated lymphoid tissue and lymphatics.[75] Although the relationship of multiple AR and their effect on CR has not been systematically investigated in CTA, a rat hind-limb allograft model was developed in which repetitive AR was able to reproduce expected histopathologic changes of CR. Included were hair loss (**Fig. 6**) and adnexal epithelial, skin, and muscle atrophy; GVD; and upregulation of profibrotic gene expression and fibrosis. In

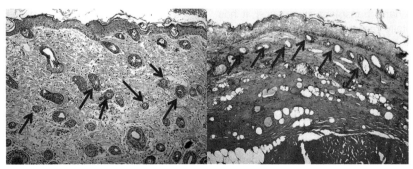

Fig. 6. Effect of multiple acute rejections on adnexa such as hair follicles. Hair follicles (*left panel; black arrows*). Loss of hair follicles with multiple AR episodes (*right panel; black arrows*). (*Courtesy of* Dr Jignesh Unadkat.)

addition, allograft bone became sclerotic, weak, and exhibited a high incidence of malunion and nonunion. Interestingly, vasculopathy was a relatively late finding, whereas muscle atrophy with macrophage infiltration was seen early, after only a few AR. Thus, multiple AR led to vasculopathy and specific-tissue pathologic condition in CTA. This was the first evidence of composite tissue vasculopathy and degeneration in limb transplants, as might be expected.

The best modality to confirm AR or CR is by histopathology. Biopsies, however, used to sample targeted structures are invasive, might not be directed at clinically suspicious areas, and are associated with morbidity. Indirect evidence of immune activation can be obtained with biomarkers such as Fas ligand, perforin, or granzyme B. Two pathways of immune activation have been proposed. The TH1 (inflammatory CD4+ T cells) pathway was thought to be associated with AR, whereas the TH2 (helper CD4+ T cells) pathway was an attribute of tolerance. Recent evidence, however, suggests that the TH2 pathway in fact favors alloantibodies, cytokines, and growth factors typically seen in CR.[76]

In SOT, quality of function early posttransplantation is a strong predictor of allograft survival. AR and, ultimately, CR have been shown to affect function with CR being the most important cause of late-graft loss in SOTs, especially kidney in which donor disease and preexisting vascular disease are already contributing to suboptimal renal function in the donor. However, correlation between early function and long-term survival is unclear in hand transplants. Motor return in hand transplants is mostly dependent on the anatomic level of the allotransplant (distal transplants fare better than proximal transplants) and the postoperative rehabilitation regime. Sensory return is dictated by nerve regeneration. Moreover, the most frequent CTA that have been performed (forearm and hand) are relatively athero-resistant vascular beds, with significant preexisting donor arterial disease less likely, in contrast to renal allografts. In the hand transplant experience, it has been anecdotally reported that functional return has not been curtailed by ongoing cellular rejection. It is not yet known what is the impact of persistent AR in hand transplants on long-term function and eventual risk of CR.

The effect of the number of HLA mismatches in the development of CR has been debated in SOT[65,66] and generally requires large cohorts for analysis; magnitudes more than current total CTA experience. It is premature, therefore, to discuss any potential effects in detail. The number of HLA mismatches in most hand transplants is six

out of six. Interestingly, the first Chinese patient who had a three out of six mismatch rejected his hand, warranting amputation at 39 months.[23] Some studies in solid organ transplants suggest that the TH2 pathway favors immune skewing toward CR.[76] In the first Chinese patient, a notable increase in IL-10 (a TH2 cytokine) was seen at 6 months after transplantation.[77] This patient eventually lost his hand to rejection. It is not yet known if CR was cause of late graft loss in this patient.

Medication noncompliance[73,74] and inadequate immunosuppression are important causes of late graft loss in SOT. The same expectations exist for CTA. Such allografts demonstrate an initial late-onset AR that eventually leads to CR. The first French patient represents a unique opportunity to study late-onset AR and CR in hand transplants in the setting of noncompliance or inadequate immunosuppression. The patient stopped taking immunosuppressive medications because of dissatisfaction with a nonfunctioning allograft. The transplanted hand was amputated at 29 months after surgery, by which time the patient had been off medications for more than 3 months. The amputated allograft showed skin to be the preferential target of rejection without less significant involvement of underlying tissues. There is, however, ambiguity in terminology used by the French team to describe the findings. One paper states that at 16 months after transplant the patient suffered from "an episode of skin rejection, which was diagnosed as chronic graft rejection." In another paper, it is stated that at 28 months, "histologic study of the amputated hand showed lichenoid graft-versus-host disease lesions."[78] It is well known that in graft-versus-host disease (GVHD), reactive donor T cells generated by the donor bone marrow attack the skin and internal organs of the recipient. They might have meant host-versus-graft disease. In other articles describing the findings in their first patient, the French team then uses the term "chronic rejection" while avoiding reference to GVHD.[79–81] More recent articles in the series of published studies describe the detailed histopathologic findings[14,33] which would be expected. Included were epidermal ischemic changes with foci of frank ulceration; deep dermal periadnexal changes; endothelialitis; and perivascular infiltration in the subcutaneous fat, comprised predominantly of lymphocytes with sparse eosinophilia. Deeper subcutaneous tissues (fat, muscle) showed vascular arteriopathy (intimal hyperplasia [IH]) with subintimal foam cells (foamy histiocytes), muscle atrophy, and interstitial fibrosis associated with lymphocytic infiltration in the muscle, as expected from the experience in other organs and the animal model. In hand transplants, however, it should be realized that some muscle atrophy can occur because of disuse or poor rehabilitation and trauma.

Hand transplant recipients, to date, have been monitored for CR by clinical and functional examinations, skin biopsies, DSA, and standard vascular imaging. The Louisville team has reported[24] the loss of the transplant in their fourth patient to ischemia secondary to progressive IH confirmed on histopathology (**Fig. 7**). Conventional testing failed to reveal any evidence of CR but deep tissue biopsies were positive for IH in all of their other patients (Dr Warren Breidenbach, personal communication, December 2010). The team concluded that the incidence and severity of IH was inversely proportional to the immunosuppressive load but did not correlate well with cellular and humoral parameters. This is the first conclusive report of CR-related findings in clinical HT. There is also a similar report of IH leading to loss of CTA wherein chronic allograft vasculopathy was seen in vascularized knee transplantation (**Fig. 8**).[82] One hundred percent of the grafts were lost within 5 years. Histopathology confirmation of the cases revealed, "diffuse concentric fibrous intimal thickening and occlusion of graft vessels." The investigators agree that the "lack of adequate tools for monitoring graft rejection might have allowed multiple untreated episodes of acute rejection, triggering myointimal proliferation and occlusion of graft vessels" and that "adequate tools for monitoring need to be developed." It seems clear that these extremities were lost secondary to IH, and this must be considered as probable CR. The inability of conventional techniques to monitor and diagnose IH as the primary predictor of CR is

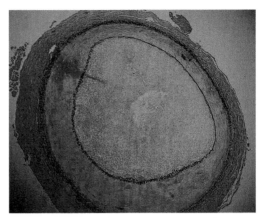

Fig. 7. Intimal hyperplasia in hand transplant recipient. Elastin stain reveals internal elastic lamina and extent of IH. Lumen is yellow. (*Courtesy of* Dr Warren Breidenbach.)

concerning and has implications for long-term outcomes after HT.

Therefore, although biopsies might be less than ideal to capture the early phases of graft vasculopathy affecting larger arteries, this limitation is no different than in other SOTs. In contrast, unlike SOT, CTA biopsies are much less invasive, have low morbidity, and can be done more frequently under direct vision. These advantages make biopsy and clinical monitoring the gold standard in hand transplantation for detection of AR or late AR (and eventually CR), particularly when conducted in conjunction with other methods of immunologic monitoring and with clinical correlation.

Nonimmunologic factors implicated in CR[83] include older donor age, donor atherosclerosis,

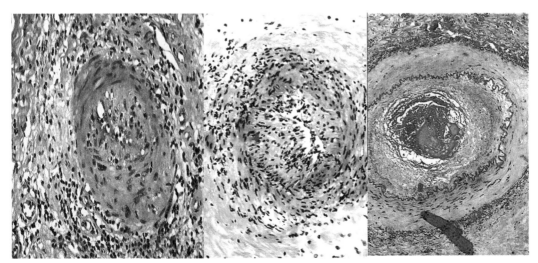

Fig. 8. Vascular intimal hyperplasia after total vascularized knee joint transplantation. Left, skin; middle, synovium; right, soft tissue.[82] (*Courtesy of* M. Diefenbeck, Friedrich-Schiller-Universität Jena, Germany.)

cadaver donor, prolonged cold ischemia, and conventional risk factors for atherosclerosis in the recipient (eg, hypertension, diabetes, hyperlipidemia, obesity). Organs procured from deceased donors and those associated with prolonged cold ischemia sustain injury secondary to a cytokine storm that leads to T-cell activation and increased chemokine gene expression. Atherosclerosis in the donor organ and metabolic disease in the recipient (primary or secondary due to immunosuppressive drugs) can lead to endothelial injury that predisposes to CR. Inferior performance of organs from aged donors may, in part, be related to molecular effects of senescence, which tilts repair responses within the organs toward profibrogenic pathways. Thus, it is important to note that CR is multifactorial in etiology and any one risk factor does not stand in isolation.

Considering the importance of GVD in the manifestation as well as evolution of CR in CTA, it is prudent to question whether there might be additional factors contributing to this phenomenon that are at least relatively unique to CTA. One possibility is arterial skeletonization or adventitial trauma and lymphatic obstruction or destruction, which is particularly evident in CTA early after transplantation. It is known that arterial adventitial stripping can cause IH in the same vessel[84] and arterial fibrointimal hyperplasia has occurred following digital auto-replantation.[85] The combination, therefore, of mechanical (eg, iatrogenic trauma) factors and immunologic (eg, rejection-related) factors might contribute more to GVD pathogenesis in CTA than in other organs. There may be considerable arterial (adventitial) trauma due to mobilization of donor or recipient vessels for anastomosis, extensive lymphatic obstruction due to loss of lymphatic channels and/or inadequate venous drainage by poor or unavailable venous networks, and inflammation associated with repeated rejection episodes.[86,87]

At this point, it is not conclusively known if factors that play a role in genesis of CR in SOT also mediate the phenomenon in CTA hand transplants, but the expectation is that the pathophysiology will be similar and immunologic injury will play the predominant role. With prolonged survival of hand transplants beyond 10 years, more grafts will inevitably develop signs of CR or succumb to CR, resulting in better definition, diagnosis, and staging of this condition. Meanwhile, physicians are limited to minimizing the known risk factors (from solid organ experience) that may contribute to a postulated increase of CR in hand transplants and also invest collective scientific intellect into identifying novel diagnostic tools and therapeutic strategies to monitor and possibly treat CR.

SUMMARY

Hand transplant and CTA have introduced exciting new possibilities in reconstructive and transplant surgery. These procedures offer new hope that was not available to patients just a few years ago. Current technology is clearly sufficient to allow for successful transplantation and maintenance of these complex grafts, but controversy continues concerning the ethics of these procedures. Potentially endangering the life of a patient with immunosuppression to maintain what is often referred to as a "quality of life" graft continues to provoke debate. Advancements in immunosuppressive therapy and, particularly, in the induction of transplant tolerance will reduce and possibly eliminate the controversy and open a window of opportunity for many patients deserving of such reconstruction.

ACKNOWLEDGMENTS

We thank the important contributions of key team members in making our upper extremity transplant program successful. We acknowledge the following for their leadership, intellectual and scientific contributions, technical expertise and valuable insights during the inception and implementation of the program: Dr W.P. Andrew Lee, Dr Gerald Brandacher, Dr Stefan Schneeberger, Dr Adriana Zeevi, Dr John Lunz and Daniel Foust. We also thank Dr Warren Breidenbach for providing important input and information for this manuscript.

REFERENCES

1. Gorantla V, Maldonado C, Frank J, et al. Composite tissue allotransplantation (CTA): current status and future insights. Eur J Trauma 2001;27(6):267–74.
2. Lee WP, Yaremchuk MJ, Pan YC, et al. Relative antigenicity of components of a vascularized limb allograft. Plast Reconstr Surg 1991;87(3):401–11.
3. Bos JD. The skin as an organ of immunity. Clin Exp Immunol 1997;107(Suppl 1):3–5.
4. Swann G. The skin is the body's largest organ. J Vis Commun Med 2010;33(4):148–9.
5. Jensen JM, Proksch E. The skin's barrier. G Ital Dermatol Venereol 2009;144(6):689–700.
6. Bos JD, Luiten RM. Skin immune system. Cancer Treat Res 2009;146:45–62.
7. Bos JD, Zonneveld I, Das PK, et al. The skin immune system (SIS): distribution and immunophenotype of lymphocyte subpopulations in normal human skin. J Invest Dermatol 1987;88(5):569–73.
8. Steinman RM. The dendritic cell system and its role in immunogenicity. Annu Rev Immunol 1991;9:271–96.

9. Nestle FO, Di Meglio P, Qin JZ, et al. Skin immune sentinels in health and disease. Nat Rev Immunol 2009;9(10):679–91.

10. Roediger B, Ng LG, Smith AL, et al. Visualizing dendritic cell migration within the skin. Histochem Cell Biol 2008;130(6):1131–46.

11. Aoki T, Fujinami T. Demonstration of tissue-specific soluble antigens in human skin by immunodiffusion. J Immunol 1967;98(1):39–45.

12. Steinmuller D, Wakely E, Landas SK. Evidence that epidermal alloantigen Epa-1 is an immunogen for murine heart as well as skin allograft rejection. Transplantation 1991;51(2):459–63.

13. Fuchimoto Y, Gleit ZL, Huang CA, et al. Skin-specific alloantigens in miniature swine. Transplantation 2001;72(1):122–6.

14. Kanitakis J, Jullien D, Petruzzo P, et al. Clinicopathologic features of graft rejection of the first human hand allograft. Transplantation 2003;76(4):688–93.

15. Cendales LC, Kirk AD, Moresi JM, et al. Composite tissue allotransplantation: classification of clinical acute skin rejection. Transplantation 2006;81(3):418–22.

16. Mathes DW, Randolph MA, Solari MG, et al. Split tolerance to a composite tissue allograft in a swine model. Transplantation 2003;75(1):25–31.

17. Brandacher G, Gorantla VS, Lee WP. Hand allotransplantation. Semin Plast Surg 2010;24(1):11–7.

18. Gorantla VS, Barker JH, Jones JW Jr, et al. Immunosuppressive agents in transplantation: mechanisms of action and current anti-rejection strategies. Microsurgery 2000;20(8):420–9.

19. Schneeberger S, Gorantla VS, Hautz T, et al. Immunosuppression and rejection in human hand transplantation. Transplant Proc 2009;41(2):472–5.

20. Shores JT, Brandacher G, Schneeberger S, et al. Composite tissue allotransplantation: hand transplantation and beyond. J Am Acad Orthop Surg 2010;18(3):127–31.

21. Petruzzo P, Lanzetta M, Dubernard JM, et al. The international registry on hand and composite tissue transplantation. Transplantation 2010;90(12):1590–4.

22. Breidenbach WC, Gonzales NR, Kaufman CL, et al. Outcomes of the first 2 American hand transplants at 8 and 6 years posttransplant. J Hand Surg Am 2008;33(7):1039–47.

23. Pei G. Long term follow up of hand allografts. J Reconstr Microsurg 2004;1(21):111. Part II.

24. Kaufman C. Vasculopathy in vascularized composite allotransplantation. Presented at the 10th IHCTAS Meeting. Atlanta, April 7–10, 2011.

25. Schneeberger S, Gorantla VS, van Riet RP, et al. Atypical acute rejection after hand transplantation. Am J Transplant 2008;8(3):688–96.

26. Cendales LC, Kanitakis J, Schneeberger S, et al. The Banff 2007 working classification of skin containing composite tissue allograft pathology. Am J Transplant 2008;8(7):1396–400.

27. Bejarano PA, Levi D, Nassiri M, et al. The pathology of full-thickness cadaver skin transplant for large abdominal defects. Am J Surg Pathol 2004;28(5):67075.

28. Kanitakis J, Petruzzo P, Jullien D, et al. Pathological score for the evaluation of allograft rejection in human hand (composite tissue) allotransplantation. Eur J Dermatol 2005;15(4):235–8.

29. Schneeberger S, Kreczy A, Brandacher G, et al. Steroid and ATG-resistant rejection after double forearm transplantation responds to Campath 1-H. Am J Transplant 2004;4(8):1372–4.

30. Cendales L, Kleiner D. Proposed classification of human composite tissue allograft acute rejection. Am J Transplant 2003;3(Suppl 5):S154.

31. Hautz T, Zelger B, Grahammer J, et al. Molecular markers and targeted therapy of skin rejection in composite tissue allotransplantation. Am J Transplant 2010;10(5):1200–9.

32. Ravindra KV, Buell JF, Kaufman CL, et al. Hand transplantation in the United States: experience with 3 patients. Surgery 2008;144:638–43 [discussion: 643–4].

33. Petruzzo P, Kanitakis J, Badet L, et al. Long-term follow-up in composite tissue allotransplantation: in-depth study of five (hand and face) recipients. Am J Transplant 2011;11(4):808–16.

34. Schneeberger S, Landin L, Jableki J, et al. Achievements and challenges in composite tissue allotransplantation. Transpl Int 2011;24(8):760–9.

35. Kanitakis J. The challenge of dermatopathological diagnosis of composite tissue allograft rejection: a review. J Cutan Pathol 2008;35(8):738–44.

36. Tobin G, Breidenbach W, Pidwell D, et al. Transplantation of hand, face, and composite structures: evolution and current status. Clin Plast Surg 2007;34:271.

37. Cavadas PC, Landin L, Ibañez J. Bilateral hand transplantation: result at 20 months. J Hand Surg Eur Vol 2009;34:434–43.

38. Colvin R, Smith R. Antibody mediated organ allograft rejection. Nat Rev Immunol 2005;5:807–17.

39. Colvin RB. Pathology of chronic humoral rejection. Contrib Nephrol 2009;162:75–86.

40. Lucas JG, Co JP, Nwaogwugwu UT, et al. Antibody-mediated rejection in kidney transplantation: an update. Expert Opin Pharmacother 2011;12(4):579–92.

41. Mauiyyedi S, Crespo M, Collins AB, et al. Acute humoral rejection in kidney transplantation: II. Morphology, immunopathology, and pathologic classification. J Am Soc Nephrol 2002;13(3):779–87.

42. Crespo M, Pascual M, Tolkoff-Rubin N, et al. Acute humoral rejection in renal allograft recipients: I. Incidence, serology and clinical characteristics. Transplantation 2001;71(5):652–8.

43. Racusen LC, Colvin RB, Solez K, et al. Antibody-mediated rejection criteria - an addition to the Banff 97 classification of renal allograft rejection. Am J Transplant 2003;3(6):708–14.

44. Herzenberg AM, Gill JS, Djurdjev O, et al. C4d deposition in acute rejection: an independent long-term prognostic factor. J Am Soc Nephrol 2002; 13(1):234–41.

45. Takemoto S, Zeevi A, Feng S, et al. National conference to assess antibody-mediated rejection in solid organ transplantation. Am J Transplant 2004;4:1033–41.

46. Ionescu D, Girnita AL, Zeevi A, et al. C4d deposition in lung allografts is associated with circulating anti-HLA alloantibody. Transpl Immunol 2005;15(1):63–8.

47. Krukemeyer M, Moeller J, Morawietz L, et al. Description of B lymphocytes and plasma cells, complement, and chemokines/receptors in acute liver allograft rejection. Transplantation 2004;78:65–70.

48. Melcher M, Olson JL, Baxter-Lowe LA, et al. Antibody mediated rejection of a pancreas allograft. Am J Transplant 2006;6:423–8.

49. John R, Lietz K, Schuster M, et al. Immunologic sensitization in recipients of left ventricular assist devices. J Thorac Cardiovasc Surg 2003;125:578–91.

50. Michaels P, Espejo ML, Kobashigawa J, et al. Humoral rejection in cardiac transplantation: risks factors, hemodynamic consequences and relationship to transplant coronary artery disease. J Heart Lung Transplant 2003;22:58–69.

51. Murata K, Baldwin WM 3rd. Mechanisms of complement activation, C4d deposition, and their contribution to the pathogenesis of antibody-mediated rejection. Transplant Rev (Orlando) 2009;23(3): 139–50.

52. Haas M. C4d-negative antibody-mediated rejection in renal allografts: evidence for its existence and effect on graft survival. Clin Nephrol 2011;75(4): 271–8.

53. Landin L, Cavadas PC, Ibanez J, et al. CD3+-mediated rejection and C4d deposition in two composite tissue (bilateral hand) allograft recipients after induction with alemtuzumab. Transplantation 2009; 87:776–81.

54. Kanitakis J, McGregor B, Badet L, et al. Absence of C4d deposition in human composite tissue (hands and face) allograft biopsies: an immunoperoxidase study. Transplantation 2007;84:265.

55. Haas M. The significance of C4d staining with minimal histologic abnormalities. Curr Opin Organ Transplant 2010;15(1):21–7.

56. Stegall MD, Gloor JM. Deciphering antibody-mediated rejection: new insights into mechanisms and treatment. Curr Opin Organ Transplant 2010; 15(1):8–10.

57. Stegall MD, Raghavaiah S, Gloor JM. The (re) emergence of B cells in organ transplantation. Curr Opin Organ Transplant 2010;15(4):451–5.

58. Colvin RB, Hirohashi T, Farris AB, et al. Emerging role of B cells in chronic allograft dysfunction. Kidney Int Suppl 2010;119:S13–7.

59. Adeyi OA, Girnita AL, Howe J, et al. Serum analysis after transplant nephrectomy reveals restricted antibody specificity patterns against structurally defined HLA class I mismatches. Transpl Immunol 2005; 14(1):53–62.

60. Balk AHMM, Weimar W. Chronic heart graft rejection in the clinical setting. In: Paul LC, Solez K, editors. Organ transplantation: long-term results. New York: Marcel Dekker; 1992. p. 187–95.

61. Wahlers T, Haverich A, Schafers HJ, et al. Chronic rejection following lung transplantation. Incidence, time pattern and consequences. Eur J Cardiothorac Surg 1993;7(6):319.

62. Wiesner RH, Batts KP, Krom RA. Evolving concepts in the diagnosis, pathogenesis, and treatment of chronic hepatic allograft rejection. Liver Transpl Surg 1999;5:388.

63. Sarris GE, Smith JA, Shumway NE, et al. Long-term results of combined heart-lung transplantation: the Stanford experience. J Heart Lung Transplant 1994;13(6):940.

64. Murase N, Demetris AJ, Matsuzaki T, et al. Long survival in rats after multivisceral versus isolated small-bowel allotransplantation under FK 506. Surgery 1991;110:87.

65. Terasaki PI. Histocompatibility testing in transplantation. Arch Pathol Lab Med 1991;115(3):250.

66. Kerman RH, Kimball PM, Lindholm A, et al. Influence of HLA matching on rejections and short- and long-term primary cadaveric allograft survival. Transplantation 1993;56(5):1242.

67. Demetris AJ, Murase N, Lee RG, et al. Chronic rejection. A general overview of histopathology and pathophysiology with emphasis on liver, heart and intestinal allografts. Ann Transplant 1997;2(2): 27–44.

68. Rubin RH. Impact of cytomegalovirus infection on organ transplant recipients. Rev Infect Dis 1990; 12(S7):S754.

69. Rubin R. Infection in organ transplant recipients. In: Rubin RH, Young LS, editors. Clinical approach to infection in the compromised host. 3rd edition. New York and London: Plenum Medical Book Company; 1994. p. 629–35.

70. Matas A. Chronic rejection in renal transplant recipients—risk factors and correlates. Clin Transplant 1994;8(3):332.

71. Michaels PJ, Fishbein MC, Colvin RB. Humoral rejection of human organ transplants. Springer Semin Immunopathol 2003;25(2):119.

72. Junge G, Tullius SG, Klitzing V. The influence of late acute rejection episodes on long-term graft outcome after liver transplantation. Transplant Proc 2005; 37(4):1716.

73. Baines LS, Joseph JT, Jindal RM. Compliance and late acute rejection after kidney transplantation: a psychomedical perspective. Clin Transplant 2002;16:69.
74. Chapman JR. Compliance: the patient, the doctor, and the medication? Transplantation 2004;77(5):782.
75. Demetris AJ, Murase N, Starzl TE, et al. Pathology of chronic rejection: an overview of common findings and observations about pathogenic mechanisms and possible prevention. Graft 1998;1(2): 52–9.
76. Shirwan H. Chronic allograft rejection. Do the Th2 cells preferentially induced by indirect alloantigen recognition play a dominant role? Transplantation 1999;68(6):715.
77. Zheng X, Pei G, Qiu Y, et al. Dynamic observation of serum cytokines in the patients with hand transplantation. Transplant Proc 2002;34(8):3405.
78. Petruzzo P, Dubernard JM. Hand transplantation: Lyon experience. In: Dubernard JM, editor. Composite tissue allgrafts. Paris: John Libbey Eurotext; 2001. p. 63–8.
79. Lefrancois N. Immunosuppression in hand allograft. In: Dubernard JM, editor. Composite tissue allgrafts. Paris: John Libbey Eurotext; 2001. p. 71–4.
80. Hakim N. Immunosuppression in composite tissue allgraft. In: Dubernard JM, editor. Composite tissue allgrafts. Paris: John Libbey Eurotext; 2001. p. 17.
81. Kanitakis J, Jullien D. Pathology of the skin after hand allografting. In: Dubernard JM, editor. Composite tissue allgrafts. Paris: John Libbey Eurotext; 2001. p. 71.
82. Diefenbeck M, Nerlich A, Schneeberger S, et al. Allograft vasculopathy after allogeneic vascularized knee transplantation. Transpl Int 2011;24(1): 1432–2277.
83. Chertow GM, Brenner BM, Mackenzie HS, et al. Non-immunologic predictors of chronic renal allograft failure: data from the United Network of Organ Sharing. Kidney Int Suppl 1995;52:S48.
84. Chignier E, Eloy R. Adventitial resection of small artery provokes endothelial loss and intimal hyperplasia. Surg Gynecol Obstet 1986;163(4):327–34.
85. Meuli-Simmen C, Eiman T, Alpert BS, et al. Fibromuscular proliferation in finger arteries after hand replantation: a case report. Microsurgery 1996; 17(10):551–4.
86. Xu X, Lu H, Lin H, et al. Aortic adventitial angiogenesis and lymphangiogenesis promote intimal inflammation and hyperplasia. Cardiovasc Pathol 2009; 18(5):269–78.
87. Demetris AJ, Murase N, Ye Q, et al. Analysis of chronic rejection and obliterative arteriopathy. Possible contributions of donor antigen-presenting cells and lymphatic disruption. Am J Pathol 1997; 150(2):563–78.

Clinical Strategies to Enhance Nerve Regeneration in Composite Tissue Allotransplantation

Simone W. Glaus, MD, Philip J. Johnson, PhD*,
Susan E. Mackinnon, MD

KEYWORDS

- Peripheral nerve • Nerve regeneration
- Composite tissue allotransplantation
- Hand transplantation • Axon • Schwann cell

Since the first successful case was reported in September 1998, at least 50 hand transplantation procedures have been performed worldwide.[1] Successful transplantation had initially been limited by availability of an immunosuppressant regimen able to prevent rejection of the composite tissue allograft (CTA). Now, realization of hand transplantation as a permanent tool in the reconstructive armamentarium and expansion of its clinical indications will no doubt depend on further breakthroughs in immunomodulation, such as development of new protocols that minimize maintenance immunosuppression or induce a state of graft tolerance. Just as important to the ultimate success of hand transplantation, however, is improving its long-term functional results. With the ever-increasing cost of health care and with the growing pressure on health care providers to justify expenditures with published evidence of substantial clinical benefit, improving functionality must remain as high a priority as lessening risk and decreasing cost.

PERIPHERAL NERVE INJURY AND REGENERATION

Axonal disruption in the peripheral nerve activates a highly regulated and sophisticated sequence of events.[2] Wallerian degeneration occurs distal to the site of injury, with early changes revolving around the removal of cellular debris and degenerating distal axon segments by local macrophages and Schwann cells (SCs).[2–5] Mitogenic cytokines released by the injured axons induce SCs to change from a myelinating phenotype to a proliferative phenotype.[6–10] These cytokine signals, as well as those secreted by infiltrating macrophages, induce SCs to line up into columns along the basement membrane of endoneurial tubes. These columns of SCs, termed bands of Büngner, secrete neurotrophic factors that stimulate axonal sprouting and guide axonal regeneration.[11–14]

Proximal to the site of injury, axons are pruned back by one or two nodes of Ranvier.[15] Each axon then sprouts multiple growth cones, each growth cone giving rise to a daughter axon, with

The authors have nothing to disclose. No benefits or funding in any form have been received or will be received in relation to this article.
Division of Plastic and Reconstructive Surgery, Washington University School of Medicine, 660 South Euclid Avenue, St Louis, MO 63110, USA
* Corresponding author.
E-mail address: johnsonp@wudosis.wustl.edu

Hand Clin 27 (2011) 495–509
doi:10.1016/j.hcl.2011.07.002
0749-0712/11/$ – see front matter © 2011 Elsevier Inc. All rights reserved.

a ratio of approximately five daughter axons per parent axon.[16–18] The axon cell body changes the focus of its protein production from synthesis of neurotransmitters to structural proteins, which are used to lengthen axon projections. Each daughter axon searches to reconnect with a neuromuscular junction under the guidance of the endoneurial microstructure, regenerative SCs, and neurotrophic factors—all derived from the distal nerve stump. Regeneration proceeds slowly, at approximately 1 mm per day in humans.[19] Daughter axons that fail to reach the appropriate target organ undergo pruning. Time to reinnervation of the neuromuscular junctions be months or, in cases of very proximal nerve injury, even years.

When nerve continuity cannot be restored after transection by a tension-free repair, a nerve graft must be interposed between the proximal and distal nerve stumps to act as a scaffold for axonal regeneration. Nerve autografts, harvested from the patient's own noncritical sensory nerves, have served as the gold standard by providing both endoneurial microstructure and supportive SCs to aid regeneration. However, when the supply of available autografts is insufficient, such as in the repair of large, segmental, or complex nerve injuries, cadaveric or donor-related allografts provide a readily accessible alternative.[20] Experimental studies on rodents, large animals, and nonhuman primates, as well as the senior author's clinical experience, have shown that nerve allografts in the presence of immunosuppression provide equal regeneration and functional recovery as autografts, if not slightly better owing to the use of the regeneration-enhancing immunosuppressant tacrolimus.[21–25] Understanding the interaction between host tissues and nerve allografts and the unique regenerative challenges that are present in this clinical model is essential to predicting and optimizing nerve regeneration in the peripheral nerves of hand transplants. This article discusses the clinical scenario of a nerve allograft alone, without the other CTA components, followed by the differences in nerve regeneration when the nerve allograft is part of a CTA.

WHAT HAVE WE LEARNED FROM NERVE ALLOTRANSPLANTATION?

Whereas its axonal content will degenerate following harvest, the fresh unprocessed nerve allograft contains both endoneurial architecture and supportive SCs to promote host axonal regeneration across the graft. SCs are the most immunogenic component of human nerve.[26–32] Nerve allotransplantation, therefore, requires immunosuppression during the period of host axonal regeneration across the allograft to ensure donor SC support. The entire length of the graft must ultimately become populated with host SCs; however, in such a way that immunosuppression can be safely withdrawn once host axons have regenerated through the graft.[21] Should large portions of the graft remain populated solely by donor SCs, removal of immunosuppression will result in massive donor SC loss and debilitating conduction block. Nerve conduction will only be supported long-term if regenerated host axons have been myelinated by host SCs that have migrated into the graft.

At the time of implantation, host and donor SCs exist in two distinct populations—donor SCs within the allograft and host SCs in the proximal and distal nerve stumps. In the presence of immunosuppression, donor and host SCs proliferate and support axonal regeneration. Even with adequate traditional immunosuppression, however, the donor SC population will initially be depleted by short subclinical episodes of rejection, providing a stimulus for host SC migration from both the proximal and distal host nerve stumps (**Fig. 1**).[33] Interestingly, in a nerve autograft situation, Aguayo and colleagues[34,35] have shown that SCs do not migrate, but rather stay in their original location, whether that be within the graft or within the proximal and distal nerve stumps.

Host SCs have been shown to migrate into the allograft from both the proximal and distal stumps of the recipient nerve.[36–39] In vivo imaging of SC migration demonstrated a greater proportion of migration from the distal host nerve stump. In an acellularized nerve graft model (processed to remove immunogenic cells, including SCs), host SCs quickly repopulated the graft, within 10 days, while axonal regeneration lagged behind by an additional 10 to 15 days.[37] In a fresh, unprocessed nerve allograft model, a delay in host SC migration was observed, during which time donor SCs seemed to assist axonal regeneration across the graft. Host SCs later migrated into the graft. This was likely in response to episodes of subclinical acute rejection that diminished donor SC numbers, until what was observed was a coexisting population of host and donor SCs in the graft. Once axonal regeneration through the graft was complete and immunosuppression was withdrawn, host SCs immediately attempted to fill any gaps left by the loss of the remaining donor SCs.[33]

WHAT IS DIFFERENT ABOUT SC MIGRATION IN A CTA VERSUS A NERVE ALLOGRAFT?

The nerve components of a transplanted hand are similar in many ways to a nerve allograft—they

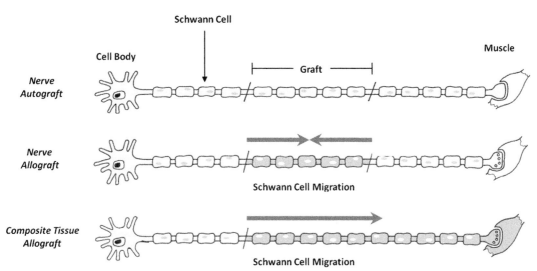

Fig. 1. SC migration. In the nerve autograft (*top*), autologous SCs support axonal regeneration through the graft and there is no migration of SCs from within the graft or from the proximal and distal stumps. In the nerve allograft (*middle*), donor SCs initially support axonal regeneration but may be replaced as the graft is repopulated by inward migration of host SCs from the proximal and distal nerve stumps. In the composite tissue allograft (*bottom*), only unidirectional host SC migration is possible. It is unknown whether host SCs are capable of replicating and migrating enough to repopulate the distal-most extent of the nerve. (*Adapted from* Moore AM, Ray WZ, Chenard KE, et al. Nerve allotransplantation as it pertains to composite tissue transplantation. Hand 2009;4:239–44; with permission.)

provide the same intact nerve architecture and supportive, albeit immunogenic, donor SCs. Many of the same mechanisms for SC turnover described above likely apply in the CTA model. However, significant differences between the two models exist that could make nerve regeneration in a CTA model inferior to a "stand-alone" nerve allograft. First, in a hand transplant, there is no host distal nerve stump and no distal source of host SCs. The entire distal neuromuscular unit is comprised of donor tissue, and repopulation of the donor nerve with host SCs relies solely on proximal host SC proliferation and migration (see **Fig. 1**). It is unknown whether host SCs will be capable of meeting this demand and populating the most distal extents of the transplanted nerve, especially as the level of transplantation moves proximally up the arm.[40]

A second difference between allografts and CTA involves the impetus for SC migration. In nerve allografts, multiple subclinical rejection events in which the donor SC population is trimmed back but not eliminated likely provide the cue for host SC migration into the graft. In the hand transplant, other tissues, such as skin and muscle, have even greater antigenicity than SCs and require a more stringent suppression of the immune system.[41] Without the mini rejection episodes that are permissible and probably even desirable in nerve

allografting alone, it is unknown to what extent host SCs will be triggered to proliferate and migrate into the graft. Should the graft remain exclusively populated by donor SCs, axonal regeneration will still occur. Donor SCs are intrinsically no different from host SCs in their support of regeneration. However, if a significant rejection episode occurs later that significantly impacts the donor SC population, the patient will be left with a long, unsupported segment of nerve and a devastating nerve conduction block that will render the hand transplant nonfunctional (**Fig. 2**). Demyelination, which occurs with loss of SC support, is a major stimulus for SC migration. However, the authors know from their work with SC migration into acellularized nerve grafts that migration is limited to about 5 cm, even with SC migration occurring from both proximal and distal nerve stumps (Ying Yan, unpublished data, 2011). Until immunosuppressive strategies are developed that consistently induce tolerance of all donor tissue, the late loss of donor SCs due to unexpected episodes of rejection is a significant concern. Therefore, strategies to enhance nerve regeneration in CTA must take into account the delicate interplay between donor and host SCs, by promoting eventual complete repopulation of the donor nerve by host SCs, by keeping donor SCs alive long enough to support axonal regeneration until host SCs arrive, and by

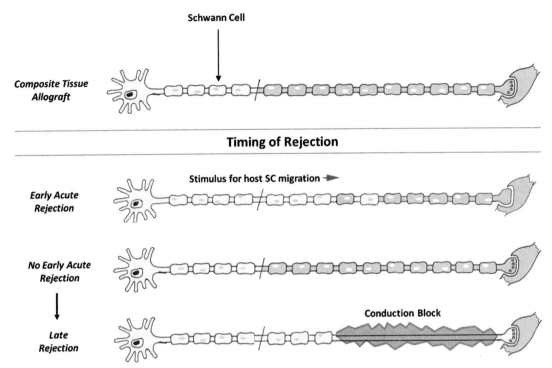

Fig. 2. SC fate in relation to timing of rejection in composite tissue allotransplantation. Minor early acute rejection episodes provide a stimulus for proximal host SC migration into the donor nerve. Without early rejection episodes, donor SCs will support axonal regeneration as well as host SCs. However, should late rejection occur without repopulation of the regenerated nerve by host SCs, the patient will be left with a debilitating conduction block. In this scenario, the host axon will not be supported by the rejected donor SCs, and host SCs cannot repopulate the entire length of the nerve from the proximal stump alone. (*Adapted from* Moore AM, Ray WZ, Chenard KE, et al. Nerve allotransplantation as it pertains to composite tissue transplantation. Hand 2009;4:239–44; with permission.)

avoiding any damage to or rejection of the composite tissue transplant during accomplishment of these objectives.

CRITICAL WINDOW OF TIME FOR REGENERATION

There is a critical window of time in which regeneration must occur for optimal recovery to be achieved. With regeneration proceeding at approximately 1 mm per day, many months may pass before target neuromuscular junctions are reinnervated.[42–45] As the months pass, with distal SCs lacking axonal contact and target muscle remaining denervated, irreversible changes begin that are detrimental to functional recovery. First, SCs that previously dedifferentiated from a myelinating phenotype to a regenerative phenotype settle back into a quiescent mode.[46–48] The SCs disarrange themselves from the bands of Büngner, decrease secretion of growth factors, and stop replication. Early reports suggest that SCs may even disappear altogether.[49] The result is inadequate support of regenerating axons. It is unknown

exactly how long it takes denervated SCs to become quiescent in humans. Clinical experience with proximal nerve injuries in humans seems to indicate that little additional motor functional recovery can be achieved by a patient beyond 1 year after injury.[50] Sensory recovery does not appear to be as time-dependent.

The second irreversible change that occurs with prolonged denervation is atrophy and fibrosis in the chronically denervated muscle.[51–54] In humans, these changes begin several months after denervation.[19] After this point, even if the muscle should become reinnervated, it can no longer achieve the same bulk or contractile force as preinjury. To ensure optimal functional recovery, regeneration must occur during the critical window of time. As the level of transplantation moves more and more proximally—from the hand to the forearm to the upper arm—one must be cognizant of these time constraints. Therefore, strategies to enhance nerve regeneration in CTA should include: (1) speeding the rate of axonal regeneration while ensuring quality of regeneration, (2) maintaining perfect SC support during the entire course of axonal regeneration, and (3) preserving the distal muscle until it can be reinnervated; all while preventing rejection of the composite tissue graft. This article highlights the experimental and clinical research that pertains to optimizing axonal regeneration and SC support in a CTA model.

SPEEDING AXONAL REGENERATION WHILE ENSURING QUALITY OF REGENERATION

A large proportion of the axon's axoplasmic volume is amputated when it undergoes transection. This traumatic event will, at the least, lead to structural and functional changes in the neuronal cell body and may even lead to cell death.[55,56] At the start of regeneration, therefore, there may be fewer available axons than were originally present in the nerve, highlighting the need to ensure successful regeneration of all remaining axons. Within hours after injury, the neuronal cell body has altered its metabolic machinery to focus on structural protein synthesis and has begun producing numerous growth cones, or terminal sprouts.[4,57,58] These represent the first wave of sprouts and are followed by a second wave within the first 2 days after injury.[15,59] The second wave of sprouts contains the definitive sprouts that proceed to regeneration, while the early sprouts degenerate. The time until appearance of the definitive sprouts is referred to as the initial delay.[60] The time is variable and may be increased or decreased because of stress, activity, or drugs. The advancing sprouts must cross the critical interstump zone,[2] the area of repair between the proximal and distal nerve stumps. The sprouts cross in a staggered fashion, and the final success of the nerve regeneration relies in great part on all regenerating axons successfully crossing this critical area. This highlights the importance of the growth-supportive milieu and architectural cues provided by the SCs of the distal nerve stump. In the absence of appropriate neurotrophic and structural guidance, the regenerative axons may lose their way and form a neuroma, a disorganized collection of connective tissue and nerve fibers.[60] Strategies to promote perfect SC support will be discussed later in this article.

FK-506, also known as tacrolimus, is a potent calcineurin phosphatase inhibitor that is an essential part of immunosuppression regimens for a variety of organ transplants. Its immunosuppressive mechanism ultimately inhibits the activation of T-cell proliferation through binding and inhibition of calcineurin. In 1995, Gold and colleagues[61] first described the ability of FK-506 to enhance peripheral nerve regeneration in a rat model. Since that time, experimental studies have shown that

FK-506 enhances regeneration after crush,[62,63] transection,[64] and chronic axotomy[65] injuries and in isograft[66] and allograft[21,67] models. Its ability to accelerate functional recovery has been shown in small and large animal models. Although the exact molecular pathways leading to its enhanced regeneration are not completely clear, evidence of calcineurin-independent pathway of action suggests that mediators such as FKBP-52, growth associated protein 43 (GAP43), heat shock protein 90 (HSP-90), and cytoskeletal dynamics may be involved in its neuro-regenerative properties.[68–73] FK-506 has been shown to increase the number of regenerated myelinated and unmyelinated nerve fibers,[63] stimulate even chronically axotomized motoneurons,[65] and block neuronal apoptosis.[74,75]

Correct timing of FK-506 administration is essential to its efficacy. Animal studies have shown that the neuroregenerative effect of FK-506 is decreased with delayed administration in both crush[76] injury and transection[77] models. Specifically, neuroregenerative benefit was diminished when administration was delayed by 3 days in a transection and immediate repair model, and was lost when administration was delayed by 5 days.[77] Therefore, as long as there is no individual contraindication to therapy, FK-506 should be provided as part of immunosuppression induction, as it was for all hand transplant patients between 1998 and 2006.[20] Ideally, the patient would receive FK-506 preloading for 3 days before nerve transection; this has been shown experimentally to further enhance FK-506's neuroregenerative effect[78] and has been implemented clinically in elective cases of reconstructive nerve allotransplantation.[79] Whereas this duration of preloading is not possible in hand transplantation due to the unpredictable nature of transplant availability, there is often a window of time of approximately 12 hours, in which the recipient is being notified of and prepared for surgery but the transplant is still being procured and prepared. Though it has not been definitively shown, the authors hypothesize that FK-506 preloading during this window of time, given as a loading dose to reach therapeutic levels similar to those achieved with 3 days preloading, will similarly optimize the regenerative effects of FK-506.

Consideration should be given also to including FK-506 in the patient's immunosuppressive maintenance regimen. (Ying Yan, Unpublished data, 2011) from our laboratory demonstrates that FK-506 continues to provide regenerative benefits for as long as it is administered. Specifically, for nerve transection injuries that posit a real regenerative challenge, FK-506 administration for a portion of the regenerative period shows better recovery than controls, but administration for the entire predicted regenerative period produces superior recovery. This corroborates with previous data that showed FK-506 to be advantageous even in the case of chronically axotomized axons.[65] The regenerating nerves in hand transplants, especially those of transplants at more proximal levels, are chronically axotomized for the many months they spend waiting to reach their distal targets. During this prolonged period, the patient will likely transition to a pared-back immunosuppressive regimen. Incorporating FK-506 into this maintenance regimen will provide not only immunosuppressive graft protection, but also continued regenerative support.

Much research is being performed on how to minimize immunosuppression or, ideally, induce graft tolerance in CTA. As progress is made awareness should be maintained that changing immunosuppressive regimens may differentially affect FK-506's ability to stimulate regeneration. Animal studies have examined the regenerative impact of combining FK-506 administration with anti-CD40 ligand costimulatory blockade (CSB). Combining therapeutic doses of CSB with immunosuppressive doses of FK-506 significantly eliminated FK-506's regenerative benefit. Using therapeutic CSB with a low dose of FK-506, however, maintained the same regenerative benefit as therapeutic FK-506 alone.[80] Other studies have shown that FK-506 maintains neuroregenerative benefit at low doses,[63,81–84] with a dose-benefit relationship that may not be strictly linear.[85] Although not specifically studied, it was hypothesized that the full immunosuppressive doses of each drug interfered with the mechanism of action of the other drug, each making the other less effective. Further understanding of the mechanisms by which these immunosuppressive agents potentiate and abrogate each other will progress our ability to create immunosuppressive or tolerance regimens that effectively protect the transplant while including the right dosing of FK-506 to promote regeneration.

In addition to impacting the rate of axonal regeneration, varying immunosuppressive regimens differentially impacted donor SC fate. In a study using transgenic mice with SCs expressing green fluorescent protein under the S-100b (expressed by well-differentiated SCs) or nestin promoters (expressed after a denervation stimulus), donor SC survival and phenotype in an allograft model were evaluated using different immunosuppressive regimens via serial imaging.[86] Mice immunosuppressed with FK-506 demonstrated mild acute rejection as well as somewhat hindered myelin formation and maturation of donor SCs

(from a proliferative to myelinating phenotype) after axonal regeneration was complete. Mice treated with CSB, on the other hand, experienced virtually no graft rejection, and showed optimal myelin formation and maturation of SCs after axonal regeneration. However, despite the improved restoration of mature SC-axonal relationships in CSB-treated mice, FK-506-treated mice demonstrated more robust regeneration of myelinated and unmyelinated axons, greater motor endplate reinnervation, and earlier functional recovery. Although this study did not evaluate a combined FK-506 and CSB regimen, it would be useful to know whether an optimal combination could be found that blended the best of both regimens—the enhanced axonal regeneration of FK-506 treatment and the improved myelin formation of CSB treatment. The impact of this ideal combination regimen on host SC migration needs to be studied to determine the distribution and ratio of donor-to-host SCs that remain after axonal regeneration and what risk this might pose should late rejection occur.

ENSURING PERFECT SC SUPPORT

As previously discussed, SCs are induced after nerve injury to change from a myelinating phenotype to a proliferative phenotype. Proliferative SCs are intimately involved in the process of axonal regeneration, through provision of structural guidance via bands of Büngner and secretion of neurotrophic factors. Without axonal contact, however, SCs will not indefinitely maintain their new proliferative phenotype or their injury-induced increase in number.[46–48] An experimental study in a rat model demonstrated the detrimental effect of chronic denervation on SC ability to support axonal regeneration.[87] The common peroneal branch of the rat sciatic nerve was transected and the distal stump subjected to 0 to 24 weeks of chronic denervation. After the denervation period, the tibial branch of the sciatic nerve was transected and the proximal tibial stump repaired end-to-end to the chronically denervated peroneal distal stump. Retrograde labeling 12 months later demonstrated that denervation of SCs for up to 4 weeks did not negatively impact axonal regeneration, but axonal regeneration rapidly decreased when distal nerve SCs were denervated for 8 weeks or more. With SC chronic denervation for 24 weeks, the number of regenerating axons was diminished to less than 10%. Interestingly, the 10% of regenerated axons were well myelinated. Therefore, although chronically denervated SCs may not retain their ability to support regeneration, they retain their ability to myelinate, likely due to reversion back to a myelinating phenotype from a proliferative phenotype.

Perfect proliferative SC support is required, therefore, to optimize axonal regeneration. Perfect SC support is threatened, however, in a CTA model. As mentioned previously, episodes of rejection threaten donor SCs, which are crucial to early nerve regeneration. Lack of short episodes of rejection, however, may remove the cue for migration of host SCs into the transplanted nerve, with the potential for a devastating conduction block if residual donor SCs are later rejected. Even if adequate cues for host SC migration are provided, lack of a distal host SC source may leave too large a proliferation and migration burden on proximal host SCs—proximal host SCs may not be able to populate the distal-most extent of the transplanted nerve.

Strategies to optimize SC support include reactivating SCs that have reverted from their proliferative phenotype to their original myelinating phenotype, or preventing this reversion. Alternatively, supplementation with cultured SCs or stem-cell derived SC-like cells after a period of chronic denervation might provide fresh support for regenerating axons, in essence "resetting the clock."

Interaction of SCs with invading macrophages is important for subsequent SC support of regeneration. After nerve injury, transforming growth factor β (TGF-β) is secreted into the nerve by invading macrophages[88] as well as resident SCs.[89] Several in vitro studies have shown TGF-β to be essential in the transformation of SCs to a nonmyelinating, proliferative phenotype.[90–94] Additionally, TGF-β is involved in mediating the neurotrophic effect of several other neurotrophic factors, such as glial cell line-derived neurotrophic factor (GDNF), a very potent neurotrophic factor for motoneurons.[95,96] An experimental study in a rat model of chronic SC denervation showed that TGF-β was able to attenuate the adverse effects of chronic denervation in vivo.[97] SCs were isolated from rat distal nerve stumps that had been chronically denervated for 24 weeks. After incubation in culture medium with or without TGF-β, the SCs were placed into Silastic tubes that were grafted into a freshly transected rat tibial nerve. Retrograde labeling 3 months later showed a fourfold increase in the number of distally regenerated motoneurons in the group that had received SC incubation with TGF-β.[87,97] It appears that TGF-β has the capability to reverse the detrimental effect of chronic denervation on SC ability to support axonal regeneration. Studies using local delivery of TGF-β in a prolonged or chronic denervation model would be useful to assess its potential as a therapeutic

in cases of human proximal nerve injury or hand transplantation, where prolonged denervation of distal SCs is anticipated.

If reawakening SCs into a proliferative mode is not possible or practical in vivo, supplementation with autologous cultured SCs or stem-cell–derived SC-like cells may function to the same end. Supplementation also would be indicated in hand transplantation, for replacement of donor SCs that die off because of rejection episodes. Alternatively, prophylactic "replacement" of donor SCs with host SCs could be performed at the time of transplant to seed the entire donor nerve with preoperatively cultured cells, thereby creating a mixed population of host and donor SCs. In all cases, except complete immune tolerance, this mixed population would be beneficial to better withstand rejection episodes.

ALTERNATIVE SOURCES FOR HOST SCS

Isolation and culture of human SCs has been described in the peripheral nerve literature since 1991[98] but has been fraught with many difficulties in achieving good primary cell yields and in adequately excluding fibroblasts. Even though significant strides have been made, with a recently published protocol describing a relatively fast (21 day) and efficient (90%–95% pure) culture of primary human SCs,[99] cultured SCs have failed to achieve clinical translation over the past 20 years. Additionally, culture of human SCs requires invasive nerve biopsy with subsequent sensory loss and the risk of neuroma formation and neuropathic pain. More accessible and less morbid sources of SCs, therefore, have been sought.

Bone marrow, adipose tissue, and skin with its associated structures have arisen as sources of stem cells that may be induced to SC-like character. Bone marrow stromal cells (BMSCs), harvested from the long bones, have been studied by several groups and have shown to differentiate into an adherent SC-like phenotype when cultured in media with appropriate cytokines.[100–102] Though they have shown some promise in rodent and nonhuman primate experimental models of nerve conduits[101–104] and acellular grafts,[100] there is increased interest in less invasive sources of stem cells.

Adipose tissue has been identified as a source of multipotent stromal stem cells with the ability to differentiate into SC phenotype in appropriate culture conditions. These adipose tissue-derived stem cells (ADSCs) have been shown to promote motor neurite outgrowth in vitro.[105] Two recent studies have evaluated cultured primary SCs, differentiated BMSCs, differentiated ADSCs, and undifferentiated ADSCs for supplementation of a 1 cm fibrin nerve conduit in a rat sciatic nerve model.[106,107] Evaluation of regenerative distance 2 weeks after conduit implantation showed that (1) supplementation with either cultured primary SCs, differentiated BMSCs, or differentiated ADSCs significantly increased the distance of axonal regeneration over that of conduits with media alone, (2) primary SCs were superior to both differentiated BMSCs and ADSCs, and (3) differentiated BMSCs and ADSCs were equivalent in their regeneration enhancement.[106] In a separate study, undifferentiated ADSCs seeded into the fibrin conduit were also able to increase regeneration distance over media alone. However, cell tracking 14 days after transplantation showed almost no remaining implanted cells.[107] This raises questions about the longevity of implanted cells that are undifferentiated versus differentiated, about the mechanisms by which these cells work, and about the relationship between stem cell lifespan and regenerative benefit.

Finally, the skin dermis contains neural crest-related precursor cells, termed skin-derived precursor cells (SKPs), which have shown to differentiate into SC-like cells in vitro when supplied with appropriate cues, in rodents[108,109] and in humans.[110,111] Recent studies have tested the ability of SKPs to enhance regeneration in rodent acute injury and chronic denervation models. In a rat 12 mm sciatic nerve gap model, acellularized nerve allografts (ANAs) were seeded with cultured SCs or SKPs and compared with autografts (positive control) and ANAs with vehicle (negative control). Time points of 4 and 8 weeks showed (1) continued survival of SKPs, (2) significantly better regeneration with SKP-seeded ANAs than with vehicle alone, (3) equivalent regeneration between SKP-seeded ANAs and autografts, and (4) equivalent or slightly better regeneration in SKP-seeded ANAs than SC-seeded ANAs.[112] Skin-derived precursor cells were tested in a chronic denervation model and found to significantly enhance regeneration of motoneurons compared with vehicle control, in essence re-awakening the regenerative capability of the chronically denervated distal stump.[113] The mechanism behind this phenomenon—whether this improved support is directly due to the influence of SKPs on regenerating axons or secondary to interactions between SKPs and host SCs—has yet to be elucidated.

There are a few practical considerations concerning the use of stem cells in peripheral nerve repair.[114] To optimize stem cell therapy, more research on the number, method, and timing of stem cell delivery is needed. Seeded stem cell numbers have varied widely across studies and injury models, and the optimal dosing regimen is unknown. Additionally, the degree of predifferentiation before seeding is being worked out. Although it seems that survival is improved with predifferentiation,[110] supplementation with naïve stem cells might better maintain the cells' proliferative capacity, while allowing in vivo signals to prompt differentiation.[115] Survival should also be improved, as most studies to date have shown only between 0.5% and 38% survival of implanted stem cells.[114] Finally, the tumorigenic capabilities of these stem cells must be explored, especially before consideration in an immunosuppressed transplant population because capacity for malignant transformation is a potential negative consequence of using multipotent precursors. Although these parameters require further study before clinical translation, the use of stem cells for augmenting axonal regeneration is, nevertheless, an exciting area of research with the potential to significantly further peripheral nerve surgery outcomes.

Optimizing Surgical Technique

Several surgical techniques can be used to enhance motor and sensory recovery following hand transplantation. First, a thorough understanding of the motor and sensory topography of the ulnar and median nerves must guide their repair. This understanding will lead to proper alignment of ulnar nerve motor and sensory components, ultimately promoting appropriate reinnervation of motor and sensory targets. Second, with the realization that 95% of the median nerve at the wrist is sensory, nerve transfer of the distal anterior interosseous nerve to the median nerve deep motor branch optimizes motor reinnervation of the thenar musculature, enhancing specific functional recovery. Finally, because regenerating nerves will slow at areas of known nerve entrapment, decompression of nerve entrapment points distal to the nerve repair sites should be performed. Both the carpal tunnel and the ulnar nerve through Guyon canal can be decompressed through the same incision.

The intraneural topography of the ulnar nerve has been understood since Jabaley and colleagues[116] first described a preliminary report in 1980. Specifically, distal to the takeoff of the dorsal cutaneous branch of the ulnar nerve (DCU), the sensory component that innervates the volar aspect of the hand makes up about 60% of the nerve cross-sectional area, and the motor component that continues as the deep motor branch makes up the remaining 40% (**Fig. 3**). Proximal

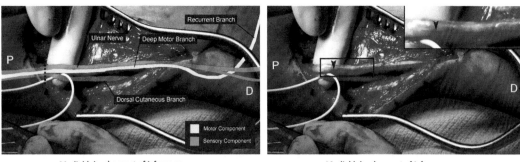

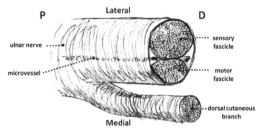

Fig. 3. Ulnar nerve topography within the distal forearm. (*Left*) The motor (*yellow*) and sensory (*green*) fascicles should be identified at the time of transplantation to facilitate appropriate alignment during repair. Proximally, the ulnar nerve topography is sensory-motor-sensory, until the dorsal cutaneous branch separates from the remainder of the nerve approximately 10 cm proximal to the wrist crease. To confirm the identity of the motor fascicle, the deep motor branch should be identified within Guyon canal distally (not shown), then followed visually to where it joins the main sensory fascicular group proximally. (*Right*) A prominent longitudinally oriented vessel (*arrow*) is frequently present, marking the natural cleavage plane between the sensory and motor fascicular groups of the ulnar nerve. (*bottom*) Ulnar nerve in cross-section (*dashed lines*). Below the take-off of the dorsal cutaneous branch, the sensory fascicle comprises approximately 60% of the ulnar nerve, and the motor fascicle 40%. D, distal; P, proximal. (*Adapted from* Brown JM, Yee A, Mackinnon SE. Distal median to ulnar nerve transfers to restore ulnar motor and sensory function within the hand. Neurosurgery 2009;65:966–78; with permission.)

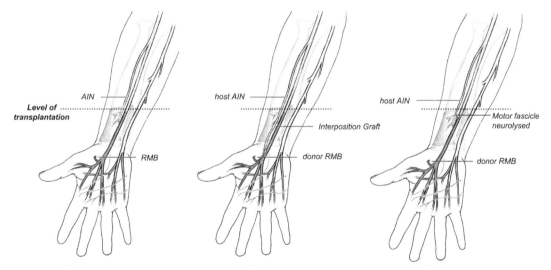

Fig. 4. Distal AIN to median RMB transfer. For hand transplants at or below the level of the pronator quadratus muscle (*left*), the host AIN may serve as a reliable donor of motor axons to the thenar muscles, via nerve transfer to the RMB. The AIN may be transferred to the RMB either with the use of an interposing nerve graft (*middle*) or after more proximal motor fascicle dissection of the donor nerve (*right*). (*Adapted from* Colbert SH, Mackinnon SE. Nerve transfers in the hand and upper extremity. Tech Hand Up Extrem Surg 2008;12:20–33; with permission; and *From* Brown JM, Mackinnon SE. Nerve transfers in the forearm and hand. Hand Clin 2008;24:319–40; with permission.)

to the takeoff of the DCU, the motor fascicular group is sandwiched between the DCU medially and the main sensory component of the ulnar nerve laterally. The DCU branches off from the main ulnar nerve about 10 cm above the wrist crease. As it travels distally, the motor component turns into the deep motor branch (DMB) of the ulnar nerve and moves from lying medial to the sensory portion of the ulnar nerve, to travelling under the sensory component as it turns around the hook of the hamate, where it finally assumes a position lateral to the sensory component. There is an intraneural cleavage plane between the motor and sensory groups, as well as between the main ulnar nerve and the DCU, that is easily discernible using micro-pickups. Tapping across the surface of the nerve, micro-pickups will "fall" into the intraneural cleavage plane. Often, there is also a streak of fatty tissue or a microvessel that delineates this cleavage plane (see **Fig. 3**).[117] Certainly, in the donor hand, the motor and sensory components can be clearly delineated by tracing the DMB proximally to identify the motor fascicular group. In the recipient forearm, at or proximal to the level of the wrist, the larger sensory component of the ulnar nerve will lie most laterally (ie, most radially) compared with the motor component and, above 10 cm proximal to wrist level, there will also be a smaller fascicular group present on the most medial (ulnar) aspect that is the DCU. Appropriate alignment of motor and sensory fascicular components at the time of hand transplantation will optimize appropriate re-innervation of motor and sensory targets.

With respect to the median nerve, 95% of the nerve at wrist level is comprised of sensory axons. Topographic mapping of the recipient median nerve at this level during nerve repair is, therefore, not as feasible. Although guidance of regenerating sensory axons to their sensory targets is practically assured, the ability to direct the remaining 5% of motor axons to the thenar muscles is tenuous. It is straight-forward, however, to identify the recurrent motor branch (RMB) of the median nerve in the donor hand and to trace the motor fascicle proximally to the proposed repair site. Consideration can then be given to reinnervating the median nerve's RMB to the thenar muscles with a nerve transfer from the distal portion of the anterior interosseous nerve (AIN) (**Fig. 4**).

The successful transfer of the distal AIN to the RMB was first demonstrated in 1992 by Huang[118] with rhesus monkeys and, subsequently, was reported in a case series of 17 patients in 1997.[119] Vernadakis and colleagues[120] also reported the use of this nerve transfer to restore thenar muscle function after resection of a median nerve

neuroma-in-continuity. The distal AIN provides a suitable donor for transfer of motor axons to the RMB of the median nerve because, anatomically, the AIN and the RMB are comparable in diameter (AIN?1.3–1.5 mm, RMB?1.4–1.7 mm) and number of myelinated fibers (AIN?866–912, RMB?1020–1120).[121–124] Also, although the AIN is a mixed nerve, it consists primarily of motor fibers.[117] The only limitation to this nerve transfer is the location of the AIN at 60 mm proximal to the distal wrist crease.[123] Either a nerve graft is necessary for successful tension-free nerve transfer or the motor branch of the donor median nerve needs to be neurolysed proximally enough in the donor forearm to facilitate a tension-free direct repair (see **Fig. 4**).

To perform the nerve transfer, the RMB can be identified in the carpal tunnel and traced back proximally to the repair site. The authors use a technique we call "neurolysing with our eyes." We physically identify the recurrent motor branch as it enters the thenar muscles and simply follow it proximally with micro-pickups until we can mark its position on the median nerve with blue ink. This allows us to determine the site at which we will transfer the AIN without the added operative time or unnecessary risks of physical neurolysis. The AIN may be identified as it enters the pronator quadratus, transected just proximal to its branches at the midportion of the muscle, and either transferred to the RMB with the use of an interposing nerve graft or transferred to the more proximal motor fascicle dissection on the donor nerve. If a nerve graft is used, the authors recommend use of an autologous nerve graft because it provides immediate SC support and the potential to provide host SCs for migration and repopulation of donor nerves. Please refer to these articles for more detailed descriptions of the AIN harvest[117,125] and transfer to the RMB.[120]

The authors' final recommendation is to perform decompression of the carpal tunnel and Guyon canal with specific release of the DMB to prevent slowing of regeneration at these common areas of nerve entrapment. Both of these decompressions may be performed through a single longitudinal incision made approximately 6 mm ulnar to the thenar crease.

SUMMARY

Reinnervation of a hand transplant ultimately dictates functional recovery but provides a significant regenerative challenge. In addition to high quality of regeneration, rapidity of regeneration is essential because there is a critical window of time for regeneration before detrimental changes occur in the distal nerve and target muscle.

Interventions to enhance nerve regeneration include acceleration of axonal regeneration via FK-506 administration and augmentation of SC support, either by reactivation of chronically axotomized SCs or by SC supplementation. Optimizing surgical technique at the time of transplantation also better supports intrinsic muscle recovery. Appropriate alignment of ulnar nerve motor and sensory components and prophylactic release of potential entrapment points should be performed. Transfer of the distal anterior interosseous nerve to the recurrent motor branch of the median nerve should be considered. Improving long-term functional recovery through the previously discussed interventions will ultimately help determine the success and longevity of the field of hand transplantation.

REFERENCES

1. International Registry on Hand and Composite Tissue Transplantation. Available at: http://www.handregistry.com/. Accessed July 30, 2011. A running tally of the number of single and double hand transplants is provided under the "world experience" tab.
2. Geuna S, Raimondo S, Ronchi G, et al. Chapter 3: Histology of the peripheral nerve and changes occurring during nerve regeneration. Int Rev Neurobiol 2009;87:27–46.
3. Bigbee JW, Yoshino JE, DeVries GH. Morphological and proliferative responses of cultured Schwann cells following rapid phagocytosis of a myelin-enriched fraction. J Neurocytol 1987;16:487–96.
4. Fu SY, Gordon T. The cellular and molecular basis of peripheral nerve regeneration. Mol Neurobiol 1997;14:67–116.
5. Stoll G, Jander S. The role of microglia and macrophages in the pathophysiology of the CNS. Prog Neurobiol 1999;58:233–47.
6. Rogister B, Delree P, Leprince P, et al. Transforming growth factor beta as a neuronoglial signal during peripheral nervous system response to injury. J Neurosci Res 1993;34:32–43.
7. Mews M, Meyer M. Modulation of Schwann cell phenotype by TGF-beta 1: inhibition of P0 mRNA expression and downregulation of the low affinity NGF receptor. Glia 1993;8:208–17.
8. Heumann R. Regulation of the synthesis of nerve growth factor. J Exp Biol 1987;132:133–50.
9. Thoenen H, Bandtlow C, Heumann R, et al. Nerve growth factor: cellular localization and regulation of synthesis. Cell Mol Neurobiol 1988;8:35–40.
10. Funakoshi H, Frisen J, Barbany G, et al. Differential expression of mRNAs for neurotrophins and their receptors after axotomy of the sciatic nerve. J Cell Biol 1993;123:455–65.
11. Brushart TM. Preferential reinnervation of motor nerves by regenerating motor axons. J Neurosci 1988;8:1026–31.
12. Lundborg G, Dahlin LB, Danielsen N, et al. Tissue specificity in nerve regeneration. Scand J Plast Reconstr Surg 1986;20:279–83.
13. Lundborg Gr, Dahlin L, Danielsen N, et al. Trophism, tropism and specificity in nerve regeneration. J Reconstr Microsurg 1994;10:345–54.
14. Mackinnon SE, Dellon AL, Lundborg G, et al. A study of neurotrophism in a primate model. J Hand Surg Am 1986;11:888–94.
15. Cajal SR. Degeneration and regeneration of the nervous system. New York: Oxford University Press; 1928.
16. Toft PB, Fugleholm K, Schmalbruch H. Axonal branching following crush lesions of peripheral nerves of rat. Muscle Nerve 1988;11:880–9.
17. Aitken JT, Sharman M, Young JZ. Maturation of regenerating nerve fibres with various peripheral connexions. J Anat 1947;81:1–22.
18. Mackinnon SE, Dellon AL, O'Brien JP. Changes in nerve fiber numbers distal to a nerve repair in the rat sciatic nerve model. Muscle Nerve 1991;14:1116–22.
19. Mackinnon SE, Dellon AL. Surgery of the peripheral nerve. New York: Thieme; 1988.
20. Siemionow M, Sonmez E. Nerve allograft transplantation: a review. J Reconstr Microsurg 2007;23:511–20.
21. Mackinnon SE, Doolabh VB, Novak CB, et al. Clinical outcome following nerve allograft transplantation. Plast Reconstr Surg 2001;107:1419–29.
22. Bain JR, Mackinnon SE, Hudson AR, et al. Preliminary report of peripheral nerve allografting in primates immunosuppressed with cyclosporin A. Transplant Proc 1989;21:3176–7.
23. Midha R, Mackinnon SE, Evans PJ, et al. Comparison of regeneration across nerve allografts with temporary or continuous cyclosporin A immunosuppression. J Neurosurg 1993;78:90–100.
24. Nakao Y, Mackinnon SE, Mohanakumar T, et al. Monoclonal antibodies against ICAM-1 and LFA-1 (CD11A) induce specific tolerance to peripheral nerve allograft in rats. Transplant Proc 1995;27:373–7.
25. Strasberg SR, Hertl MC, Mackinnon SE, et al. Peripheral nerve allograft preservation improves regeneration and decreases systemic cyclosporin a requirements. Exp Neurol 1996;139:306–16.
26. Gulati AK. Immune response and neurotrophic factor interactions in peripheral nerve transplants. Acta Haematol 1998;99:171–4.
27. Gulati AK, Cole GP. Nerve graft immunogenicity as a factor determining axonal regeneration in the rat. J Neurosurg 1990;72:114–22.
28. Pollard JD, Gye RS, McLeod JG. An assessment of immunosuppressive agents in experimental

peripheral nerve transplantation. Surg Gynecol Obstet 1971;132:839–45.

29. Trumble TE, Shon FG. The physiology of nerve transplantation. Hand Clin 2000;16:105–22.

30. Lassner F, Schaller E, Steinhoff G, et al. Cellular mechanisms of rejection and regeneration in peripheral nerve allografts. Transplantation 1989; 48:386–92.

31. Mackinnon S, Hudson A, Falk R, et al. Nerve allograft response: a quantitative immunological study. Neurosurgery 1982;10:61–9.

32. Yu LT, Rostami A, Silvers WK, et al. Expression of major histocompatibility complex antigens on inflammatory peripheral nerve lesions. J Neuroimmunol 1990;30:121–8.

33. Whitlock EL, Myckatyn TM, Tong AY, et al. Dynamic quantification of host Schwann cell migration into peripheral nerve allografts. Exp Neurol 2010;225: 310–9.

34. Aguayo AJ, Charron L, Bray GM. Potential of Schwann cells from unmyelinated nerves to produce myelin: a quantitative ultrastructural and radiographic study. J Neurocytol 1976;5:565–73.

35. Aguayo AJ, Epps J, Charron L, et al. Multipotentiality of Schwann cells in cross-anastomosed and grafted myelinated and unmyelinated nerves: quantitative microscopy and radioautography. Brain Res 1976;104:1–20.

36. Fornaro M, Tos P, Geuna S, et al. Confocal imaging of Schwann-cell migration along muscle-vein combined grafts used to bridge nerve defects in the rat. Microsurgery 2001;21:153–5.

37. Fukaya K, Hasegawa M, Mashitani T, et al. Oxidized galectin-1 stimulates the migration of Schwann cells from both proximal and distal stumps of transected nerves and promotes axonal regeneration after peripheral nerve injury. J Neuropathol Exp Neurol 2003;62:162–72.

38. Tseng CY, Hu G, Ambron RT, et al. Histologic analysis of Schwann cell migration and peripheral nerve regeneration in the autogenous venous nerve conduit (AVNC). J Reconstr Microsurg 2003;19:331–40.

39. Hayashi A, Koob JW, Liu DZ, et al. A double-transgenic mouse used to track migrating Schwann cells and regenerating axons following engraftment of injured nerves. Exp Neurol 2007;207:128–38.

40. Moore AM, Ray WZ, Chenard KE, et al. Nerve allotransplantation as it pertains to composite tissue transplantation. Hand (N Y) 2009;4:239–44.

41. Hettiaratchy S, Melendy E, Randolph MA, et al. Tolerance to composite tissue allografts across a major histocompatibility barrier in miniature swine. Transplantation 2004;77:514–21.

42. Wang MS, Zeleny-Pooley M, Gold BG. Comparative dose-dependence study of FK506 and cyclosporin A on the rate of axonal regeneration in the

rat sciatic nerve. J Pharmacol Exp Ther 1997;282: 1084–93.

43. Pan YA, Misgeld T, Lichtman JW, et al. Effects of neurotoxic and neuroprotective agents on peripheral nerve regeneration assayed by time-lapse imaging in vivo. J Neurosci 2003;23:11479–88.

44. Gutmann E, Guttmann L, Medawar PB, et al. The Rate of Regeneration of Nerve. J Exp Biol 1942; 19:14–44.

45. Mackinnon SE. Surgical management of the peripheral nerve gap. Clin Plast Surg 1989;16:587–603.

46. Li H, Terenghi G, Hall SM. Effects of delayed reinnervation on the expression of c-erbB receptors by chronically denervated rat Schwann cells in vivo. Glia 1997;20:333–47.

47. Roytta M, Salonen V. Long-term endoneurial changes after nerve transection. Acta Neuropathol 1988;76:35–45.

48. You S, Petrov T, Chung PH, et al. The expression of the low affinity nerve growth factor receptor in long-term denervated Schwann cells. Glia 1997; 20:87–100.

49. Weinberg HJ, Spencer PS. The fate of Schwann cells isolated from axonal contact. J Neurocytol 1978;7:555–69.

50. Sulaiman OA, Gordon T. Role of chronic Schwann cell denervation in poor functional recovery after nerve injuries and experimental strategies to combat it. Neurosurgery 2009;65:A105–14.

51. Fu SY, Gordon T. Contributing factors to poor functional recovery after delayed nerve repair: prolonged denervation. J Neurosci 1995;15:3886–95.

52. Fu SY, Gordon T. Contributing factors to poor functional recovery after delayed nerve repair: prolonged axotomy. J Neurosci 1995;15:3876–85.

53. Finkelstein DI, Dooley PC, Luff AR. Recovery of muscle after different periods of denervation and treatments. Muscle Nerve 1993;16:769–77.

54. Kobayashi J, Mackinnon SE, Watanabe O, et al. The effect of duration of muscle denervation on functional recovery in the rat model. Muscle Nerve 1997;20:858–66.

55. Horch K. Central responses of cutaneous sensory neurons to peripheral nerve crush in the cat. Brain Res 1978;151:581–6.

56. Kristensson K. Retrograde signalling of nerve cell body response to trauma. In: Gorio A, Millesi H, Mingrino S, editors. Posttraumatic peripheral nerve regeneration. New York: Raven Press; 1981. p. 115–28.

57. Ducker TB, Kempe LG, Hayes GJ. The metabolic background for peripheral nerve surgery. J Neurosurg 1969;30:270–80.

58. Lieberman AR. The axon reaction: a review of the principal features of perikaryal responses to axon injury. Int Rev Neurobiol 1971;14:49–124.

59. Grafstein B, McQuarrie IG. Role of the nerve cell body in axonal regeneration. In: Cotman CW,

editor. Neuronal plasticity. New York: Raven Press; 1978. p. 155–95.

60. Sunderland SS. Nerve and nerve injuries. 2nd edition. Edinburgh (United Kingdom): Churchill Livingstone; 1978.

61. Gold BG, Katoh K, Storm-Dickerson T. The immunosuppressant FK506 increases the rate of axonal regeneration in rat sciatic nerve. J Neurosci 1995; 15(11):7509–16.

62. Lee M, Doolabh VB, Mackinnon SE, et al. FK506 promotes functional recovery in crushed rat sciatic nerve. Muscle Nerve 2000;23:633–40.

63. Udina E, Ceballos D, Gold BG, et al. FK506 enhances reinnervation by regeneration and by collateral sprouting of peripheral nerve fibers. Exp Neurol 2003;183:220–31.

64. Jost SC, Doolabh VB, Mackinnon SE, et al. Acceleration of peripheral nerve regeneration following FK506 administration. Restor Neurol Neurosci 2000;17:39–44.

65. Sulaiman OA, Voda J, Gold BG, et al. FK506 increases peripheral nerve regeneration after chronic axotomy but not after chronic Schwann cell denervation. Exp Neurol 2002;175:127–37.

66. Doolabh VB, Mackinnon SE. FK506 accelerates functional recovery following nerve grafting in a rat model. Plast Reconstr Surg 1999;103:1928–36.

67. Feng FY, Ogden MA, Myckatyn TM, et al. FK506 rescues peripheral nerve allografts in acute rejection. J Neurotrauma 2001;18:217–29.

68. Gold BG, Zeleny-Pooley M, Wang MS, et al. A nonimmunosuppressant FKBP-12 ligand increases nerve regeneration. Exp Neurol 1997;147:269–78.

69. Klettner A, Baumgrass R, Zhang Y, et al. The neuroprotective actions of FK506 binding protein ligands: neuronal survival is triggered by de novo RNA synthesis, but is independent of inhibition of JNK and calcineurin. Brain Res Mol Brain Res 2001;97:21–31.

70. Tanaka K, Fujita N, Higashi Y, et al. Neuroprotective and antioxidant properties of FKBP-binding immunophilin ligands are independent on the FKBP12 pathway in human cells. Neurosci Lett 2002;330:147–50.

71. Gold BG, Villafranca JE. Neuroimmunophilin ligands: the development of novel neuroregenerative/ neuroprotective compounds. Curr Top Med Chem 2003;3:1368–75.

72. Gold BG, Zhong YP. FK506 requires stimulation of the extracellular signal-regulated kinase 1/2 and the steroid receptor chaperone protein p23 for neurite elongation. Neurosignals 2004;13:122–9.

73. Gold BG, Yew JY, Zeleny-Pooley M. The immunosuppressant FK506 increases GAP-43 mRNA levels in axotomized sensory neurons. Neurosci Lett 1998;241:25–8.

74. Dawson TM, Steiner JP, Dawson VL, et al. Immunosuppressant FK506 enhances phosphorylation of nitric oxide synthase and protects against glutamate neurotoxicity. Proc Natl Acad Sci U S A 1993;90:9808–12.

75. Yardin C, Terro F, Lesort M, et al. FK506 antagonizes apoptosis and c-jun protein expression in neuronal cultures. Neuroreport 1998;9:2077–80.

76. Gold BG, Gordon HS, Wang MS. Efficacy of delayed or discontinuous FK506 administrations on nerve regeneration in the rat sciatic nerve crush model: lack of evidence for a conditioning lesion-like effect. Neurosci Lett 1999;267:33–6.

77. Sobol JB, Lowe IJ, Yang RK, et al. Effects of delaying FK506 administration on neuroregeneration in a rodent model. J Reconstr Microsurg 2003;19: 113–8.

78. Snyder AK, Fox IK, Nichols CM, et al. Neuroregenerative effects of preinjury FK-506 administration. Plast Reconstr Surg 2006;118:360–7.

79. Fox IK, Mackinnon SE. Experience with nerve allograft transplantation. Semin Plast Surg 2007;21: 242–9.

80. Brenner MJ, Mackinnon SE, Rickman SR, et al. FK506 and anti-CD40 ligand in peripheral nerve allotransplantation. Restor Neurol Neurosci 2005; 23:237–49.

81. Chunasuwankul R, Ayrout C, Dereli Z, et al. Low dose discontinued FK506 treatment enhances peripheral nerve regeneration. Int Surg 2002;87: 274–8.

82. Ellis RA, Brenner MJ, Mackinnon SE, et al. Use of mixed lymphocyte reaction to identify subimmunosuppressive FK-506 levels in mice. Microsurgery 2003;23:276–82.

83. Udina E, Voda J, Gold BG, et al. Comparative dose-dependence study of FK506 on transected mouse sciatic nerve repaired by allograft or xenograft. J Peripher Nerv Syst 2003;8:145–54.

84. Yang RK, Lowe JB 3rd, Sobol JB, et al. Dose-dependent effects of FK506 on neuroregeneration in a rat model. Plast Reconstr Surg 2003;112: 1832–40.

85. Udina E, Ceballos D, Verdu E, et al. Bimodal dose-dependence of FK506 on the rate of axonal regeneration in mouse peripheral nerve. Muscle Nerve 2002;26:348–55.

86. Hayashi A, Moradzadeh A, Tong A, et al. Treatment modality affects allograft-derived Schwann cell phenotype and myelinating capacity. Exp Neurol 2008;212:324–36.

87. Sulaiman OA, Gordon T. Effects of short- and long-term Schwann cell denervation on peripheral nerve regeneration, myelination, and size. Glia 2000;32: 234–46.

88. Assoian RK, Fleurdelys BE, Stevenson HC, et al. Expression and secretion of type beta transforming growth factor by activated human macrophages. Proc Natl Acad Sci U S A 1987;84:6020–4.

89. Ridley AJ, Davis JB, Stroobant P, et al. Transforming growth factors-beta 1 and beta 2 are mitogens for rat Schwann cells. J Cell Biol 1989;109:3419–24.

90. Chandross KJ, Chanson M, Spray DC, et al. Transforming growth factor-beta 1 and forskolin modulate gap junctional communication and cellular phenotype of cultured Schwann cells. J Neurosci 1995;15:262–73.

91. Einheber S, Hannocks MJ, Metz CN, et al. Transforming growth factor-beta 1 regulates axon/Schwann cell interactions. J Cell Biol 1995;129:443–58.

92. Guenard V, Gwynn LA, Wood PM. Transforming growth factor-beta blocks myelination but not ensheathment of axons by Schwann cells in vitro. J Neurosci 1995;15:419–28.

93. Guenard V, Rosenbaum T, Gwynn LA, et al. Effect of transforming growth factor-beta 1 and -beta 2 on Schwann cell proliferation on neurites. Glia 1995;13:309–18.

94. Rosner BI, Hang T, Tranquillo RT. Schwann cell behavior in three-dimensional collagen gels: evidence for differential mechano-transduction and the influence of TGF-beta 1 in morphological polarization and differentiation. Exp Neurol 2005;195:81–91.

95. Krieglstein K, Henheik P, Farkas L, et al. Glial cell line-derived neurotrophic factor requires transforming growth factor-beta for exerting its full neurotrophic potential on peripheral and CNS neurons. J Neurosci 1998;18:9822–34.

96. Schober A, Hertel R, Arumae U, et al. Glial cell line-derived neurotrophic factor rescues target-deprived sympathetic spinal cord neurons but requires transforming growth factor-beta as cofactor in vivo. J Neurosci 1999;19:2008–15.

97. Sulaiman OA, Gordon T. Transforming growth factor-beta and forskolin attenuate the adverse effects of long-term Schwann cell denervation on peripheral nerve regeneration in vivo. Glia 2002; 37:206–18.

98. Morrissey TK, Kleitman N, Bunge RP. Isolation and functional characterization of Schwann cells derived from adult peripheral nerve. J Neurosci 1991;11:2433–42.

99. Haastert K, Mauritz C, Chaturvedi S, et al. Human and rat adult Schwann cell cultures: fast and efficient enrichment and highly effective non-viral transfection protocol. Nat Protoc 2007;2:99–104.

100. Keilhoff G, Stang F, Goihl A, et al. Transdifferentiated mesenchymal stem cells as alternative therapy in supporting nerve regeneration and myelination. Cell Mol Neurobiol 2006;26:1235–52.

101. Dezawa M, Takahashi I, Esaki M, et al. Sciatic nerve regeneration in rats induced by transplantation of in vitro differentiated bone-marrow stromal cells. Eur J Neurosci 2001;14:1771–6.

102. Tohill M, Mantovani C, Wiberg M, et al. Rat bone marrow mesenchymal stem cells express glial markers and stimulate nerve regeneration. Neurosci Lett 2004;362:200–3.

103. Chen CJ, Ou YC, Liao SL, et al. Transplantation of bone marrow stromal cells for peripheral nerve repair. Exp Neurol 2007;204:443–53.

104. Wakao S, Hayashi T, Kitada M, et al. Long-term observation of auto-cell transplantation in non-human primate reveals safety and efficiency of bone marrow stromal cell-derived Schwann cells in peripheral nerve regeneration. Exp Neurol 2010;223:537–47.

105. Kingham PJ, Kalbermatten DF, Mahay D, et al. Adipose-derived stem cells differentiate into a Schwann cell phenotype and promote neurite outgrowth in vitro. Exp Neurol 2007;207:267–74.

106. di Summa PG, Kingham PJ, Raffoul W, et al. Adipose-derived stem cells enhance peripheral nerve regeneration. J Plast Reconstr Aesthet Surg 2010;63:1544–52.

107. Erba P, Mantovani C, Kalbermatten DF, et al. Regeneration potential and survival of transplanted undifferentiated adipose tissue-derived stem cells in peripheral nerve conduits. J Plast Reconstr Aesthet Surg 2010;63:e811–7.

108. Fernandes KJ, McKenzie IA, Mill P, et al. A dermal niche for multipotent adult skin-derived precursor cells. Nat Cell Biol 2004;6:1082–93.

109. Toma JG, Akhavan M, Fernandes KJ, et al. Isolation of multipotent adult stem cells from the dermis of mammalian skin. Nat Cell Biol 2001;3:778–84.

110. McKenzie IA, Biernaskie J, Toma JG, et al. Skin-derived precursors generate myelinating Schwann cells for the injured and dysmyelinated nervous system. J Neurosci 2006;26:6651–60.

111. Toma JG, McKenzie IA, Bagli D, et al. Isolation and characterization of multipotent skin-derived precursors from human skin. Stem Cells 2005;23:727–37.

112. Walsh S, Biernaskie J, Kemp SW, et al. Supplementation of acellular nerve grafts with skin derived precursor cells promotes peripheral nerve regeneration. Neuroscience 2009;164:1097–107.

113. Walsh SK, Gordon T, Addas BM, et al. Skin-derived precursor cells enhance peripheral nerve regeneration following chronic denervation. Exp Neurol 2010;223:221–8.

114. Walsh S, Midha R. Practical considerations concerning the use of stem cells for peripheral nerve repair. Neurosurg Focus 2009;26:E2.

115. Brannvall K, Corell M, Forsberg-Nilsson K, et al. Environmental cues from CNS, PNS, and ENS cells regulate CNS progenitor differentiation. Neuroreport 2008;19:1283–9.

116. Jabaley ME, Wallace WH, Heckler FR. Internal topography of major nerves of the forearm and hand: a current view. J Hand Surg Am 1980;5: 1–18.

117. Brown JM, Yee A, Mackinnon SE. Distal median to ulnar nerve transfers to restore ulnar motor and sensory function within the hand: technical nuances. Neurosurgery 2009;65:966–77 [discussion: 977–68].

118. Huang G. Experimental reconstruction on intrinsic hand muscle function by anterior interosseous nerve transference. 318. Zhonghua Yi Xue Za Zhi 1992;72:269–72 [in Chinese].

119. Wang Y, Zhu S. Transfer of a branch of the anterior interosseus nerve to the motor branch of the median nerve and ulnar nerve. Chin Med J (Engl) 1997;110:216–9.

120. Vernadakis AJ, Humphreys DB, Mackinnon SE. Distal anterior interosseous nerve in the recurrent motor branch graft for reconstruction of a median nerve neuroma-in-continuity. J Reconstr Microsurg 2004;20:7–11.

121. Novak CB, Mackinnon SE. Distal anterior interosseous nerve transfer to the deep motor branch of the ulnar nerve for reconstruction of high ulnar nerve injuries. J Reconstr Microsurg 2002;18:459–64.

122. Ustun ME, Ogun TC, Buyukmumcu M, et al. Selective restoration of motor function in the ulnar nerve by transfer of the anterior interosseous nerve. An anatomical feasibility study. J Bone Joint Surg Am 2001;83:549–52.

123. Ustun ME, Ogun TC, Karabulut AK, et al. An alternative method for restoring opposition after median nerve injury: an anatomical feasibility study for the use of neurotisation. J Anat 2001;198:635–8.

124. Wang Y, Zhu S, Zhang B. Anatomical study and clinical application of transfer of pronator quadratus branch of anterior interosseous nerve in the repair of thenar branch of median nerve and deep branch of ulnar nerve. Zhongguo Xiu Fu Chong Jian Wai Ke Za Zhi 1997;11:335–7 [in Chinese].

125. Brown JM, Mackinnon SE. Nerve transfers in the forearm and hand. Hand Clin 2008;24:319–40, v.

Favoring the Risk–Benefit Balance for Upper Extremity Transplantation—The Pittsburgh Protocol

Vijay S. Gorantla, MD, PhD[a],*, Gerald Brandacher, MD[b],
Stefan Schneeberger, MD[c], Xin Xiao Zheng, MD[d],
Albert D. Donnenberg, PhD[e], Joseph E. Losee, MD[d],
W.P. Andrew Lee, MD[f]

KEYWORDS

- Upper extremity transplantation • Transplant tolerance
- The Pittsburgh Protocol

In the period between 1988 and 1996, there were a total of 134,421 upper extremity amputations reported in the United States, of which 5399 were anatomically located between the elbow and the wrist.[1] In 2005, 1.6 million people were living with the loss of a limb.[2] There is currently no national database or registry regarding devastating upper extremity injuries requiring significant reconstruction in the civilian population. It is reasonable to estimate that management of these disfiguring, disabling, and debilitating tissue injuries/losses costs the US health care system billions of dollars each year. To date, approximately 1.7 million troops have served in the 2 theaters of conflict in Iraq and Afghanistan. Data from these ongoing conflicts indicate that combat trauma to the upper extremity region constitutes 39% of injuries.[3]

Current surgical procedures after major trauma rely on conventional reconstruction with autogenous flaps/grafts or free tissue transfers. These procedures are not only limited by available tissues for reconstruction, but also despite the best efforts, functional and esthetic outcomes are limited to poor. Additionally, morbidity high from extensive surgery, and recovery/rehabilitation is long. In this regard, reconstructive transplantation (RT) of composite tissue allografts such as hand or face can achieve near-perfect restoration of tissue defects with improved functional and aesthetic outcomes and avoidance of multiple, expensive surgeries.[4]

[a] Pittsburgh Reconstructive Transplantation Program, Division of Plastic Surgery, Department of Surgery, 3550 Terrace Street, Pittsburgh, PA 15261, USA
[b] Department of Plastic and Reconstructive Surgery, Johns Hopkins University School of Medicine, Ross Research Building 749D, 720 Rutland Avenue, Baltimore, MD 21205, USA
[c] Department of Plastic and Reconstructive Surgery, Johns Hopkins University School of Medicine, Baltimore, MD 21287, USA
[d] Division of Plastic Surgery, Department of Surgery, University of Pittsburgh School of Medicine, Pittsburgh, PA, USA
[e] Pittsburgh Cancer Institute, University of Pittsburgh Medical Center, 5115 Centre Avenue, Pittsburgh, PA 15232-1301, USA
[f] Department of Plastic and Reconstructive Surgery, Johns Hopkins University School of Medicine, 601 North Caroline Street, Baltimore, MD 21287, USA
* Corresponding author.
E-mail address: gorantlavs@upmc.edu

Hand Clin 27 (2011) 511–520
doi:10.1016/j.hcl.2011.08.008

UPPER EXTREMITY ALLOTRANSPLANTATION: BENEFIT VERSUS RISK

During the past decade, upper extremity and face transplantation has become a clinical reality. In case of the human upper extremity, RT represents a superior alternative to restore the appearance, anatomy, and function in amputees who do not benefit from or decide not to choose prostheses.

In the past decade, more than 70 upper extremity transplants have been performed around the world, confirming that this procedure is not only feasible but represents a valuable option to reconstruct limb loss secondary to devastating injuries (www.handregistry.com). Overall functional outcomes have been good, with results superior to prostheses. Graft survival, immunologic, and quality of life outcomes have also been highly encouraging.[5] Yet, if the aggregate of transplants performed were considered, it would be reasonable to argue that the numbers performed per year remain low around the world. However, wider application is restricted by the risks of prolonged (life-long), high-dose, multidrug (a combination of 2 to 3 agents) immunosuppression necessary to prevent graft rejection. Initial treatment with an antibody targeting recipient immune cells followed by triple-drug maintenance therapy represents the current standard in hand transplantation. Such a regimen has occasionally been supplemented with additional boosts in drug dosage to treat rejection episodes, and has successfully prevented loss of allografts.[6]

Triple-drug regimens (including a combination of drugs like tacrolimus, mycophenolic acid mofetil, rapamycin, or steroids) used in hand transplantation have resulted in diabetes mellitus, nephrotoxicity, bilateral hip osteonecrosis, leucopenia, hypertension, and hyperlipidemia. Opportunistic infections have been observed that include *Staphylococcus aureus* osteitis, mycoses, herpes simplex, molluscum contagiosum, and cytomegalovirus (CMV). CMV infection is serious, can trigger acute rejection, and could be life-threatening. In summary, when the collective risk of complications like infection, fracture, neoplasia, drug toxicity, and metabolic derangement is considered, lifelong immunosuppression can be thought of as a chronic disease characterized by its own set of risks.[7] Taken together, although no serious life-threatening complications have been noted, the morbidity of immunosuppression after upper extremity transplantation threatens to affect the quality-of-life outcomes, alter the risk profile, and jeopardize the benefits of such procedures.[8] Maintaining graft survival while reducing drug adverse effects and improving or optimizing functional outcomes stands to significantly impact the benefit–risk equation of the procedure, enabling its widespread application as a reconstructive option.

MINIMIZING AND WEANING IMMUNOSUPPRESSION: PREMISE AND IMPLICATIONS

Immunosuppressive drugs like calcineurin inhibitors such as tacrolimus have improved short-term outcomes, but failed to improve long-term outcomes after solid organ transplants.[9] In addition to their adverse effects as discussed previously, immunosuppressive agents can also contribute to late allograft loss.[10] Thus, several trials have attempted immunosuppression minimization months after the transplant when there is a lower risk of rejection or completely weaned patients off drugs, but have had variable success at improving long-term outcomes.[11–17] One of the few studies with favorable outcomes was that by Starzl and colleagues[18] from the University of Pittsburgh. Eighty-two patients undergoing kidney, liver, pancreas, or small bowel transplantation were treated with rabbit antithymocyte globulin (5 mg/kg) followed by carefully adjusted frequency and dosing of tacrolimus monotherapy as post-transplant maintenance therapy (except in case of breakthrough rejection when additional drugs were used). Patients were considered for dose spacing to alternate day or longer after 4 months. Immunosuppression-related morbidity was minimal, with graft survival at 88% close to 2 years. Sixty percent of recipients could be maintained on spaced doses of tacrolimus monotherapy. The Starzl group also reported for the first time immunosuppressive withdrawal in 23 patients with liver transplants. Initially, some patients had incidental withdrawal due to noncompliance, life-threatening infectious complications requiring termination of immunosuppression, or were weaned by their physician.[19] Later, the group weaned in a controlled manner recipients with stable function and no evidence of rejection at least 5 years after transplantation. Of 59 patients who commenced weaning, 16 (27%) were withdrawn from immunosuppression.[20] Subsequently, several groups have reported successful weaning of immunosuppression,[21–26] with approximately 22% of over 350 patients being weaned. However, these were selected patients who had good graft outcome before weaning and represent something less than 10% of the total number of all liver transplant patients.[27] In other studies, steroid weaning protocols have been associated with increased acute rejection.[28–30] While it is still unclear if drug-weaning regimens can improve long-term outcomes, there is surely a concern that such manipulation may adversely affect the immunologic balance between the host and donor graft (**Fig. 1**). Thus, there is a need for a new paradigm for long-term maintenance of allografts.

OPERATIONAL TOLERANCE: PROMISE AND PROGRESS

Operational tolerance is defined as prolonged survival of a transplanted organ in the absence of immunosuppression, without signs of a destructive response while retaining normal reactivity to infections and tumors. Lifelong operational tolerance is difficult to achieve, especially without risk of chronic rejection. Also, complete absence of immunosuppression poses some risk of graft damage or loss as a result of low-grade chronic processes, especially as these cannot be effectively monitored at present. The seminal observations of Billingham, Brent and Medawar[31] in 1953, that H-2 disparate donor bone marrow-derived cells could bring about lifelong specific acquired immunologic tolerance to skin allografts in fetal or newborn murine recipients laid the foundation for the goal of establishing donor-specific tolerance in organ transplantation. It was not until over 20 years later that it was first observed that multiple nonspecific and subsequently donor-specific blood transfusions often led to improved acceptance of human kidney transplants.[32,33] It was then also demonstrated that peritransplant infusion of donor bone marrow (DBM) cells together with total lymphoid irradiation (TLI) or antilymphocyte/thymocyte serum (ie, T cell depletion) prolonged and sometimes brought about indefinite allograft survival in adult murine, canine, and primate recipients in the absence of chronic immunosuppression.[34–37] The development of DBM protocols used for infusion/augmentation is interesting and is integral to understanding approaches to immunomodulation and immunosuppression minimization, development of chimerism, and induction of operational tolerance.[38]

DONOR BONE MARROW INFUSION/ AUGMENTATION IN SOLID ORGAN TRANSPLANTATION: EVOLUTION AND EARLY INSIGHTS

The early developments that served as the foundations of modern tissue transplantation are credited to the US Navy Tissue Bank, which was established in 1949 by George Hyatt, an orthopedic surgeon at the Naval Medical Center in Bethesda, Maryland. The US Navy Tissue Bank pioneered standards and criteria for tissue donation as well as procurement and processing, documentation, and clinical evaluation of a variety of tissues including DBM. Indeed, it was the US Navy Tissue Bank that was the vanguard in the establishment of the National Marrow Donor Program and the American Association of Tissue Banks in the United States. Five decades of research in their laboratories were key to establishment of methods such as cryopreservation, freeze drying, and sterilization of tissues, but also advanced the field of organ preservation and cadaveric DBM recovery, isolation, storage, and transplantation.[39]

In the 1980s, Sharp and colleagues[40] demonstrated that DBM procured from freshly resected donor vertebral bodies (VBs) provided the best source of bone marrow, with average yields double that from entire ilia. A study of 46 surgical specimens and 9 cadaveric tissue donors confirmed that such DBM is less heavily contaminated with peripheral blood lymphocytes, a known source of mature T cells when compared with bone marrow (BM) obtained by iliac crest aspiration. Mugushima and colleagues[41] determined in 17 cadaver donors the T cell load of iliac crest BM. They showed that DBM processed from iliac crests removed en bloc contained lower T cell loads than that procured via aspiration in living donors.

Although Monaco was the first to test the effects of iliac crest DBM in cadaver kidney transplants,[42] the 1990s witnessed a remarkable progress in the understanding, applications, and immunomodulatory implications of DBM

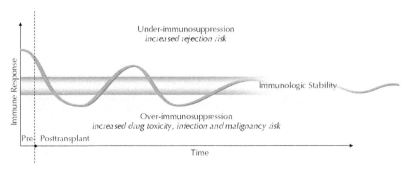

Fig. 1. The importance of optimal immunosuppression and immunologic stability.

infusion/augmentation in clinical organ transplantation. In 1991, Barber and colleagues[43] published the results of a controlled prospective study of cryopreserved DBM infusion in 57 patients receiving cadaveric kidney transplants under Minnesota antilymphocyte globulin (ALG) induction (10–14 days) and cyclosporine, azathioprine, and prednisone maintenance. Fifty-four patients served as controls without DBM but were transplanted under the same immunosuppressive regimen. In the DBM group, the infusion was given on day 7 after the last dose of ALG. The study found that the numbers of rejection episodes were similar across both groups, but DBM improved overall allograft survival (90% at 1 year compared with 71% in controls) with diminished donor-specific responsiveness on mixed lymphocyte cultures. They concluded that there was a need for a more effective induction protocol to reduce overall number of rejection episodes.

Around the same time, the Bone Marrow Transplant Program at the Pittsburgh Cancer Institute was reviving the application of VB-derived DBM in organ transplantation. Rybka and colleagues[44] quantified hematopoietic progenitor cell (HPC) content of DBM obtained from donor VB as well as iliac crests and found that it was similar. Notably, the numbers of viable nucleated cells were significantly greater in the VB group compared with the iliac crest group despite testing at 12 to 72 hours after procurement. This was one of the earliest studies to establish VB-derived DBM for infusion/augmentation after solid organ transplantation. Between 1992 and 1995, the Pittsburgh group lead by Starzl and colleagues investigated a combined solid organ (liver or kidney or kidney plus pancreas or kidney plus islets or heart or lung) with or without DBM augmentation. One hundred thirty-eight study patients were compared with 57 controls. Whole DBM from VB was infused intravenous at a dose of 3 to 5×10^8 cells/kg after transplantation followed by a regimen of tacrolimus and prednisone in both groups. No other induction was given. Overall, there were no significant differences between the groups in graft survival or rejection, and no graft versus host disease (GVHD) was noted in the DBM group despite the large doses of unfractionated cell infusion. The DBM infusion was associated with donor cell chimerism in all organ patients, with twofold increase in donor-specific hyporesponsiveness (DSH) seen in liver and lung recipients. All DBM-augmented recipients who also had DSH had improved long-term outcomes. This was one of the early studies to demonstrate the safety and potential positive immunomodulatory effects of DBM in solid organ transplantation.[45,46]

The Miami group reported (between 1994 and 2000) 350 deceased donor liver (or liver/intestinal), 111 kidney, 25 kidney/pancreas, and 5 kidney/islet transplant recipients that were given VB DBM,[47–53] as well as 47 living-related donor (LRD) haploidentical kidney recipients infused with iliac crest DBM.[49,52,54,55] In deceased donor kidney transplant recipients, higher graft survival was observed compared with (nonrandomized) noninfused controls.[51,56–59] These and other studies highlighted the immunomodulatory effects of DBM cells, which included strong down-regulation of antidonor immune responses.[55,60–66]

DONOR BONE MARROW AUGMENTATION IN SOLID ORGAN TRANSPLANTATION: INDUCTION OF CHIMERISM AND OPERATIONAL TOLERANCE

Medawar established the concept of chimerism[67] based on the observations of Owen[68] in Freemartin calf dizygotic twins, describing a mixture of blood cells due to cross-circulation in the common placenta in utero. Such fetal chimerism is associated with lifelong unresponsiveness to donor alloantigens. Ildstad and Sachs described the phenomenon of mixed allogeneic chimerism, which was induced by inoculation of both syngeneic and allogeneic bone marrow into sublethally irradiated adult hosts, and associated with long-term donor-specific tolerance.[69,70] Terminology such as macrochimerism, microchimerism, and finally nanochimerism, has been suggested to refer to various tolerance or immunomodulatory states. Macrochimerism connotes high level (>1% of donor derived cells, detectable by flow cytometry) while microchimerism indicates (<1% of donor derived cells, detectable only by molecular assays such as short tandem repeats or polymerase chain reaction [PCR]) in the recipient. Nanochimerism is a term used to refer to donor cells that are virtually undetectable but hypothetically present. Over the past 20 years there has been controversy with regard to the role, durability, extent, and threshold of chimerism needed, especially in the clinical situation to achieve drug-free organ transplant acceptance.[71] Some groups have used the terms central versus peripheral tolerance to describe the relevance of the thymus in tolerance induction. Macrochimerism resulting from central (deletional/thymic/Medawarian) mechanisms is purported to ensure a more robust and reliable tolerance state. This is when ongoing production of both donor and recipient dendritic cells and other antigen presenting cells by BM stem cells results in the continuous deletion of newly produced alloreactive T and B cells.

There is strong support for specific and nonspecific immunoregulatory effects of various subsets of cells in DBM infusions. Preclinical studies in animal models including dogs and primates have demonstrated the induction of chimerism and operational tolerance to organ transplants.[34,36,37,72] Similar findings have been reported in patients receiving combined kidney and DBM transplantation.[73–75] Starzl and colleagues[76,77] reported in separate studies microchimerism of DBM-derived cells observed in several transplant recipients who had stopped immunosuppression for several years with functioning grafts. The vascularized BM environments of the body have been shown to support engraftment of donor stem cells in kidney transplant recipients receiving DBM. These patients have shown no GVHD[48–50] and have low risk of chronic rejection.[51] These findings could be manifestations of a functional immune equilibrium that could have been possible due to induction of anergy,[78,79] by incomplete antigen presentation in the absence of costimulatory molecules,[80] by tolerogenic allopeptides,[81] or even by microchimerism in the vascular bone marrow microenvironments of the iliac crest or elsewhere transferring infectious tolerance by development of (autologous) suppressor T cells in the recipient.[82] There are also arguments against this dynamic peripheral immune regulation, which is supposedly less reliable and can be broken by infection or inflammation. Although DBM has been shown to result in operational tolerance, enabling tapering or withdrawal of immunosuppression in transplant recipients, it is argued to be a metastable state that is susceptible to immune danger signals (eg, incidental bacterial or viral infections).[83] Acute and chronic rejections have been reported in operationally tolerant organ recipients who maintained stable graft function over extended periods of time.[84]

NONMYELOABLATIVE DEPLETIONAL INDUCTION: PROSPECTS FOR PROPE TOLERANCE

The use of lymphodepleting induction therapy to eliminate early detrimental immune signals and promote clonal deletion of effector cells has been extensively studied and was pioneered by Roy Calne.[85] Studies have demonstrated the possible regulatory effects of antithymocyte globulin and the anti-CD52 antibody alemtuzumab in deleting alloreactive effector cells while preserving regulatory cells and their components.[86] Limited but emerging data suggest that such induction approaches may favor or enable immunosuppressive minimization.[18,25] Alternatively, these approaches may not be conducive to immuosuppressive withdrawal. For example, ATG induction with early tacrolimus withdrawal in liver recipients resulted in high rates of rejection and prevented minimization.[87] This may be due to the presence of memory effector cells that are more resistant to lymphodepletional therapy.[88] Although tolerance would be the ideal goal, the heterogeneity of donor recipient combinations, immune status, underlying disease, and unpredictable consequences of infection might make stable tolerance extremely difficult to achieve for all patients. This is where low-dose maintenance monotherapy may be a realized in patients undergoing short-course depletional induction, ensuring that no patient is put at risk of rejection should graft acceptance be broken by intercurrent infection or other danger triggers. This is the fundamental concept of prope tolerance.

NOVEL IMMUNOMODULATORY THERAPIES: THE BIDIRECTIONAL PARADIGM

The pioneering studies of Medawar and Owen showed the association with donor leucocyte chimerism with acquired tolerance.[31,67,68] However, early attempts at inducing chimerism with donor leucocyte infusions even after ablation of recipients uniformly failed ending with either lethal GVHD or rejection. Experimentally, macrochimerism was successful in inducing tolerance without GVHD under select protocols of recipient conditioning. When donor cells fell to microchimeric levels (<1%), these protocols failed. However, the role of macrochimerism as a requirement for organ engraftment was challenged when organ transplantation was successfully performed with conventional immunosuppression. No leucocyte infusions were used in these unconditioned patients. There was evidence of neither chimerism nor GVHD. Starzl and colleagues[76] discovered in 1991 that long-surviving organ recipients had evidence of multilineage donor chimerism. It was postulated that this was possible because the cells from the organ (passenger leucocytes) migrated and survived in the host (similar to a leucocyte or DBM infusion). However, these cells were present at levels less than 1% (microchimerism). This gave credence to the hypothesis that sustained donor microchimerism was responsible for promoting graft survival in these patients and thereby led to the bidirectional paradigm.[89–91]

The mechanistic basis of such a bidirectional paradigm is described in **Fig. 2**.

High dose immunosuppression of the recipient (as conventionally used) is deleterious, because it blunts T-cell surveillance of neoplasms and infections. Importantly, heavy post-transplant

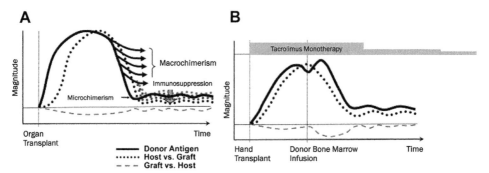

Fig. 2. The bidirectional paradigm-the mechanistic dogma of the pittsburgh protocol. (*A*) Two immunologic responses occur following organ or tissue transplantation: the host-versus-graft (HVG) response driven by host effector (cytotoxic) T cells and a graft-versus-host (GVH) response caused by passenger leucocytes, which are delivered together with the graft.[93] If these 2 activities are not reciprocal and balanced, 1 cell population will predominate over the other, resulting in either rejection or graft-versus-host disease (GVHD). The reciprocal GVH response is shown in the hashed line. Following organ transplantation, the donor antigen (*bold black line*) increases in the host lymphoid system as the passenger leucocytes migrate to immune sites. This is what triggers the HVG (rejection response, as shown in the dotted line). If the donor cells retain dominance over the recipent T lymphocytes, the latter response may be exhausted and deleted.[94] If the donor cells persist in large numbers, this macrochimerism can maintain such exhaustion/deletion and prevent rejection of the graft. Such effects can happen even when the donor cells are in lower numbers (microchimerism), when low degrees of host immunosuppression can help this process.[95] (*B*) Although the balance between mobile donor antigen (microchimerism) and antigen-reactive T cells is important, maintenance immunosuppression in small amounts can help sustain the stable HVG and GVH equilibrium in spite of in vitro evidence of ongoing antidonor reactivity. Such a stable equilibrium could be achieved faster if a second donor antigenic stimulus (boost) is provided to the recipient to augment the clonal exhaustion and deletion response. This is facilitated by a donor bone marrow infusion around 2 weeks after the surgery to follow the peaking of the mobile donor load derived from the graft. (*Modified from* Marcos A, Lakkis F, Starzl TE. Tolerance for organ recipients: a clash of paradigms. Liver Transpl 2006;12(10):1449; with permission.)

immunosuppression reduces the window for early clonal exhaustion–deletion that coincides with the burst of donor antigen after transplant. Attempts to minimize drug therapy in such patients are not successful, because the persistent cell clones recover and lead to late rejection. Thus, based on the previously mentioned bidirectional dogma, Starzl and colleagues developed the Pittsburgh Protocol, which relies on recipient pretreatment (by nonmyeloablative depletional conditioning) followed by minimal post-transplant immunosuppression. These principles have been applied since 2001 in solid organ and hand transplantation recipients at Pittsburgh.

Fig. 2B shows the application of the Pittsburgh Protocol in hand transplantation.

RECONSTRUCTIVE TRANSPLANTATION: IMMUNOMODULATION VERSUS IMMUNOSUPPRESSION

The overarching goal of the application of the Pittsburgh Protocol in hand transplantation was to enhance the risk to benefit ratio by minimizing the number, dose, and duration of drugs used, and in turn improve the safety, efficacy, and applicability of this reconstructive modality.

When the Pittsburgh Protocol was used by Starzl and colleagues in living-related organ transplants, BM was obtained from the iliac crests of donors who were pretreated in vivo with stimulating factors to increase the yield of cells (**Fig. 3**). To use the Pittsburgh Protocol in hand transplantation wherein only deceased donors are available, the authors first manipulated the logistics of the cadaveric donor situation (**Fig. 4**). Notably, this involved obtaining BM from VBs of cadaver donors and calibrating/standardizing/validating it for use in hand transplant recipients.[92] All patients are leukapheresed before transplantation to cryopreserve T cells for later transfusion in even of an inadvertent GVH response.

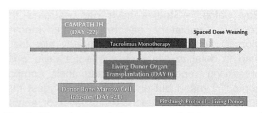

Fig. 3. The pittsburgh immunomodulatory protocol for living related organ transplantation.

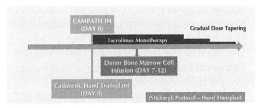

Fig. 4. The pittsburgh immunomodulatory protocol for upper extremity reconstructive transplantation.

Application of the Pittsburgh Protocol is facilitated in hand transplantation due to several reasons:

It is possible to continuously monitor the skin component of a hand allograft for early clinical signs of acute rejection. Early diagnosis of rejection allows timely intervention with drug therapy titrated to the minimum levels necessary to treat rejection.

The skin offers the possibility of transdermal (topical) drug application as an alternative or adjunct to systemic treatment.

Biopsies can easily be taken per protocol as well as upon clinical suspicion. Thus the sensitivity of directed biopsies in detecting rejection is optimized with minimal or no morbidity. Immunosuppressive treatment can be continuously fine-tuned in real-time to the clinical situation without the risk of missing rejection. Subtle dosing adjustments can be made without altering systemic levels significantly, thus keeping toxicity low.

In the past 2 years, the authors have implemented this novel immunomodulatory protocol in 8 hand/forearm transplants performed in 5 patients at the University of Pittsburgh. Initial and emerging data suggest that the protocol is safe, efficacious, and well tolerated. It has allowed graft survival under low-dose monotherapy with infrequent immunologic sequelae and easily reversed, minimal complications. All patients are progressing in motor and sensory recovery with intensive occupational therapy. Some patients have returned to employable or vocational status. The authors' experience is the world's first successful implementation of an immunomodulatory therapy in clinical reconstructive transplantation.

In summary, the Pittsburgh Protocol could primarily enable reduction of the number and dose of drugs needed to sustain a highly immunogenic allograft like a hand by enabling

The transition from conventionally used triple or double therapy of maintenance immunosuppression to low-dose mono-therapy (a significant first step in risk reduction)

Manipulation of host alloresponses through cell-based immunomodulation (deletional induction followed by DBM infusion), allowing tapering or minimization of drug therapy (a necessary goal for widespread application of hand transplantation)

SUMMARY

Upper extremity transplantation is an innovative reconstructive strategy with potential of immediate clinical application and the most near-term pay-off for select amputees, allowing reintegration into employment and society. In this context, reducing the need and risk of immunosuppressive drugs needed for graft survival is a key and immediate goal.

Routine applicability and widespread impact of such strategies for the upper extremity amputees with devastating limb loss could be enabled by implementation of cellular therapies that integrate and unify the concepts of transplant tolerance induction with those of RT. Such therapies when combined with novel high-efficacy immunosuppression regimens devoid of toxicities offer the promise of dramatic improvement in long-term survival. The clinical impact of such immunomodulatory approaches in optimizing outcomes of these reconstructive modalities cannot be underestimated.

REFERENCES

1. Ziegler-Graham K, MacKenzie EJ, Ephraim PL, et al. Estimating the prevalence of limb loss in the United States: 2005 to 2050. Arch Phys Med Rehabil 2008; 89(3):422–9.

2. Dillingham TR, Pezzin LE, MacKenzie EJ. Limb amputation and limb deficiency: epidemiology and recent trends in the United States. South Med J 2002;95(8):875–83.

3. Dougherty AL, Mohrle CR, Galarneau MR, et al. Battlefield extremity injuries in Operation Iraqi Freedom. Injury 2009;40(7):772–7.

4. Shores JT, Brandacher G, Schneeberger S, et al. Composite tissue allotransplantation: hand transplantation and beyond. J Am Acad Orthop Surg 2010;18(3):127–31.

5. Petruzzo P, Lanzetta M, Dubernard JM, et al. The International Registry on Hand and Composite Tissue Transplantation. Transplantation 2010;90 (12):1590–4.

6. Gorantla VS, Barker JH, Jones JW Jr, et al. Immunosuppressive agents in transplantation: mechanisms

of action and current antirejection strategies. Micro-surgery 2000;20(8):420–9.

7. Baumeister S, Kleist C, Döhler B, et al. Risks of allo-geneic hand transplantation. Microsurgery 2004; 24(2):98–103.

8. Jones NF. Concerns about human hand transplanta-tion in the 21st century. J Hand Surg Am 2002;27(5): 771–87.

9. Opelz G, Dohler B. Influence of immunosuppressive regimens on graft survival and secondary outcomes after kidney transplantation. Transplantation 2009; 87:795.

10. Nankivell BJ, Borrows RJ, Fung CL, et al. The natural history of chronic allograft nephropathy. N Engl J Med 2003;349:2326.

11. Abramowicz D, Del Carmen Rial M, Vitko S, et al. Cyclosporine withdrawal from a mycophenolate mofetil-containing immunosuppressive regimen: results of a five-year, prospective, randomized study. J Am Soc Nephrol 2005;16:2234.

12. Dudley C, Pohanka E, Riad H, et al. Mycophenolate mofetil substitution for cyclosporine a in renal trans-plant recipients with chronic progressive allograft dysfunction: The creeping creatinine study. Trans-plantation 2005;79:466.

13. Ekberg H, Tedesco-Silva H, Demirbas A, et al. Reduced exposure to calcineurin inhibitors in renal transplantation. N Engl J Med 2007;357:2562.

14. Schena FP, Pascoe MD, Alberu J, et al. Conversion from calcineurin inhibitors to sirolimus maintenance therapy in renal allograft recipients: 24-month effi-cacy and safety results from the CONVERT trial. Transplantation 2009;87:233.

15. Vincenti F, Ramos E, Brattstrom C, et al. Multicenter trial exploring calcineurin inhibitors avoidance in renal transplantation. Transplantation 2001;71: 1282.

16. Flechner SM, Goldfarb D, Modlin C, et al. Kidney transplantation without calcineurin inhibitor drugs: a prospective, randomized trial of sirolimus versus cyclosporine. Transplantation 2002;74:1070.

17. Larson TS, Dean PG, Stegall MD, et al. Complete avoidance of calcineurin inhibitors in renal trans-plantation: a randomized trial comparing sirolimus and tacrolimus. Am J Transplant 2006;6:514.

18. Starzl TE, Murase N, Abu-Elmagd K, et al. Tolero-genic immunosuppression for organ transplantation. Lancet 2003;361(9368):1502–10.

19. Reyes J, Zeevi A, Ramos H, et al. Frequent achieve-ment of a drug-free state after orthotopic liver-trans-plantation. Transplant Proc 1993;25:3315.

20. Ramos HC, Reyes J, Abuelmagd K, et al. Weaning of immunosuppression in long-term liver transplant recipients. Transplantation 1995;59:212.

21. Mazariegos GV, Reyes J, Marino IR, et al. Weaning of immunosuppression in liver transplant recipients. Transplantation 1997;63:243.

22. Devlin J, Doherty DG, Thomson LJ, et al. Defining the outcome of immunosuppression withdrawal after liver transplantation. Hepatology 1998;27:926.

23. Takatsuki M, Uemoto S, Inomata Y, et al. Weaning of immunosuppression in living donor liver transplant recipients. Transplantation 2001;72:449.

24. Tryphonopoulos P, Tzakis AG, Weppler D, et al. The role of donor bone marrow infusions in withdrawal of immunosuppression in adult liver allotransplantation. Am J Transplant 2005;5:608.

25. Eason JD, Cohen AJ, Nair S, et al. Tolerance: Is it worth the risk? Transplantation 2005;79:1157–9.

26. Tisone G, Orlando G, Cardillo A, et al. Complete weaning off immunosuppression in HCV liver trans-plant recipients is feasible and favourably impacts on the progression of disease recurrence. J Hepatol 2006;44:702.

27. McCaughan GW. Withdrawal of immunosuppression in liver transplant recipients: Is this as good as it gets? Liver Transpl 2002;8:408.

28. Schold JD, Santos A, Rehman S, et al. The success of continued steroid avoidance after kidney transplantation in the US. Am J Transplant 2009;9:2768.

29. Woodle ES, First MR, Pirsch J, et al. A prospective, randomized, double-blind, placebo-controlled multi-center trial comparing early (7 day) corticosteroid cessation versus long-term, low-dose corticosteroid therapy. Ann Surg 2008;248:564.

30. Knight SR, Morris PJ. Steroid avoidance or with-drawal after renal transplantation increases the risk of acute rejection but decreases cardiovascular risk. A meta-analysis. Transplantation 2010;89:1.

31. Billingham RE, Brent L, Medawar PB. Actively acquired tolerance of foreign cells. Nature 1953; 172:603–6.

32. Opelz G, Terasaki PI. Improvement of kidney graft survival with increased numbers of blood transfu-sions. N Engl J Med 1978;299:799–803.

33. Salvatierra O Jr, Vincenti F, Amend W, et al. Delib-erate donor-specific blood transfusions prior to living-related renal transplantation. Ann Surg 1980; 192:543–52.

34. Slavin S, Fuks Z, Strober S, et al. Transplantation tolerance across major histocompatibility barriers after total lymphoid irradiation. Transplantation 1979;28:359–61.

35. Monaco AP, Wood ML. Studies on heterologous anti-lymphocyte serum in mice: VII. Optimal cellular antigen for induction of immunologic tolerance with ALS. Transplant Proc 1970;2:489–96.

36. Caridis DT, Liegeois A, Barrett I, et al. Enhanced survival of canine renal allografts of ALS-treated dogs given bone marrow. Transplant Proc 1973;5: 671–4.

37. Thomas JM, Carver FM, Foil MB. Renal allograft tolerance induced with ATG and donor bone marrow

in out-bred rhesus monkeys. Transplantation 1983; 36:104–6.

38. Wood K, Sachs DH. Chimerism and transplantation tolerance: cause and effect. Immunol Today 1996; 17:584–7.

39. Strong DM. The US Navy Tissue Bank: 50 years on the cutting edge. Cell Tissue Bank 2000;1:9–16.

40. Sharp TG, Sachs DH, Matthews JG, et al. Harvest of human bone marrow directly from bone. J Immunol Methods 1984;69(2):187–95.

41. Mugishima H, Terasaki P, Sueyoshi A. Bone marrow from cadaver donors for transplantation. Blood 1985;65(2):392–6.

42. Monaco AP, Clark AW, Wood ML, et al. Possible active enhancement of a human cadaver renal allograft with antilymphocyte serum (ALS) and donor bone marrow: case report of an initial attempt. Surgery 1976;79:384–92.

43. Barber WH, Mankin JA, Laskow DA, et al. Long-term results with transfusion of donor-specific bone marrow in 57 cadaveric renal allograft recipients. Transplantation 1991;51(1):70–5.

44. Rybka WB, Fontes PA, Rao AS, et al. Hematopoietic progenitor cell content of vertebral body marrow used for combined solid organ and bone marrow transplantation. Transplantation 1995;59(6):871–4.

45. Zeevi A, Pavlick M, Banas R, et al. Three years of follow-up of bone marrow-augmented organ transplant recipients: the impact on donor-specific immune modulation. Transplant Proc 1997;29:1205–6.

46. Shapiro R, Rao AS, Fontes P, et al. Kidney/bone marrow transplantation. Dial Transplant 1996;25(5): 282–7.

47. Ricordi C, Karatzas T, Selvaggi G, et al. Multiple bone marrow infusions to enhance acceptance of allografts from the same donor [review]. Ann N Y Acad Sci 1995;770:345–50.

48. Garcia-Morales R, Carreno M, Mathew J, et al. The effects of chimeric cells following donor bone marrow infusions as detected by PCR-flow assays in kidney transplant recipients. J Clin Invest 1997; 99:1118–29.

49. Garcia-Morales R, Carreno M, Mathew J, et al. Continuing observations on the regulatory effects of donor-specific bone marrow cell infusions and chimerism in kidney transplant recipients. Transplantation 1998;65:956–65.

50. Miller J, Mathew J, Garcia-Morales R, et al. The human bone marrow as an immunoregulatory organ [review]. Transplantation 1999;68:1079–90.

51. Ciancio G, Miller J, Garcia-Morales RO, et al. Six-year clinical effect of donor bone marrow infusions in renal transplant patients. Transplantation 2001; 71:827–35.

52. Ciancio G, Burke GW, Garcia-Morales R, et al. Effect of living-related donor bone marrow infusion on chimerism and in vitro immunoregulatory activity in kidney transplant recipients. Transplantation 2002; 74:488–96.

53. Chatzipetrou MA, Mathew JM, Kenyon NS, et al. Analysis of post-transplant immune status in recipients of liver/bone marrow allografts. Hum Immunol 1999;60:1281–8.

54. Ciancio G, Burke GW, Moon J, et al. Donor bone marrow infusion in deceased and living donor renal transplantation. Yonsei Med J 2004;45: 998–1003.

55. Mathew JM, Garcia-Morales RO, Carreno M, et al. Immune responses and their regulation by donor bone marrow cells in clinical organ transplantation. Transpl Immunol 2003;11:307–21.

56. Cirocco RE, Carreno MR, Mathew JM, et al. FoxP3 mRNA transcripts and regulatory cells in renal transplant recipients 10 years after donor marrow infusion. Transplantation 2007;83:1611–9.

57. Gammie JS, Colson YL, Griffith BP, et al. Chimerism and thoracic organ transplantation [review]. Semin Thorac Cardiovasc Surg 1996;8:149–55.

58. Gammie JS, Pham SM. Simultaneous donor bone marrow and cardiac transplantation: can tolerance be induced with the development of chimerism? Curr Opin Cardiol 1999;14:126–32.

59. Salgar SK, Shapiro R, Dodson F, et al. Infusion of donor leukocytes to induce tolerance in organ allograft recipients. J Leukoc Biol 1999;66:310–4.

60. Mathew JM, Carreno M, Fuller L, et al. Modulatory effects of human donor bone marrow cells on allogeneic cellular immune responses. Transplantation 1997;63:686–92.

61. Mathew JM, Carreno M, Fuller L, et al. In vitro immunogenicity of cadaver donor bone marrow cells used for the induction of allograft acceptance in clinical transplantation. Transplantation 1999;68: 1172–80.

62. Mathew JM, Carreno M, Zucker K, et al. Cellular immune responses of human cadaver donor bone marrow cells and their susceptibility to commonly used immunosuppressive drugs in transplantation. Transplantation 1998;65:947–55.

63. Mathew JM, Fuller L, Carreno M, et al. Involvement of multiple subpopulations of human bone marrow cells in the regulation of allogeneic cellular immune responses. Transplantation 2000;70:1752–60.

64. Mathew JM, Carreno M, Fuller L, et al. Regulation of alloimmune responses (GvH reactions) in vitro by autologous donor bone marrow cell preparation used in clinical organ transplantation. Transplantation 2002;74:846–55.

65. Lagoo-Deenadayalan S, Lagoo AS, Lemons JA, et al. Donor-specific bone marrow cells suppress lymphocyte reactivity to donor antigens and differentially modulate TH1 and TH2 cytokine gene expression in the responder cell population. Transpl Immunol 1995;3:124–34.

66. Rachamim N, Gan J, Segall H, et al. Tolerance induction by megadose hematopoietic transplants: donor-type human CD34 stem cells induce potent specific reduction of host antidonor cytotoxic T lymphocyte precursors in mixed lymphocyte culture. Transplantation 1998;65:1386–93.

67. Anderson D, Billingham RE, Lampkin GH, et al. The use of skin grafting to distinguish between monozygotic and dizygotic twins in cattle. Heredity 1952;6: 201–21.

68. Owen RD. Immunogenetic consequences of vascular anastomoses between bovine twins. Science 1945; 102:400–1.

69. Ildstad ST, Wren SM, Bluestone JA, et al. Characterization of mixed allogeneic chimeras. Immunocompetence, in vitro reactivity, and genetic specificity of tolerance. J Exp Med 1985;162:231–44.

70. Sharabi Y, Sachs DH. Mixed chimerism and permanent specific transplantation tolerance induced by a nonlethal preparative regimen. J Exp Med 1989; 169:493–502.

71. Elwood ET, Larsen CP, Maurer DH, et al. Microchimerism and rejection in clinical transplantation. Lancet 1997;349(9062):1358–60.

72. Gozzo JJ, Wood ML, Monaco AP. Use of allogenic, homozygous bone marrow cells for the induction of specific immunologic tolerance in mice treated with antilymphocyte serum. Surg Forum 1970;21: 281–4.

73. Salama AD, Womer KL, Sayegh MH. Clinical transplantation tolerance: many rivers to cross. J Immunol 2007;178:5419–23.

74. Fudaba Y, Spitzer TR, Shaffer J, et al. Myeloma responses and tolerance following combined kidney and nonmyeloablative marrow transplantation: in vivo and in vitro analyses. Am J Transplant 2006;6:2121–33.

75. Scandling JD, Busque S, Dejbakhsh-Jones S, et al. Tolerance and chimerism after renal and hematopoietic cell transplantation. N Engl J Med 2008;358: 362–8.

76. Starzl TE, Demetris AJ, Trucco M, et al. Cell migration and chimerism after whole-organ transplantation: the basis of graft acceptance. J Hepatol 1993;17:1127–52.

77. Starzl TE, Demetris AJ, Trucco M, et al. Chimerism and donor-specific nonreactivity 27 to 29 years after kidney allotransplantation. Transplantation 1993;55: 1272–7.

78. Burlingham WJ, Grailer AP, Fechner JH Jr, et al. Microchimerism linked to cytotoxic T lymphocyte functional unresponsiveness (clonal anergy) in a tolerant renal transplant recipient. Transplantation 1995;59: 1147–55.

79. Mathew JM, Miller J. Immunoregulatory role of chimerism in clinical organ transplantation. Bone Marrow Transplant 2001;28:115–9.

80. Howland KC, Ausubel LJ, London CA. The roles of CD28 and CD40 ligand in T cell activation and tolerance. J Immunol 2000;164:4465–70.

81. Jiang S, Tugulea S, Pennesi G, et al. Induction of MHC-class I restricted human suppressor T cells by peptide priming in vitro. Hum Immunol 1998;59: 690–9.

82. Cortesini R, LeMaoult J, Ciubotariu R, et al. CD8+CD28– T suppressor cells and the induction of antigen-specific, antigen-presenting cell-mediated suppression of Th reactivity. Immunol Rev 2001;182: 201–6.

83. Ildstad ST, Shirwan H, Leventhal J. Is durable macrochimerism key to achieving clinical transplantation tolerance? Curr Opin Organ Transplant 2011;16(4): 343–4.

84. Levitsky J. Operational tolerance: past lessons and future prospects. Liver Transpl 2011;17:222–32.

85. Calne R. "Prope" tolerance: induction, lymphocyte depletion with minimal maintenance. Transplantation 2005;80(1):6–7.

86. Lopez M, Clarkson MR, Albin M, et al. A novel mechanism of action for antithymocyte globulin: induction of CD4+CD25+Foxp3+ regulatory T cells. J Am Soc Nephrol 2006;17:2844–53.

87. Benítez CE, Puig-Pey I, López M, et al. ATG-fresenius treatment and low-dose tacrolimus: results of a randomized controlled trial in liver transplantation. Am J Transplant 2010;10:2296–304.

88. Neujahr D, Turka LA. Lymphocyte depletion as a barrier to immunological tolerance. Contrib Nephrol 2005;146:65–72.

89. Starzl TE. Organ transplantation: a practical triumph and epistemological collapse. Proc Am Philos Soc 2003;147(3):226–45.

90. Marcos A, Lakkis F, Starzl TE. Tolerance for organ recipients: a clash of paradigms. Liver Transpl 2006;12(10):1448–51.

91. Starzl TE, Zinkernagel R. Transplantation tolerance from a historical perspective. Nat Rev Immunol 2001;1:233–9.

92. Gorantla VS, Schneeberger S, Moore LR, et al. Development and validation of a procedure to isolate viable bone marrow cells from the vertebrae of cadaveric organ donors for composite organ grafting. Cytotherapy 2011. [Epub ahead of print].

93. Starzl TE, Demetris AJ. Transplantation milestones: viewed with one- and two-way paradigms of tolerance. JAMA 1995;273:876–9.

94. Starzl TE, Zinkernagel R. Antigen localization and migration in immunity and tolerance. N Engl J Med 1998;339:1905–13.

95. Bonilla WV, Geuking MB, Aichele P, et al. Microchimerism maintains deletion of the donor cell-specific CD8+ T cell repertoire. J Clin Invest 2006; 116:156–62.

Surgical and Technical Aspects of Hand Transplantation: Is it Just Another Replant?

Tristan L. Hartzell, MD[a],*, Prosper Benhaim, MD[a],
Joseph E. Imbriglia, MD[b], Jaimie T. Shores, MD[c],
Robert J. Goitz, MD[b], Marshall Balk, MD[b],
Scott Mitchell, MD[a], Roee Rubinstein, MD[a],
Vijay S. Gorantla, MD, PhD[d], Stefan Schneeberger, MD[e],
Gerald Brandacher, MD[f], W.P. Andrew Lee, MD[e],
Kodi K. Azari, MD[g]

KEYWORDS

- Hand allotransplantation
- Composite tissue transplantation • Replantation

Before 1962 individuals suffering a traumatic amputation of the hand or arm were left with no option but to live without the part, devoid of its function and appearance. That changed on May 23, 1962 when Ronald Malt performed the world's first replantation at the Massachusetts General Hospital. The patient was a 12 year-old boy who had his right arm amputated at the level of the humeral neck in a train accident.[1] Since this first replant, thousands of individuals have benefited from the reattachment of amputated parts, with restoration of form and function. However, for the next several decades those who were not candidates for replantation were left with a prosthetic as the only option.

Forty years after the first replant, long-term amputees were given new hope by a team of surgeons in Lyon, France. On September 23, 1998 a New Zealander became the world's first hand transplant recipient in the modern era of immunosuppression (the graft was amputated 2 years later after an episode of rejection following patient noncompliance with immunosuppression medication).[2,3] This operation was followed by the first long-term success when a team in Louisville, Kentucky performed a transplant on a 24-year-old man

The authors have nothing to disclose.

[a] Division of Plastic Surgery, Department of Orthopedic Surgery, David Geffen School of Medicine at University of California Los Angeles,10945 Le Conte Avenue, Suite 3355, Los Angeles, CA 90095, USA

[b] Division of Hand and Upper Extremity Surgery, Department of Orthopedic Surgery, University of Pittsburgh Medical Center, 180 Fort Couch Road, Suite 400, Pittsburgh, PA 15241, USA

[c] Division of Plastic and Reconstructive Surgery, Department of Surgery, University of Pittsburgh Medical Center, Falk Medical Building 3601 Fifth Avenue, Suite 6B, Pittsburgh, PA 15213, USA

[d] Pittsburgh Reconstructive Transplantation Program, Division of Plastic Surgery, Department of Surgery, 3550 Terrace Street, Pittsburgh, PA 15261, USA

[e] Department of Plastic and Reconstructive Surgery, Johns Hopkins University School of Medicine, 601 North Caroline Street, Baltimore, MD 21287, USA

[f] Department of Plastic and Reconstructive Surgery, Johns Hopkins University School of Medicine, Ross Research Building 749D, 720 Rutland Avenue, Baltimore, MD 21205, USA

[g] Department of Orthopedic Surgery, University of California, 10945 Le Conte Avenue, Room 33-55G PVUB, Los Angeles, CA 90095, USA

* Corresponding author.

E-mail address: tristanhartzell@gmail.com

who had lost his hand in a firework accident.[4] The Louisville patient lives on to this day with his new hand, enjoying a restoration of function and appearance once deemed impossible.

More than 40 patients have now been the recipients of hand, forearm, and arm transplants in the modern era of immunosuppression.[3] Three hands have been amputated in the United States and Europe (due to bacterial infection, intimal hyperplasia, and rejection from noncompliance), 7 hands in China have been removed (due to nonprovidence or noncompliance with immunosuppressive therapy), and one patient has died of cerebral anoxia due to airway obstruction (the patient underwent a concurrent face transplant).[5] Similar to the experience with replantations,[6] the functional outcomes of hand allotransplantation have been promising.[5,7–13] All patients have developed protective sensibility, 90% tactile sensibility, and 82% discriminative sensibility, and motor outcomes have generally been good enough to allow performance of daily activities. Many patients have returned to work. The quality of life scores have improved in 75% of patients after transplant.[5]

The ultimate goal of hand allotransplantation is to achieve graft survival and useful long-term function. To achieve these goals, selection of the appropriate patient, detailed preoperative planning, and precise surgical technique are of paramount importance.

Allotransplantation is not a suitable treatment for everyone with an upper extremity amputation. This modality should be reserved for motivated consenting adults who are in good general heath, psychologically stable, and have failed a trial of prosthetic use. Ideal candidates are those with favorable amputation mechanisms and levels. The more distal amputation levels (eg, wrist and metacarpal hand) are ideal, as the nerve anastomosis will be closer to the target end organ and the intrinsic muscles innervated sooner. More proximal amputations such as the proximal one-third of the forearm and above the elbow remain controversial at present. Furthermore, patients with sharp guillotine-style amputation mechanisms are preferable to those with injuries involving avulsions, crush mechanisms, or burns.

Two years after his successful replant, Malt reported his technique. The replantation was performed by first repairing both communicating brachial veins, then the brachial artery. An intramedullary steel rod was placed for internal fixation, muscles were coapted, and the skin was closed.[1] While the key surgical steps of transplantation are similar, there are major differences. The aim of this article is to describe the steps in hand allotransplantation, and the importance of patient selection as well as preoperative and postoperative care.

SURGICAL TECHNIQUE

The surgical techniques used for hand allotransplantation share their roots with replantation surgery.[6] Hand allotransplantation is performed under tourniquet control[2,4] and general anesthesia, with regional anesthetic augmentation for vasodilation and postoperative pain control. The sequence of events is similar to that in major upper extremity replantations, as are many of the nuances of microsurgery and tendon repair.

In general, the surgical sequence begins with bone preparation and osteosynthesis. Next, revascularization is accomplished by anastomosis of one main artery and two veins. Tendon/muscle repair, nerve repair, and skin closure follow.

As for replantation, the operative sequence of hand transplantation varies based on the amount of muscle carried by the graft. Distal transplantations (distal to the distal one-third of the radius) carry very little muscle mass and can tolerate a longer period of ischemia. Proximal forearm transplantations, with the concomitant increased muscle bulk, require rapid revascularization to avoid ischemic injury and prevent subsequent muscle fibrosis. Prolonged warm ischemia was believed to be a leading reason for the flexion contracture and forearm muscle fibrosis in a forearm allograft performed in Spain.[7] Hence, when transplantation proximal to the mid-forearm is performed, revascularization is of utmost importance.[11]

Based on the group's experience with 9 hand/forearm transplantations at the University of Pittsburgh Medical Center and UCLA, the authors have modified the operative sequence of events for transplantations distal to the mid-forearm so that revascularization is performed later in the operative sequence. As before, the procedure starts with osteosynthesis but instead of arterial revascularization, the extensor tendons are next repaired followed by rapid anastomosis of 1 to 2 dorsal veins. The forearm is then rotated over and the nerves are repaired. At this point, both radial and ulnar arteries are coapted, followed by more veins. Finally, the flexor tendons are repaired and the skin is closed.

This sequence modification was used for transplantations distal to the mid-forearm for several reasons. The primary reason is that the repair of the dorsal veins and major nerves is easier under a bloodless field; this is particularly true with the median and ulnar nerves, where precise group fascicular repair of the individual motor and sensory branches can be performed in hopes of a better return of function (**Fig. 1**). After reperfusion, group fascicular repair is much more difficult, due to severe nerve edema and blood staining. These modifications were made possible by the authors' group because the same surgical team did the operation each time, thus providing comfort and familiarity with the surgical sequence as well as shorter operative times. In addition, with more distal amputations, longer ischemia times are considered to be more tolerable.

In addition to these variations in operative sequence, there are 3 key conceptual differences that exist between replantation and allotransplantation, which must be accounted for: (1) availability of tissues; (2) relative tendon tension; and (3) bone length.

With replantation there is a paucity of tissue, and efforts are made to conserve tissue. Limited bone shortening is done to alleviate tension on the neurovascular and tendon repairs. However, the relative tension and balance between the flexor and extensor tendons is generally left intact. Conversely, with allotransplantation an excess of tissue is available and one must judge exactly what is needed to suit the recipient's unique requirements (**Fig. 2**). As a result, the relative tension between the flexor and extensor tendons must be reestablished. The third major difference between replantation and transplantation is forearm length. Barring major traumatic bone loss, forearm length is generally preserved with replantations. With transplantation the appropriate forearm length must be reconstructed to match the contralateral side (**Fig. 3**).

Preoperative Planning

Absolute and relative contraindications to replantation are well established,[14] whereas guidelines for the transplantation of a hand are still being

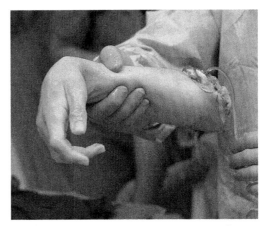

Fig. 2. The donor limb, with an excess of tissue harvested.

formulated. In general, patients must be in good health, psychologically stable, willing and able to tolerate a lifelong immunosuppressant regimen, and accepting of a deceased nonautologous part. The authors select for patients who have failed prosthetics. Patients with bilateral or dominant hand amputations and a favorable amputation mechanism are generally preferable. Ideal levels of amputation are the metacarpal head, wrist, and distal forearm, whereas proximal forearm and above-elbow transplantations remain controversial.

Prospective donors are matched to the recipient for size, sex, and skin tone, as well as blood group, cytomegalovirus, and Epstein-Barr virus status. The recipient also undergoes electromyography,

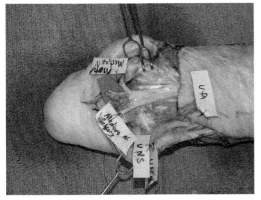

Fig. 1. Identification of the group fascicles of the median nerve.

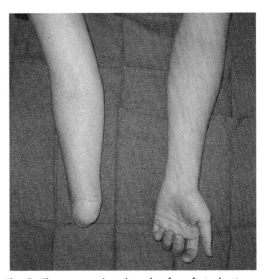

Fig. 3. The appropriate length of graft to be transplanted is determined by comparison with the normal limb in a unilateral hand transplant.

angiography, testing of nerve conduction velocity, and computed tomography/magnetic resonance imaging as indicated.

Team Coordination

A hand or finger replant can easily be performed by a single surgeon and surgical assistant. By contrast, the hand allotransplantation operation mandates a multifaceted surgical approach to keep ischemia times as short as possible. At least 2 operative teams for unilateral and 4 teams for bilateral operations are required to work simultaneously and in concert on the donor and recipient (**Fig. 4**).[12,13,15] It is ideal to have the recipient and "back table" donor teams in the same operating room so that perfect coordination of transplant timing and tissue requirements can be communicated in real time. If large enough operating rooms are not available, the donor and recipient teams should be located in adjacent operating theaters.

Timing

With replantation the amputated segment is usually prepared first on a back table, while waiting for the patient to arrive at the operating room and be anesthetized. However, many more considerations must be taken with allotransplantation. The timing of the hand transplant operation depends on the condition and geographic location of the donor limb. If the procurement team deems that the donor limb is in excellent condition then the recipient can be brought to the operating room for stump preparation prior to arrival of the donor limb. The timing obviously must be coordinated based on geographic location and travel times. Furthermore, if there is any concern about the condition of the donor limb (such as vascular injury or thrombosis from arterial lines), it is prudent to not proceed with the recipient stump dissection and exposure to immunosuppression induction. In this instance, the donor limb should be recovered in the usual fashion, brought back, and carefully examined on the back table before recipient dissection and administration of induction agent. It is possible that on-table angiogram or donor limb dissection is warranted before making the decision to proceed with transplantation.

Once a decision is made to harvest the donor limb, the brachial artery is exposed 3 cm above the elbow with a fish-mouth incision, cannulated, and flushed with preservation solution at 4°C. The limb is placed in moist sponges, transferred into triple organ transplantation bags, and placed on ice. The fish-mouth incision of the stump is closed for later prosthetic placement.

Skin Incisions

Unique to hand allotransplantation, the design of the skin incisions is of paramount importance. The goal of the incisions is the removal of unhealthy and scarred tissue, and closure in a nonconstrictive manner (**Fig. 5**). Because extensive dissection may be required, the authors have found that the 4-flap interposing incision provides optimal exposure of structures and creates a zigzag skin flap closure that does not result in a circumferential scar contracture (**Fig. 6**). The

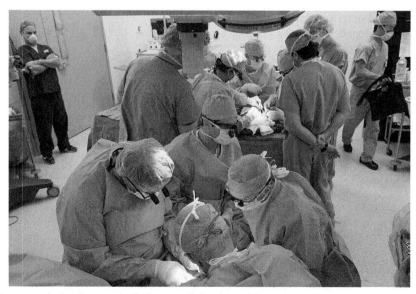

Fig. 4. Two teams work simultaneously during a unilateral hand transplant.

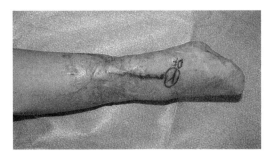

Fig. 5. A scarred recipient stump, with a paucity of local tissue.

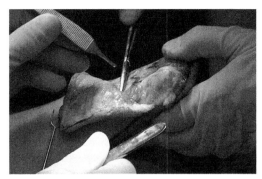

Fig. 7. Careful dissection of the recipient stump. The critical structures are often friable, tenuous, and encased in scar.

interposing 4-flap design is created by the placement of mid-lateral incisions on the recipient stump, and dorsal and volar mid-axial incisions on the donor limb. The donor limb volar mid-axial incision can easily be extended to decompress the carpal canal (see **Fig. 6**). It is important that skin flaps be designed long at the start to help obviate the need for skin graft. The tendon repairs add bulk, and it is easy to trim the flaps later at inset.

Dissection and Identification of Structures

The dissection of donor and recipient limbs should ideally be performed simultaneously in the same operating room. The preparation of the recipient stump is often difficult and must be performed carefully. The structures may be tenuous, atrophied, and encased in scar, which is particularly the case with amputations resulting from explosive injuries, burns, and meningococcal sepsis (**Fig. 7**). Dissection of the recipient stump should begin in the subcutaneous plane with careful attention to the preservation of the superficial veins that are often diminutive. The authors have found that vein mapping of the recipient using a portable ultrasound unit just before transplantation in the preoperative holding area aids in the intraoperative identification (**Fig. 8**).

Dissection of the donor limb begins proximally and ends distally from the subcutaneous tissues to the bone. It is performed on a bed of iced

sponges to minimize warm ischemia time. This dissection can be performed rather rapidly and the structures are left long, as excess tissue can easily be discarded later in the operation. Leaving the structures long is of paramount importance and cannot be overstated. This point holds particularly true for tendons, vessels, nerves, and skin flaps, as it is deceptively difficult to judge the correct tissue amounts needed. For example, the tendon repairs tend to add significant bulk to the forearm, and longer than expected skin flaps are needed for soft tissue coverage. Furthermore, the long skin flaps can be an excellent source of full-thickness skin grafts if there is too much tension on skin closure.

It is critical that each identified donor and recipient structure is individually tagged (**Fig. 9**). The authors tag each structure with a rectangular piece

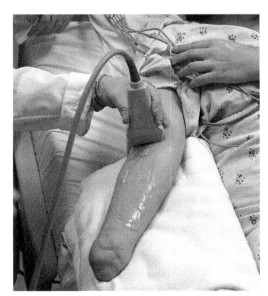

Fig. 8. Preoperative vein mapping of the recipient limb.

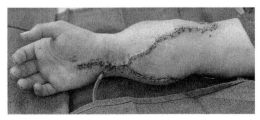

Fig. 6. The zigzag skin flap closure, preventing circumferential scar contracture. The distal extent of the incision provides access for a carpal tunnel release.

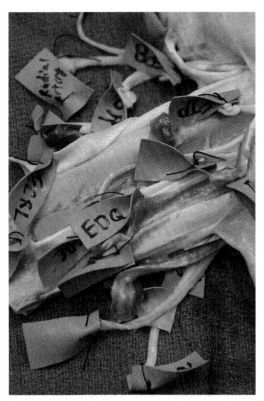

Fig. 9. Structures are tagged with an Esmarch bandage and indelible ink.

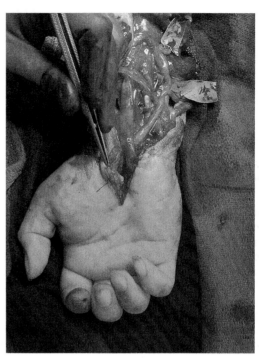

Fig. 10. Structures become much more difficult to identify once the field is edematous and bloody. Ink can easily smear off if the appropriate marker has not been used.

of Esmarch bandage marked with indelible ink markers and secured with 2-0 silk sutures (see **Fig. 9**). The elastic Esmarch bandage does not tear easily, the knots of silk sutures do not unravel, and indelible markers do not smear when placed in contact with blood. Once the graft is revascularized, the structures will become edematous, bloodstained, and difficult to identify. If appropriate tagging has not been performed, a significant and unnecessary complexity is added to the operation (**Fig. 10**).

Osteosynthesis

The objectives of osteosynthesis are to reconstruct length, restore alignment (especially distal radial-ulnar joint congruity), and obtain union. The authors have found that the 3.5-mm locking compression plate is ideal for proximal and mid-forearm transplantations, as they provide compression and a rigid construct (**Fig. 11**).[10] To promote osseous union, care must be taken to avoid aggressive periosteal stripping. In distal forearm transplantations, 2.7-mm volar locking distal radius and ulna plates can be used (**Fig. 12**).

In their practice, the authors provisionally plate the donor radius and ulna, then remove the plate

and perform the osteotomies. The osteotomies are made perpendicular to the long axis of the bone, as oblique angles have been found to be unnecessary for increased bony contact and union. The plates are then reapplied and secured in compression mode to the donor radius and ulna (**Fig. 13**).

Vessel Repair

As mentioned previously, in most cases vascular anastomosis is performed following bone fixation to reestablish flow. Up to this point, the operation is done while keeping the graft cool using ice slush. Once initial revascularization is complete, the ice is removed and the graft warmed with sterile saline irrigation to decrease vasospasm. This action is followed by tendon and nerve repair, although early revascularization can make group fascicular repair of the nerve more difficult because of edema and blood staining (the authors have recently done arterial anastomosis after nerve repair for this reason).

The authors prefer to anastomose the veins (end to end) first, as it is more easily performed in a bloodless field (**Fig. 14**). However, if the veins cannot be easily located, arterial repair (either

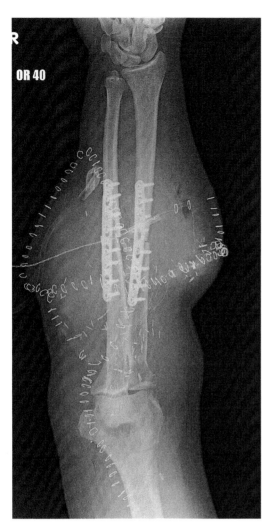

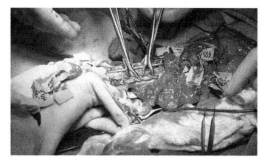

Fig. 13. The plates are secured in compression.

disruption of the proximal muscle belly nutrient branches, which can result in late muscle fibrosis. In addition, it must be noted that donor radial artery injuries are common and may necessitate an on-table angiogram. If a donor artery thrombosis is identified, a mechanical embolectomy, tissue plasminogen activator, or a bypass may be required.

Later, once the tendon and nerve structures are repaired, definitive vascular repair is performed by repairing the other artery and more veins. It is advisable to anastomose at least 4 veins from both the superficial and deep systems. An anastomotic coupler may be helpful.

Muscle/Tendon Repair

The technique for repair of muscle and tendons largely depends on the level of transplantation. For muscle repairs proximal to the myotendinous junction, individual muscle units may not be identifiable. In these instances, the only choice is epimysium and perimysium repairs. However, with distal repairs and the presence of tendon, a stronger repair can be performed and early

Fig. 11. Mid-radius and ulna osteosynthesis with 3.5-mm locking compression plates.

radial or ulnar) is performed first, which will dilate the veins and allow easier identification.

Arterial repairs should be performed end to end, distal to the mid-forearm, and with as little as possible adventitial stripping or disruption. In more proximal transplants, the arterial anastomosis should be end to side. This action will avoid

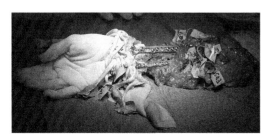

Fig. 12. Distal radius and ulna osteosynthesis with 2.7-mm locking compression plates.

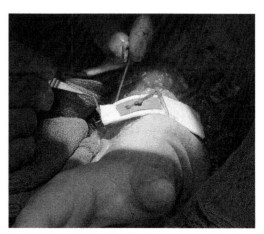

Fig. 14. Preparation of veins for anastomosis prior to tourniquet release.

active range of motion can be safely initiated. The authors' method of choice has been the Pulvertaft weave technique (**Fig. 15**). This method adds bulk and takes longer to perform than some of the end-to-end techniques such as the Tsuge method.[16] However, the authors have found that the increased strength and ability to initiate early active range of motion is worth the trade-off. Tendon transfers are performed as needed, based on the level of amputation, availability of tissue, and potential for muscle unit innervation.

Regardless of which method of muscle tendon repair is chosen or if tendon transfers are used, the ultimate goal is to reestablish the relative tension between the flexor and extensor tendons. This challenge is one of the more difficult of the hand transplant operation. Errors of judgment in reestablishing the critical flexor-extensor balance will most certainly lead to postoperative functional limitations that will be very difficult to correct.

To set the balance, the authors first begin with the extensor tendons. The wrist extensors are initially repaired followed by the digit and thumb extensors. The tension is ideally set so that the digits fully extend when the wrist is flexed 20° to 30° (**Fig. 16**). Then the forearm is supinated and the flexor tendons are repaired to a tension that restores the natural resting digital cascade.

Nerve Repair

The nerve repair is done as with a replantation. It should be performed precisely, under an operative microscope. All major forearm and hand nerves should be repaired: median, ulnar, and radial (or radial sensory and posterior interosseous nerve). In addition, if applicable, the palmar cutaneous branch of the median nerve and dorsal ulnar sensory nerve are repaired.

The repair technique depends on the level of transplantation. Distal amputations such as metacarpal hands or at the radiocarpal level afford the luxury of precise ulnar and median nerve motor and sensory branch dissection as well as group

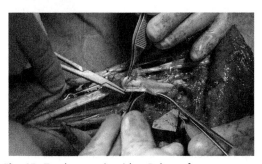

Fig. 15. Tendon repair with a Pulvertaft weave.

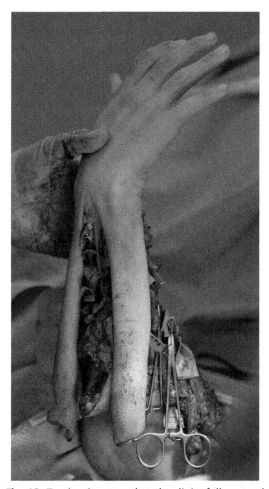

Fig. 16. Tension is set so that the digits fully extend when the wrist is flexed 20° to 30°.

fascicular anastomosis (see **Fig. 1**).[10] Proximal transplantations with mixed nerve topography can be repaired based on surgeon preference by epineurial suture or nerve conduit.

The authors routinely perform prophylactic carpal tunnel releases in their hand transplants, due to postoperative edema concerns. In their experience there has not been an instance of flexor tendon bowstringing in 9 transplanted hands, each with carpal tunnel release.

Skin Closure and Dressing

After obtaining meticulous hemostasis, the skin flaps are trimmed and loosely inset over closed suction drains. The final appearance is 4 interdigitating flaps that close in a zigzag manner. More often than not, the authors have found that there is paucity of forearm skin to loosely cover all structures. In this case, full-thickness skin grafts from the donor are preferable to tight closures (**Fig. 17**).

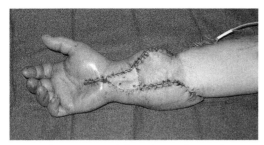

Fig. 17. If necessary, a full-thickness skin graft is used to prevent unnecessary tension on flap inset.

Dressings consist of sheets of petroleum gauze, 4 × 4 sponges, and a nonconstricting plaster splint.

Postoperative Care

Flap monitoring is performed from dual sources. An implantable Doppler monitor is wrapped around one of the vein anastomoses. In addition, one pulse oximeter is placed on one of the transplanted hand digits and another on the contralateral (nontransplanted) hand or toe (bilateral hand transplants). This double-pulse oximeter technique allows for easy postoperative monitoring by comparing the arterial wave forms and oxygen saturations between the transplanted hand and the nontransplant control.[17]

DISCUSSION

The planning and execution of hand allotransplantation requires thoughtful precision at every step. From the preoperative planning phase, when a team of health care providers is assembled and a patient is chosen, to the decades of postoperative therapy and immunosuppressant management, a meticulous approach must be maintained. Thus far, this article has expounded on the differences between replantation and hand transplantation. However, there are also key differences among surgical techniques used by different hand transplantation teams around the world.

The sequence of structure repair in transplantation is certainly debatable. While bony fixation is universally accepted as a starting point, there is wide variation in the order of subsequent steps. The early adopters of hand transplantation in Lyon and Louisville advocated early arterial revascularization to minimize ischemia time.[2,4] Supporting this was a report from Spain, detailing forearm muscle fibrosis in a transplant arm that was repaired in an artery-last sequence.[7] However, this strategy allows for edema to set in and for a bloodstained field to develop. Subsequent structure repair becomes more difficult, especially group fascicular

repair of the nerves. The authors prefer to repair the arteries later for this reason, although they do modify the strategy and repair the artery early in cases with prolonged warm ischemia, especially in proximal transplantations with forearm muscle.

While the principles employed for the repair of individual structures are maintained by all hand transplant surgeons (setting appropriate tendon tension, avoiding skin contractures with interdigitating flaps, precise repair of structures), there are nuances that have developed among different groups.[2,4,15,18,19] Of note, differences have arisen with the repair of musculotendinous structures and the level of vessel coaptation. Because availability of donor tendon is not an issue, the authors prefer a Pulvertaft weave for its strength, rather than an end-to-end repair. The bulk of this repair must be compensated for in skin-flap design. If possible, the authors repair each individual tendon to allow for independent action rather than en masse repair, and use tendon transfers only as needed.

In addition, the authors prefer an arterial anastomosis at a level that requires the least amount of donor and recipient vessel dissection to be performed safely and well. While recognizing the advantages of performing vessel repair at the elbow, where the vessels are a larger caliber and free from much of the surgical trauma at the stump site, there is the possibility that extensive vessel dissection submits the artery to unnecessary structural damage and subsequent myointimal proliferation.

Ultimately, what sets hand allotransplantation far apart from the practice of replantation is the potential for evolution. From the first attempt to transplant a human hand in 1964 in Ecuador with primitive immunosuppressants[20,21] to the first transplants in the "modern" era of immunosuppression in Lyon and Louisville, much has changed.[2,4] Although the principles and surgical technique of replantation have varied little since Malt's experience in 1962, it will be astonishing if the surgical technique of hand transplantation is not dramatically different 50 years from now, as new immunosuppressive strategies are developed and experience is gained.

SUMMARY

Similar to a replantation, the goal of hand allotransplantation is the achievement of long-term graft survival and useful function. Though alike in some key steps, there are many critical aspects of hand allotransplantation that make it dramatically different to replantation. Nevertheless, with thoughtful patient selection, detailed preoperative planning, meticulous surgical technique, and diligent follow-up care, excellent results can be achieved.

REFERENCES

1. Malt RA, McKhann CF. Replantation of severed arms. JAMA 1964;189:716–22.

2. Dubernard JM, Owen E, Herzberg G, et al. Human hand allograft: report on first 6 months. Lancet 1999;353(9161):1315–20.

3. Dubernard JM, Lanzetta M, Petruzzo P. International registry on hand and composite tissue transplantation. Available at: http://www.handregistry.com/page.asp?page=4. Accessed February 3, 2011.

4. Jones JW, Gruber SA, Barker JH, et al. Successful hand transplantation. One-year follow-up. Louisville Hand Transplant Team. N Engl J Med 2000;343(7):468–73.

5. Petruzzo P, Lanzetta M, Dubernard JM, et al. The international registry on hand and composite tissue transplantation. Transplantation 2010;90:1590–4.

6. Kleinert HE, Jablon M, Tsai TM. An overview of replantation and results of 347 replants in 245 patients. J Trauma 1980;20(5):390–8.

7. Landin L, Cavadas P, Garcia-Cosmes P, et al. Perioperative ischemic injury and fibrotic degeneration of muscle in a forearm allograft. Ann Plast Surg 2011;66:202–9.

8. Ravindra R, Buell J, Kaufman C, et al. Hand transplantation in the United States: experience with 3 patients. Surgery 2008;144:638–44.

9. Gordon C, Siemionow M. Requirements for the development of a hand transplant program. Ann Plast Surg 2009;63:262–73.

10. Cavadas PC, Landin L, Ibanez J. Bilateral hand transplantation: result at 20 months. J Hand Surg Eur Vol 2009;34(4):434–43.

11. Schneeberger S, Ninkovic M, Gabl M, et al. First forearm transplantation: outcome at 3 years. Am J Transplant 2007;7(7):1753–62.

12. Margreiter R, Brandacher G, Ninkovic M, et al. A double-hand transplant can be worth the effort! Transplantation 2002;74(1):85–90.

13. Piza-Katzer H, Ninkovic M, Pechlaner S, et al. Double hand transplantation: functional outcome after 18 months. J Hand Surg Br 2002;27(4):385–90.

14. Boulas HJ. Amputations of the fingers and hand: indications for replantation. J Am Acad Orthop Surg 1998;6:100–5.

15. Schneeberger S, Ninkovic M, Margreiter R. Hand transplantation: the Innsbruck experience. In: Hewitt CW, Lee WP, editors. Transplantation of composite tissue allografts. New York: Springer; 2008. p. 234–50.

16. Labana N, Messer T, Lautenschlager E, et al. A biomechanical analysis of the modified Tsuge suture technique for repair of flexor tendon lacerations. J Hand Surg Br 2001;26(4):297–300.

17. Chang J, Jones NF. Twelve simple maneuvers to optimize digital replantation and revascularization. Tech Hand Up Extrem Surg 2004;8(3):161–6.

18. Gorantla VS, Breidenbach WC. Hand transplantation: the Louisville experience. In: Hewitt CW, Lee WP, Gordon CR, editors. Transplantation of composite tissue allografts. New York: Springer; 2008. p. 215–33.

19. Petruzzo P, Morelon E, Kanitakis J. Hand transplantation: the Lyon experience. In: Hewitt CW, Lee WP, Gordon CR, editors. Transplantation of composite tissue allografts. New York: Springer; 2008. p. 209–14.

20. Gilbert R. Transplant is successful with a cadaver forearm. Med Trib Med News 1964;5:20.

21. Gilbert R. Hand transplanted from cadaver is reamputated. Med Trib Med News 1964;5:23.

Development of an Upper Extremity Transplant Program

Kadiyala V. Ravindra, MD[a],*, Vijay S. Gorantla, MD, PhD[b]

KEYWORDS

- Hand transplantation • Composite tissue transplantation
- Upper extremity

Hand transplantation has now been performed successfully at more than a dozen centers worldwide[1] and at 5 centers in the United States.[2] The growth has been slow, largely because of skepticism of the immunologic feasibility initially[3] and later the fear of immunosuppression-related complications.[4,5] The proof of concept of the procedure has been well established with long-term success[6,7] and few major complications.

There have been growing efforts in the United States and the rest of the world toward wider application of the procedure. Many centers are in the process of establishing vascularized composite allotransplantation (VCA) programs. This article focuses on the efforts that go into the establishment of a hand transplant program. In 2005, there were approximately 1.6 million persons living with limb loss in the United States.[8] Of these, nearly 540,000 individuals had loss of upper limb; trauma accounted for 498,000 and, of these, 34,000 were listed as major loss.[8] There is thus a vast potential for the use of hand transplantation as a treatment modality in this patient population. To place this in perspective, the United Network for Organ Sharing (UNOS) Web site states that more than 85,000 patients are on the wait-list for a kidney transplant in the United States as of September 2010, and more than 12,000 renal transplants are performed each year. It is thus clear that, even if 1% of those with major upper limb loss were deemed candidates for hand transplantation, this would entail more than 300 procedures. However, only 15 patients have undergone hand transplantation in the United States to date. There is thus an urgent need to establish new hand transplant programs in the country.

ORGANIZING A CORE HAND TRANSPLANT TEAM

Transplantation and teamwork are synonymous. Unlike most other fields of medicine, transplantation cannot succeed without the dedication of many disciplines and a wide array of personnel. The reconstructive or transplant surgeon cannot do this alone. This basic tenet must be embraced when starting a hand/VCA program. One interested individual at any center (be it a reconstructive plastic surgeon, a hand surgeon, or a transplant surgeon) should take the lead and build the team that is essential to this endeavor.

The core of the hand transplant team should include:

1. Transplant coordinator
2. Hand/reconstructive surgeons
3. Transplant physician.

The transplant coordinator plays the important role of organizing team meetings, maintaining minutes of the discussions, and following up on action points. The initial meetings help gauge the level of interest for the project in the group. In

The authors have nothing to disclose.
^a Department of Surgery, Duke University, DUMC Box 3512, Durham, NC 27710, USA
^b Pittsburgh Reconstructive Transplantation Program, Division of Plastic Surgery, Department of Surgery, 3550 Terrace Street, Pittsburgh, PA 15261, USA
* Corresponding author.
E-mail address: Kadiyala.ravindra@duke.edu

Hand Clin 27 (2011) 531–538
doi:10.1016/j.hcl.2011.07.008
0749-0712/11/$ – see front matter © 2011 Elsevier Inc. All rights reserved.

hand.theclinics.com

addition, there is opportunity to educate members about the process and the potential obstacles to taking the idea forward. The process of organ transplantation involves much regulation and many procedures, and this is new territory for the reconstructive team members.

The transplant process is well established but is bound by tight regulation. This regulation is not well known to most outside the field and often comes as a surprise to reconstructive plastic/hand surgeons who wish to start a hand program. The logistics of hand transplantation can often overwhelm them even before they get started, which is where the experience of the solid organ transplant members of the group helps in negotiating through the complex process.

The team must review the currently available literature and explore the feasibility of the program at the local level. The questions that need to be answered include (1) are the team members convinced that hand transplantation offers unique benefits to recipients? This seems a superfluous question but, unless all the members agree that this is an option worth pursuing, little progress will be made. (2) Does the effort agree with the objectives of the hospital? (3) Will there be support, including financial support from the hospital to fund the initial cost for the program? Unless these are answered in the affirmative, the efforts are unlikely to make headway.

Early in the process, it is important to liaise with a program that has successfully performed hand transplantation. It helps to learn from the experiences of an established center and apply the lessons. The entire team or some of the members can visit a center that has performed a hand transplantation procedure. At this point, there are only 5 that have successfully performed the procedure in the United States, and these include the University of Louisville; University of Pittsburgh; University of California, Los Angeles; Emory; and the Wilford Medical Center, Texas. Interaction with the members of the successful team will be helpful in addressing the concerns and diffidence of the new team. Guidance about Institutional Review board (IRB) protocols, interaction with the local organ procurement organization (OPO), and budgeting for the procedure are some of the aspects that may be covered during the visit.

IDENTIFYING A MULTIDISCIPLINARY GROUP OF SURGEONS/CLINICIANS/ANCILLARY STAFF

Eventually the core group will have to be expanded to include other members who are crucial for any transplant venture. The transplant operation itself is complex and requires 4 or more hand/plastic surgeons to be involved during the operation. This amount of surgical manpower is essential for this long procedure: one person being responsible for the procurement of the organ and the others performing the complex surgery of reestablishing the multiple anatomic connections that are a part of the hand transplant surgery. The expanded team must also include a psychologist/psychiatrist, social worker, insurance and financial advisor, and an infectious disease specialist. The role of each of the members is detailed later.

Reconstructive/Hand Surgeons

The hand surgery team leader heads the transplant team. The team leader should ideally have expertise in microsurgery and some background in transplant immunology. This expertise is important because the team leader, along with a core group of colleagues, is responsible for donor and recipient evaluation and selection, surgery, as well as the postoperative follow-up and management of the transplant.

The only similarity between reimplantation of a severed limb and allotransplantation of a hand is the surgical procedure. The other components of the procedure are new to the routine practice of the hand surgeons but are not insurmountable. The hand surgery team leader is responsible for coordinating and mobilizing the team and orchestrating the surgery and posttransplant management within the multidisciplinary team.

Transplant Team

The transplant team is a well-knit multidisciplinary group consisting of the transplant physician (so far, most of those involved in VCA have been abdominal transplant surgeons), transplant coordinator, social worker, finance specialists, and a psychologist/psychiatrist.

Transplant Physician

The transplant physician brings the knowledge and experience of solid organ transplantation to the team. The medical suitability of the candidate, including screening for occult infections (eg, viral hepatitis B and C, positive tuberculin test, past history of fungal infections), cardiovascular risk profile, age-appropriate cancer screening and so forth, will be assessed. The onerous task of informing potential recipients of the planned immunosuppression and discussing potential short-term and long-term complications of such therapy is the primary responsibility of the transplant physician. The physician also has experience with selection of deceased donors and the policies governing the local OPO.

Transplant Coordinator

The transplant coordinator is a key member who has a multipronged role of liaising between the patient and the transplant team. For a new program, appointing a person with previous experience as a solid organ transplant coordinator greatly facilitates the process. This person would have adequate knowledge of transplant medications and associated complications and would be ideally suited to assume this responsibility. The role involves coordinating every aspect of the transplant process, including screening and interviewing of potential candidates, procuring all the medical records of potential candidates, scheduling, and following up on the investigations and appointments of the candidate with the different members of the team, compiling the medical record of the patient, ensuring that the protocol is implemented in the work-up, help arrange follow-up care either with the transplant team or with the patient's local physicians, and so forth. Following transplantation, the coordinator's role is vital in continuing communication with the patient and family to ensure patient compliance with immunosuppression, follow-up blood tests, and appropriate clinic visits. The duties include monitoring daily immunosuppression levels; being watchful of potential complications, including metabolism (new onset hypertension, diabetes), drug toxicity (eg, headaches, tremors, gastrointestinal disturbance, bone marrow), and infections (fevers, leucocytosis); ensuring adequate supply of medications; and motivating the patient to pursue physical therapy. In essence, the coordinator's role extends from screening to long-term follow-up care, with attention to both the medical and social concerns of the candidate. Patients receiving transplants come to rely heavily on the coordinator to negotiate the maze of transplant medicine. Transplant coordinators play an important role (sometimes in association with research coordinators) in data collection, auditing, and reporting of outcomes to internal and external regulatory and compliance agencies such as IRBs and the Data Safety Monitoring Boards.

Psychiatrist

Loss of a limb is associated with significant physical and psychosocial morbidity and many patients are on therapy with different agents including long-term pain medication. A recent report documented the presence of a mental health disorder in two-thirds of combat amputees, with a major disorder in 25%.[9] An important part of the pretransplant evaluation of candidates for hand transplantation is a psychological assessment by a qualified individual. It may be prudent for a new program to have a psychiatrist to perform this duty. This evaluation enables the team to gain insight into how the candidate might do during and after the transplant event. Posttransplant compliance with the recommendations of the transplant team is vital to the success of the procedure. The first successful hand transplant had to be amputated following noncompliance with medication. The patient probably did not fully accept the hand as his own.[10] Besides appropriate adherence to the medication regimen, follow-up to evaluate long-term morbidity, such as cardiovascular and metabolic problems, is crucial.

The psychiatrist's role in assessing the patient's expectations with the transplant and identifying risk factors for noncompliance are extremely important. The psychiatrist is then able to formulate appropriate psychosocial interventions (such as psychotherapy or behavioral therapy) to optimize the patient's candidacy for the procedure and prevent psychiatric morbidity. Combat amputees may require additional testing/rehabilitation for associated traumatic brain injury. The psychiatrist's role extends beyond the initial screening evaluation for candidacy. Transplant recipients must undergo periodic (at least annual) assessments for compliance with medication/rehabilitation, coping with the transplanted hand, and integration into body image and personal identity. In addition to providing information regarding the psychological experience of patients with amputations and their motivation for hand transplantation, it is hoped that this information, compared with posttransplant outcome data, will help further refine the assessment of candidates for this procedure and possibly other forms of composite tissue allotransplantation.[11]

Occupational/Physical Therapist

Functional recovery in the transplanted hand is a gradual process that depends on peripheral nerve regeneration and distal muscle group reinnervation. Motor and sensory function continues to improve for many years following the transplantation.[6] Thus, unlike in solid organs, physical therapy plays a significant role in hand transplantation. A rigorous rehabilitation regimen has to be implemented in all patients, with 3 to 6 hours of supervised therapy 5 days a week during the first 3 to 6 months or even longer depending on the nature and level of the transplant. Strict compliance with such an intensive regimen and follow-up with a home therapy exercise routine is paramount to achieving functionality. The occupational therapist/physical therapist should be cognizant of passive and active range-of-motion exercises with appropriate static and dynamic splinting to allow gentle active flexion/extension, limit adhesions, and promote healing. Hand-based splints, such as dynamic outrigger splints and anticlaw splints, should be used in all patients. Compression gloves are useful in patients with lymphedema. Qualitative and quantitative tests for hand and upper extremity function, such as the Carroll[12] score, DASH[13] score, and the Hand Transplantation Score System,[14] are used to chart progress in patients. These tests, along with standard tests for evaluation of motor and sensory recovery (eg, Tinel, Semmes Weinstein monofilaments, 2PD, dynamometry, peg-board tests), enable assessment of graft functional and quality-of-life outcomes and can be incorporated into activities of daily living.

PREPARATION OF HAND TRANSPLANT PROTOCOL AND IRB APPROVAL

Although hand transplantation has been successful[15] and is likely to become standard of care in the near future, for now it is still considered experimental by most outside composite tissue allotransplantation. This position is reasonable considering that only 15 patients have had the procedure performed at 5 centers in the United States in more than a decade. Hence, it is prudent for centers starting a VCA/hand program to write up a protocol and have approval by the IRB.

The protocol should specifically address the following issues: (1) enrollment of patients, (2) financial responsibilities, (3) recipient inclusion and exclusion criteria, (4) donor inclusion and exclusion criteria, (5) donor selection and matching, (6) recipient procedures, (7) immunosuppression strategy and plans for treatment of rejection episodes, (8) postoperative management and monitoring, (9) assessment of outcomes, (10) immunologic and psychosocial monitoring, (11) benefits and potential risks, (12) stopping rules, (13) adverse event reporting, (14) roles and responsibilities of team members, (15) data safety monitoring board, and (16) confidentiality.

The protocol has to detail all the aspects of the procedure and follow-up. Approval by IRB should be easier now than during the early days of upper extremity transplantation. The ethics debate has largely dissipated and the concept of hand transplantation as an alternative option for some amputees is much better accepted. Some new centers contemplating hand transplantation are reported to be embarking on hand transplantation without an IRB submission.

RECRUITMENT OF RECIPIENTS

Identification of potential recipients and evaluation for candidacy is the primary responsibility of the core team. A Web site providing information on hand transplantation as an option to potential candidates might be helpful. The Web site should have detailed information of the procedure, review of current results, the composition of the team at the center, and links to other useful sites (such as www.handregistry.com).

Communicating with potential referring physicians in the region and elsewhere could enable recruitment of appropriate candidates. In addition, talks/seminars/workshops at the center or region by experts from active centers with prior experience in the procedure may be useful in educating the team/ancillary staff as well as providing opportunities for the public and media to participate and increasing awareness for the procedure.

EVALUATION OF RECIPIENTS

Potential recipients most often contact the center by phone, electronic mail, or regular mail. The transplant coordinator must interview the candidates by telephone and seek permission to gather and record pertinent data. After the subject signs a screening consent, medical records of the patient may be obtained to assess eligibility. If there are no obvious contraindications (eg, presence of recent cancer, significant cardiovascular morbidity), the subject will have to undergo screening tests including infectious disease serology, blood counts, and chemistry panel. The medical screening tests are listed in **Box 1**. Appropriate imaging studies of the amputated limb are performed to enable surgical planning by the hand surgeon. These studies may be performed close to the patient's home. The initial screening data are reviewed by the transplant committee and a decision made about the suitability of the subject. If approved, the subject is then invited to the center to pursue further evaluation, which involves detailed evaluation of the candidate by all the members of the team as outlined earlier. During this process, the transplant coordinator's primary goal is educating the subject about hand transplantation, the center's protocol, and immunosuppression medications. The patient must be provided with data regarding outcomes of the procedure based on current literature. In addition, other adverse events diagnosed in hand recipients (even if unpublished but verified) must be communicated to the potential recipient. This screening process can take from 1 to several months.

At the completion of all the screening procedures, if patients are considered eligible, they will

At the time of transplantation, when the recipient comes to the hospital, the transplant team will again review the procedure and possible complications with the patient. The subject may be asked to sign a new copy of the consent form at the time of transplantation.

FINANCIAL CLEARANCE AND INSURANCE NEGOTIATIONS

The costs related to procuring the limb, the surgery and hospital charges, posttransplant medications, postoperative visits, and physical therapy visits for the first 3 months have been estimated to be approximately $150,000.[6] Actual costs could differ by center because of variations in charges and billing practices. The subject will be expected to stay close to the transplant center for about 3 months to enable physical therapy, clinical monitoring, and fine-tuning of drug doses to achieve target levels. The follow-up is typically frequent (at least weekly) in the first 3 months and less frequent later. Patients are usually discharged after 3 months, to be followed by a local physician and hand therapist.

The costs of long-term immunosuppression and laboratory testing are estimated to be about $15,000 per annum. Currently, third-party insurance payers do not cover hand transplantation. Currently, the initial costs of the procedure are covered through institutional support; however, it is vital to communicate with the patient's insurance provider and discuss long-term coverage. This communication could involve negotiations with insurance providers to agree to pay for immunosuppression and the laboratory testing. In eligible patients, any long-term procedures that are accepted as standard of care could be billed to their insurance providers.

TRANSPLANT COMMITTEE APPROVAL

The transplant committee consists of the reconstructive surgeons, transplant physician, transplant coordinator, psychologist/psychiatrist, social worker, and insurance specialist. Potential candidates are presented to the committee and all aspects of the candidate are debated. Fulfillment of inclusion criteria, presence of comorbidities that might affect outcome, psychological state, surgical plan, adequacy of social support mechanisms, assessment of future compliance, and insurance coverage for long-term care are discussed. The committee may approve a candidate without reservation or make recommendations that must be met by the candidate before being placed on the transplant list. Once approved, the

go through an additional education with a focus on potential complication. The formal informed consent form for the procedure is explained to them. Some centers have videotaped the consent process, but this is not essential. Some centers[6] have involved a patient advocate who is an unbiased nonfamily member who can help subjects decide whether they should or should not participate. The patient advocate receives all of the educational materials that the subject does, including a copy of the videotaped final consenting discussion. The subject is counseled that the consent process is not static and consent may be rescinded at any time.

candidate is officially on the wait-list and awaits an organ offer.

WORKING WITH THE OPO

Deceased donor transplantation in the United States is critically dependent on the work done by the OPO. The OPO is the body that identifies and obtains consent from potential donors within its jurisdiction. Most OPOs know the requirements and procedures for solid organ transplantation but have little idea of VCA. The transplant team and the reconstructive team have to spend time and energy in educating the local OPO about VCA/hand transplantation in general and, more specifically, about the center's protocol. It is of utmost importance to gain the confidence of the OPO in this matter. Without the active cooperation and involvement of the OPO, hand transplantation cannot happen.

VCA is unlike solid organ transplantation from the donor aspect. All the internal organs may be procured without visible disfigurement. With a hand or face, there is visible change that may not be acceptable to some donor families. OPOs may be averse to requesting donation of a hand/face for the fear of alienating them and thus potentially being denied consent for the solid organs as well. Even if the potential donor volunteered to be an organ donor at the time of acquiring a driver license, it is likely that hand/face donation was not a consideration at the time of decision. Thus, it is important for the OPO to obtain a specific family consent for VCA donation even in cases of declared organ donors. The process of obtaining consent for VCA is delicate but the results have so far been encouraging.

The OPO must obtain prosthesis that may be affixed to the donor arm to replace the donated hand. This prosthesis must be planned and available ahead of time. The donor requirements for a hand transplant are similar to those of solid organ transplantation as far as medical suitability is considered. However, additional factors such as limb color and length are important for a hand transplant. Some centers are using color swatches to match the donor and recipient.

Regarding the donor management, it is vital to request the OPO to avoid placing vascular lines on the limb being procured. There have been reports of vascular thrombosis after transplantation[16] from radial arterial lines. The transplant center must have prior detailed discussions with the OPO about the sequence of steps during the organ procurement procedure. Before the procedure, it may be best to inform the solid organ donor teams about when the hand will be procured. There has been no universally accepted protocol for the donor procedure. As per the third report[1] of the International Registry on Hand and Composite Tissue Transplantation, 50% of the hands were harvested before solid organs and the rest were procured after.

When the organ becomes available, the hand transplant team must directly speak to the abdominal and thoracic organ harvest teams to coordinate the new effort. It is straightforward, and prior discussions with the concerned teams involved will facilitate a smooth procedure.

DONOR ALGORITHM AND TRANSPLANT LOGISTICS

When consent has been obtained for a hand donation, the OPO will ascertain whether the hand surgeon is ready to use the organ. The hand surgeon, along with the transplant team, needs to study the donor details and decide on the suitability of the donor. The team has about an hour to make a decision. The medical suitability and the anatomic factors have to be reviewed. If the donor is deemed suitable, the next stage of evaluation is set in motion. The next major step involves performing a crossmatch.[17]

The term crossmatch refers to the process of identifying the presence of donor specific human leukocyte antigen antibodies in the recipient. The recipient's serum is added to donor lymphocytes to determine this. Only if the crossmatch is negative can the transplant proceed. The recipient is then admitted to the hospital. The surgeons meets the patient and ensures that no contraindications are present (eg, acute infection, pregnancy) and consent is again obtained.

Once the donor organ is accepted, the hand transplant team coordinates a suitable time for the donor procedure and alerts the operating room at the team's hospital about the impending transplant procedure. The required resources and personnel are mobilized.

DONOR RETRIEVAL

The hand transplant team travels to the donor hospital. Little special equipment is needed. The team confirms the brain death certification, consent for donation, and blood group result of the donor. The limb must be inspected by the team to ensure an appropriate match. Discussions are held with the other organ procurement teams about the proposed sequence and the needs of the hand team. The simplest approach is to apply a tourniquet on the limb being procured and to dissect the vessels. The limb is then disarticulated and immediately perfused with University of Wisconsin solution or another perfusion solution of choice. The limb is wrapped in moist sterile gauze and transported in a sterile container filled with iced water at 4 to 6°C. The limb may be continuously perfused with UW solution through a brachial artery cannula during transportation back to the transplant center. A cosmetic prosthesis must be fitted following retrieval on the donor to enable funeral viewing and preserving body integrity.

RECIPIENT TRANSPLANT PROCEDURE

Two teams working simultaneously help reduce the cold ischemia time. The recipient team starts the surgery with dissection of the amputated stump and identifies and marks the blood vessels, tendons, and nerves. The donor team that procured the limb works on the back table and prepares the donor limb. The technical aspects of hand transplantation are similar to hand replantation. The order of bone-artery-few veins-tendon-nerve-remaining veins (BANTNV) is usually followed. Immunosuppression is initiated as per protocol. Induction agents (eg, thymoglobulin, basiliximab, alemtuzumab) and methylprednisolone are begun before restoring the blood flow through the graft.

Being similar to hand reimplantation, the surgical exercise should not be difficult for a center that routinely performs hand surgery. The organizational aspects mainly center on the timing of procurement and recipient procedures and gathering the required manpower for both. The role of the transplant coordinator is critical for the smooth conduct of the procedure.

POSTOPERATIVE CARE AND LONG-TERM MANAGEMENT

The monitoring of the hand for vascular integrity is important in the first few days. Much attention must be paid to implementing immunosuppression as per protocol. In addition, prophylaxis agents to prevent infection are started in the immediate post-transplant period. The transplant physician's guidance is critical in these aspects. It is important to dose the medications appropriately and achieve the target levels of specific agents, particularly the calcineurin inhibitors.

Physical therapy is initiated in the first few days after the procedure. Barring any surgical complications, the patient may be ready to be discharged by the end of a week. Before discharge, the patient and a caregiver receive a one-on-one education by the transplant coordinator about the transplant medications. This aspect is central to the long-term success of the transplanted limb. Unless

the patient understands and complies with the recommendations about medicines and follow-up, including blood tests, blood pressure, and glucose monitoring, the huge effort could be compromised.

There are numerous elements that are essential to the long-term care of the hand transplant recipients. The recipients must be highly motivated to continue long-term physical therapy and continue antirejection medication. There is no escaping the long-term side effects of immunosuppression. These unavoidable side effects of the medications must be actively looked for and treatment instituted appropriately.

Organ transplantation is a lifelong partnership between the transplant center and the organ recipient. Like any relationship, this matures with time and has its ups and downs. Most transplant recipients contact the center for all questions related to their health, largely because many primary care physicians are not experienced in dealing with problems specific to this patient population. The center, in turn, must establish a good working relationship with the organ recipient's local primary care physician to ensure long-term care of chronic problems that develop, such as diabetes and. This partnership is unique and vital to the long-term success of organ transplantation, and hand transplant surgeons must recognize this to the benefit of their patients.

DEALING WITH THE MEDIA AND PUBLIC RELATIONS

Hand transplantation remains a curiosity to the public and the media continues to have tremendous interest in the topic. When a center embarks on hand transplantation, it must be prepared to deal with potentially intense media scrutiny. The media and public relations must be handled with careful planning and preparation.

The hand transplant team should involve the hospital public relations team involved with the project from inception. One individual must be designated to schedule and attend all press meetings, give press releases, and organize interviews of transplant team personnel and recipients. The center must acknowledge the role of the OPO and the donor family after the transplant event. The team must ensure confidentiality of donor family identity and the public must be specifically requested to respect their right to remain anonymous unless they choose otherwise. To avoid misinformation, the transplant team must provide periodic updates on the successes and problems that develop. In terms of increasing public awareness of donation of VCA components and educating the public about the success and life-enhancing aspects of hand transplants, there are many benefits that might be harnessed with a proper strategy.

SUMMARY

Starting a hand transplant program poses tremendous challenges. Solid organ transplantation and hand replantation are time-tested procedures and are now standard of care. Hand transplantation is the amalgamation of the scientific principles of reconstructive surgery and the concepts of organ transplantation. Thus, for any hand transplant program to be successful, there must be collaboration within a multidisciplinary team comprising a core group of hand and transplant surgeons. Such a joint effort can overcome the challenges that are inherent in a complex therapeutic option that integrates different disciplines and organizations during the planning, procedural, and posttransplant phases.

REFERENCES

1. Petruzzo P, Lanzetta M, Dubernard JM, et al. The international registry on hand and composite tissue transplantation. Transplantation 2008;86: 487–92.
2. Jones JW, Gruber SA, Barker JH, et al. Successful hand transplantation. One-year follow-up. Louisville Hand Transplant Team. N Engl J Med 2000;343: 468–73.
3. Lanzetta M, Nolli R, Borgonovo A, et al. Hand transplantation: ethics, immunosuppression and indications. J Hand Surg Br 2001;26:511–6.
4. Pollard MS. Hand transplantation–risks of immunosuppression. J Hand Surg Br 2001;26:517.
5. Brenner MJ, Tung TH, Jensen JN, et al. The spectrum of complications of immunosuppression: is the time right for hand transplantation? J Bone Joint Surg Am 2002;84:1861–70.
6. Ravindra KV, Buell JF, Kaufman CL, et al. Hand transplantation in the United States: experience with 3 patients. Surgery 2008;144:638–43 [discussion: 643–4].
7. Petruzzo P, Badet L, Gazarian A, et al. Bilateral hand transplantation: six years after the first case. Am J Transplant 2006;6:1718–24.
8. Ziegler-Graham K, MacKenzie EJ, Ephraim PL, et al. Estimating the prevalence of limb loss in the United States: 2005 to 2050. Arch Phys Med Rehabil 2008; 89:422–9.
9. Melcer T, Walker GJ, Galarneau M, et al. Midterm health and personnel outcomes of recent combat amputees. Mil Med 2010;175:147–54.
10. Kanitakis J, Jullien D, Petruzzo P, et al. Clinicopathologic features of graft rejection of the first human hand allograft. Transplantation 2003;76:688–93.
11. Klapheke MM, Marcell C, Taliaferro G, et al. Psychiatric assessment of candidates for hand transplantation. Microsurgery 2000;20:453–7.
12. Carroll D. A quantitative test of upper extremity function. J Chronic Dis 1965;18:479–91.
13. Hudak PL, Amadio PC, Bombardier C. Development of an upper extremity outcome measure: the DASH (disabilities of the arm, shoulder and hand) [corrected]. The Upper Extremity Collaborative Group (UECG). Am J Ind Med 1996;29:602–8.
14. Lanzetta M, Petruzzo P, Dubernard JM, et al. Second report (1998-2006) of the International Registry of Hand and Composite Tissue Transplantation. Transpl Immunol 2007;18:1–6.
15. Petruzzo P, Lanzetta M, Dubernard JM, et al. The International Registry on Hand and Composite Tissue Transplantation. Transplantation 2010; 90(12):1590–4.
16. Jablecki J, Kaczmarzyk L, Domanasiewicz A, et al. Hand transplantation–Polish program. Transplant Proc 2010;42:3321–2.
17. Ting A, Terasaki PI. Lymphocyte-dependent antibody cross-matching for transplant patients. Lancet 1975;1:304–6.

Recipient Screening and Selection: Who is the Right Candidate for Hand Transplantation

Jaimie T. Shores, MD

KEYWORDS

- Hand transplantation • Selection • Screening
- Composite tissue allotransplantation

Hand and upper extremity allotransplantation is an experimental reconstructive procedure that is becoming more common as more centers begin clinical programs in composite tissue allotransplantation (CTA). The principles of balancing immunologic rejection in terms of graft versus host disease and host versus graft disease, more commonly appreciated as acute or chronic rejection, are taken from traditional visceral and bone marrow transplantation principles. However, one single and important difference persists. Hand transplantation is a completely elective operation. From a physiologic point of view, this procedure is not necessary to maintain the patient's survival. Hand transplantation is not a life-giving endeavor but a quality of life–giving one. For this reason, it is incumbent upon any center participating in CTA and hand transplantation that patients be selected properly and ethically to mitigate risk. Risk exists not only for the patient, for whom we aggressively try to protect from complications and poor outcomes, but also CTA. Because of the relatively few numbers of these procedures being performed and because CTA is not considered the standard of care in the treatment of complex injuries or deformities, treatment failures early in the development of this field can have negative ramifications that may affect other centers and their ability to perform such procedures for years to come. It is in the best interest of each individual patient and CTA to ensure the safest and best possible outcomes. This can only begin with proper patient selection.

Patient screening is a multistage process which is an all-encompassing look into the patient's life. Anatomic, physiologic, psychological, and social factor data must be collected and evaluated to determine patient eligibility.[1] The most difficult of these are those factors that lend themselves to multiple levels of complexity, such as the psychological and social screening, which are the keys to long-term success regarding patient adherence to immunologic and therapy protocols.[2] Although medical and anatomic factors may be more easily evaluated with discreet variables, psychosocial screening is less concrete and continues to be refined and emphasized in the transplant literature.[2,3] In heart, lung, and combined heart-lung transplant recipients, a review of multiple studies found a medication nonadherence rate prevalence between 11% and 54% among multiple studies, with an average first-year medication nonadherence rate of 20%.[4] In a prospective trial following up liver, lung, and heart transplant recipients for 1 year postoperatively, pretransplant nonadherence was a significant predictor of posttransplant nonadherence.[2] Having less social support and lower scores on conscientiousness personality inventories were also significant predictors. Being unmarried or not living in a stable relationship was the only predictor of graft loss between 6 and 12 months postoperatively. Patient pretransplant nonadherence also predicted those who would experience 6 or more unscheduled hospitalizations during months 6 to 12 postoperatively, whereas self-reported nonadherence before transplant predicted late acute rejection in the study.[2] Thus,

Department of Plastic and Reconstructive Surgery, Johns Hopkins University School of Medicine, 601 North Caroline Street, Suite 8140C, Baltimore, MD 21287, USA
E-mail address: jshores@jhmi.edu

Hand Clin 27 (2011) 539–543
doi:10.1016/j.hcl.2011.07.009
0749-0712/11/$ – see front matter © 2011 Elsevier Inc. All rights reserved.

multifactorial patient personality, social support, and environmental factors seem to have a significant effect on outcome as it relates to adherence or compliance. Although most organ transplant recipients face adherence problems with medications, hand transplant recipients face the same challenges in addition to the challenges of remaining adherent with postoperative hand therapy, which is critical for functional rehabilitation of their graft.

Patient screening typically begins when a patient contacts our office by letter, email, or phone call. Initial data collected include the age, gender, handedness, type and level of injury, date of limb loss, medical and surgical history, and any photos available of the affected limbs, and history of prosthesis use/rehabilitation. This data is collected and the "inquiry" is presented at a weekly CTA administrative meeting. A decision at that time is made as to whether or not the patient is declined based strictly on history or anatomic level, invited for an initial visit to better evaluate the patient to determine eligibility to enroll in screening, or whether more information collection is required to make a decision.

INITIAL VISIT

All patients who will be considered for screening are invited for an initial visit where a more thorough history and directed physical examination are performed by a CTA surgeon. The patients are asked to bring their operative reports and medical records, including prior radiographs and any previous workup for transplantation or medical comorbidity with them. A direct conversation with the patients is undertaken and the specifics of hand transplantation and the particular immunomodulatory protocol are discussed. At this point, each patient has usually met with 3 team members and, in some form, received similar information regarding process, risks, and outcomes related to the world experience multiple times. Their questions are answered.

The initial visit serves both as a way for the CTA team to collect more data to determine the patient's eligibility and for the patient to collect information first hand and decide whether they still have any interest in further pursuing transplantation. If they do, their case is then evaluated once more by the CTA executive team and an invitation to undergo screening is then offered or declined.

SCREENING VISIT

Patient screening is an institutional review board (IRB)-approved process requiring informed consent by the patient to enter. This screening process evaluates the patient anatomically, medically, functionally,

psychologically and psychiatrically, socially, as well as immunologically (**Boxes 1** and **2**). In addition to these factors, some specific inclusion/exclusion criteria exist that are similar to other published criteria (**Box 3**).[5] **Boxes 1–3** are components of the current screening protocols for the University of Pittsburgh Medical Center and the Johns Hopkins University School of Medicine Hand Transplant Programs.

Anatomic Evaluation

The patient is re-examined and interviewed by a hand transplant surgeon. Plain radiographs of both upper extremities are obtained, even in cases of unilateral involvement, for comparison and possible surgical planning. Diagnostic angiography is obtained of the affected limbs to determine arterial and venous anatomy. Venous mapping using ultrasound imaging may also be used. Magnetic resonance imaging of the remaining portion of the extremity may be performed to assess the remaining extrinsic forearm motors and amount of scar tissue present for preoperative planning purposes. Photographs of the evaluated limb and the contralateral limb, even if uninvolved, are taken for comparison regarding reconstruction of length and for possible donor match characteristics such as skin tone and size.

Functional Screening

Functionality is observed by the surgeon with and without prostheses. Patients' rehabilitative histories are explored. Patients who have not made attempts to rehabilitate with the use of prosthetics are excluded. Certified hand therapists also evaluate patients to determine their level of engagement in prior and current therapy regimens and to do baseline functionality testing. Functional magnetic resonance imaging to establish baseline motor and sensory activity within the cortical regions corresponding to the lost extremity is performed.

Medical Screening

Patients undergo screening that includes dental evaluation; gastroenterologic screening, including endoscopy; and evaluation of renal, cardiac, hematologic, and nutritional status and pulmonary function. Any specific medical problems the patient has may undergo more specific evaluation with a consultation from the appropriate specialty. Tobacco and substance use/abuse are assessed.

Box 1
Screening tests from the UPMC Hand Transplant Program

Standard screening test panels

- Hematologic panel
  - Complete blood cell count, differential, reticulocyte count, platelet count
  - ABO blood typing and Rh factor, HLA yping
  - Panel reactive antibodies
  - Prothrombin time/partial thromboplastin time with international normalized ratio
- Metabolic panel
  - Serum electrolytes and renal function panel
  - Urinalysis and creatinine clearance
  - Liver functions tests
  - Dexascan (if indicated)
- Infectious disease panel
  - Cytomegalovirus, Epstein-Barr virus, herpes simplex virus, toxoplasmosis and varicella-zoster virus (IgG and IgM when indicated), human immunodeficiency virus antigen, human T-lymphotropic virus type I/II antibody, antibodies to human immunodeficiency virus 1 and 2, hepatitis C virus, syphilis, hepatitis B core antibody, and hepatitis B surface antigen titers
  - Purified protein derivative/Mantoux skin test
- Cardiopulmonary panel
  - Electrocardiogram and multiple gated acquisition or echocardiogram to check heart
  - Pulmonary function tests with DLC02
- Radiologic panel
  - Ultrasonography of the abdomen (to rule out tumor) and ultrasound imaging of the hand/stump.
  - Computed tomographic scans (computed tomographic angiography and/or conventional angiography)/musculoskeletal magneticresonance imaging of the forearm or hand, functional magnetic resonance imaging studies, and magnetoencephalographic scans.
  - Sinus radiography (to rule out infection or tumor)
  - Chest radiography
  - Plain radiography of bilateral hand, wrist, forearm, and elbow as indicated

---

Box 2
Screening consultations and assessment from the UPMC Hand Transplant Program

Consultations

- Dentistry
- Ophthalmology
- Gastroenterology including esophagogastroduodenoscopy and colonoscopy
- Otolaryngology (ear, nose, and throat)
- Urology (in men, evaluate for prostate or testicular cancer)
- Gynecology (in women, evaluate for possible ovarian, endometrial, uterine, and cervical cancer).
- Transplant psychiatry
- Transplant psychology
- Transplant social work
- Certified hand therapist

Psychosocial screening and functional assessment standardized evaluation tools

- 36-Item Short Form Health Survey: asks patients for views about their health
- Disabilities of the Arm, Shoulder and Hand Instrument: asks patients about their current health and ability to perform certain activities[a]

Psychiatric examination together with the following questionnaires: Perlin Self-Mastery Scale, Rosenberg Self-Esteem Scale, Coping Responses Inventory, Sherwood's Self-Concept Inventory, NEO Personality Scale short form

---

Immunologic Screening

ABO blood type, HLA type, and viral infection status are performed for cytomegalovirus, Epstein-Barr virus, hepatitis C virus, hepatitis A and B viruses, and human immunodeficiency virus. Panel reactive antibodies are evaluated.

Psychiatric Screening

All patients undergo a screening evaluation by a well-experienced transplant psychiatrist to further evaluate the patient for insight into their condition, expectations, motivations, mechanisms of coping, emotional and cognitive preparedness for transplantation, body image concerns, personality organization and risk of regression, preexisting psychiatric illness, possible conditions resulting directly from the trauma of their limb loss, tobacco use, substance use/abuse, and mechanisms/options for social support. This screening may require multiple visits and is an integral part of the

---

Box 3
Exclusion/inclusion criteria from the UPMC Hand Transplant Program

Exclusion criteria

Age <18 years or >69 years

Conditions that affect the immunomodulatory protocol: chronic infections (human immunodeficiency virus infection, hepatitis C), malignancy, preexisting immunologic deficiencies

Conditions that affect surgical success/healing: coagulopathies, hematologic diseases, collagen vascular disorders, connective tissue disorders

Conditions that affect functional outcomes (such as nerve or bone healing): lipopolysaccharidosis, amyloidosis, metabolic or genetic bone diseases

Patients may be excluded for any other concerns developed during the screening process

Inclusion criteria

Ages 18–69 years

No coexisting medical condition that may affect immunomodulatory, surgical, or functional results

No coexisting psychosocial problems

No history of malignancy within the last 10 years or human immunodeficiency virus infection

Consent to cell collection, storage, and bone marrow infusion as part of treatment regimen

Time since amputation >6 months with good faith attempt at prosthesis use/rehabilitation

---

screening process, which also integrates into the patient's psychological and social screening.[6]

Psychological Screening

In addition to evaluation by the transplant psychiatrist, the patient is evaluated by the transplant psychologist, and baseline testing in psychological standard measures for the purpose of establishing measures for future posttransplant comparison is performed. Life stressors, coping mechanisms, and family/social support are explored.

Social Screening

The transplant social worker and transplant coordinator evaluate the patient's resources in terms of financial/health care payer coverage, family support, and mechanisms of accomplishing required postoperative follow-up tasks (transportation, family and friend involvement, ability to obtain lifelong postoperative medications and follow-up for nontransplant medical issues, ability to obtain outpatient therapy, safe living environment and so forth).

PATIENT SELECTION

After completion of screening, the patient's medical, functional, and anatomic data are analyzed by the transplant medical/surgical team. Patients with obvious medical contraindications to a potentially long and physiologically taxing surgery with physically demanding recovery period are excluded, such as those with preexisting liver, kidney, heart, and lung disease or substantial risk factors for such disease. Any patient found to have malignancy on screening is referred for appropriate care but excluded. Anatomic factors are then considered. Patients with nondominant unilateral amputations are considered on a cases-by-case basis with a much higher threshold for approving transplantation that those with dominant unilateral amputations and those with bilateral amputations. Anatomic levels, soft tissue quality, venous and arterial anatomy, neuroanatomy, muscle bulk and length, and skeletal anatomy, including the condition of the extremity from the shoulder to the level of amputation, are discussed. Some patients may be excluded because of these considerations, or recommendations for transplantation above the nearest retained joint to maximize function and surgical success may be made a condition of transplantation.

The medical/surgical team then considers the patient's psychiatric and psychosocial evaluations. Evidence of Axis I disorders is disqualifying, whereas patients with significant Axis II disorders may or may not be disqualified depending on their coping abilities and social support. Axis III disorders are considered on a case-by-case basis to predict how they may affect the patient's ultimate functional outcome. At this time, we believe that substantial social support in the form of verifiable friends and family members who commit to assisting the recipients with their activities of daily living and transportation to and from therapy, clinic, hospital, and laboratory visits and are willing to stay with the recipient for the first 3 months postoperatively is a mandatory component of the patient's social support system.

Those candidates who seem satisfactory from these considerations are then presented at a multidisciplinary meeting consisting of medical/surgical team members, hand therapists, transplant psychiatrist, transplant psychologist, transplant coordinators, and social workers for final case discussion. All comments are considered, and final approval is by consensus of medical/surgical/psychiatry team members. Patients may be approved and invited to participate in the IRB-approved transplantation protocol, may not be approved but remain under consideration for future approval pending change of any resolvable issue that would be an impediment to their success, or may be declined from participation further within the IRB protocol for transplantation.

SUMMARY

Hand transplantation is an elective non–life saving but quality of life–giving surgery for good candidates that is not without risk.[7] Graft loss may result in a more proximal level of amputation and may relegate the patient to a worse level of function than existed before transplant. Substantial therapy is required to obtain functional improvement after transplantation. Immunomodulation requires a high level of patient adherence to therapeutic protocols. Even with strict adherence, rejection episodes may occur, and unwanted side effects from immunosuppressive agents may develop that cause patients to be less compliant or compromise other organ systems (renal failure, diabetes mellitus, lymphoproliferative disorders, malignancy, opportunistic infection, reactivation of latent infections).[7–10] An illustrative case is the first hand transplant performed in the modern era of immunosuppression, which occurred in France in 1998.[11,12] The graft was removed 29 months after transplant with severe rejection due to long-term medication noncompliance and eventual complete cessation of immunosuppression by the patient. A total of 49 hand transplant cases were reported in 2010 worldwide (which still did not include transplants from several active centers), which documented multiple infectious and metabolic sequelae of immunosuppression.[7] Twelve additional patients from China were briefly reported in the same publication as well as elsewhere[1] with 6 recipients (50% of participants) requiring graft removal, most notably for medication adherence/availability issues. Furthermore, 5 grafts have been lost in the US and European countries at the time of publication (including both hands from the first US attempt at combined hand-face transplant), and one fatality has been reported (first world attempt at combined hand-face transplantation).[7]

For these reasons, all persons involved in CTA must be extremely judicious in patient selection, both for the benefit of those whose lives we hope to improve and for the betterment of CTA, which at this early juncture cannot tolerate substantial failures. In fact, patient screening and selection is the most critical element to successful transplantation outcomes and cannot be overemphasized in terms of importance in the overall scheme of an active CTA program. Some may view transplant failure due to patient adherence with therapy or medication regimens as failure on the part of the patient. However, these are failures in patient selection, which result from inadequate screening practices. No screening practice is perfect regarding predicting posttransplant success or failure. However, as CTA continues to develop, these practices and procedures will also continue to evolve to help mitigate risk and maximize success as the cornerstone of these life-changing transplantation programs.

REFERENCES

1. Tobin GR, Breidenbach WC 3rd, Pidwell DJ, et al. Transplantation of the hand, face, and composite structures: evolution and current status. Clin Plast Surg 2007;34:271–8, ix–x.
2. Dobbels F, Vanhaecke J, Dupont L, et al. Pretransplant predictors of posttransplant adherence and clinical outcome: an evidence base for pretransplant psychosocial screening. Transplantation 2009;87:1497–504.
3. Dobbels F, De Geest S, Cleemput I, et al. Psychosocial and behavioral selection criteria for solid organ transplantation. Prog Transplant 2001;11:121–30 [quiz: 131–2].
4. De Geest S, Dobbels F, Fluri C, et al. Adherence to the therapeutic regimen in heart, lung, and heart-lung transplant recipients. J Cardiovasc Nurs 2005;20:S88–98.
5. Ravindra KV, Buell JF, Kaufman CL, et al. Hand transplantation in the United States: experience with 3 patients. Surgery 2008;144:638–43 [discussion: 643–4].
6. Amirlak B, Gonzalez R, Gorantla V, et al. Creating a hand transplant program. Clin Plast Surg 2007;34:279–89, x.
7. Petruzzo P, Lanzetta M, Dubernard JM, et al. The international registry on hand and composite tissue transplantation. Transplantation 2010;90:1590–4.
8. Brandacher G, Ninkovic M, Piza-Katzer H, et al. The Innsbruck hand transplant program: update at 8 years after the first transplant. Transplant Proc 2009;41:491–4.
9. Kaufman CL, Blair B, Murphy E, et al. A new option for amputees: transplantation of the hand. J Rehabil Res Dev 2009;46:395–404.
10. Andrew Lee WP, Nguyen VT. Perspectives on hand transplantation. Clin Plast Surg 2005;32:463–70, v.
11. Kanitakis J, Jullien D, Petruzzo P, et al. Clinicopathologic features of graft rejection of the first human hand allograft. Transplantation 2003;76:688–93.
12. Andrew Lee WP. The debate over hand transplantation. J Hand Surg Am 2002;27:757–9.

Donor-Related Issues in Hand Transplantation

Sue V. McDiarmid, MD[a],*, Kodi K. Azari, MD[a,b]

KEYWORDS

• Hand transplantation • Donation • Procurement • Allocation

The process of transplantation is unique in medicine. It relies on the altruism of the public to donate organs, at a time of great personal turmoil, to help protect the life and well-being of another, usually an anonymous stranger. The success of hand transplantation has exactly the same dependence on the public trust. The ability to obtain consent from a family for donation in an ethical manner, while protecting their confidentiality, is the essential first step without which any transplant cannot proceed.

Although obtaining consent for donation is the critical element for a transplant of any kind, a highly specialized infrastructure is required to support the entire procurement endeavor of both solid organs and tissues. In the United States, this infrastructure is provided by the 58 organ procurement organizations (OPOs) located throughout the country. Similar organizations exist in other countries. The OPOs provide procurement and distribution services to donor hospitals and to transplant centers for procured solid organs. OPOs also procure tissues and act as conduits to tissue banks and repositories. Once a potential donor is identified, the OPO personnel are responsible for all aspects of the consent process, screening for the risk of transmission of infectious disease, management of the donor after brain death (or during the process of withdrawal of support in the case of donation after cardiac death), coordinating the donor procurement teams in the operating room, and packaging and labeling of organs and tissues. In the case of solid-organ procurement, the OPO also has the task of distributing organs in accordance with often complex allocation algorithms. Jurisdiction and oversight of OPO activities for solid-organ procurement are provided by the United Network of Organ Sharing (UNOS), which operates the Organ Procurement Transplant Network (OPTN)[1] under contract with the Human Resources and Services Administration (HRSA); the US Federal Drug Administration (FDA) oversees tissue and cell procurement.[2] The main role of the OPTN is to ensure the equitable and medically effective use of human organs. To fulfill this mandate, the OPTN has detailed procedures stipulating standards for transplant centers and OPOs and is responsible for overseeing the allocation system in general. In contrast, the FDA's jurisdiction over tissues is mostly related to tissue banks and processors, with the ultimate goal of ensuring the safety of the final tissue or cell-based product. Many of these FDA regulations are found in 2 documents: "Final rule: Eligibility and Determination of Donors of Human Cells, Tissues, and Cellular and Tissue-Based Products 21 CRF 1271" (available at www.fda.gov/cber/rules/suitdonor.pdf) and "Current Good Tissue Practice for Human Cells, Tissue and Cellular and Tissue Based Product Establishments: Inspection and Enforcement: Final Rule" (implemented in 2007 and available at www.fda.gov/cber/gdlns/tissdonor.htm). The FDA provides no guidance to OPOs with regard to donor consent, protection of the donor family, procurement practices, or allocation.

The authors have nothing to declare.

[a] Department of Pediatrics and Surgery, David Geffen School of Medicine, University of California, 10833 Le Conte Ave, Los Angeles, CA 90097, USA

[b] Department of Orthopedic Surgery, University of California, 10945 Le Conte Avenue, Room 33-55G PVUB, Los Angeles, CA 90095, USA

* Corresponding author. Division of Pediatric Gastroenterology, Hepatology and Nutrition, UCLA Medical Center Room 12-383 MDCC, 10833 Le Conte Avenue, Los Angeles, CA 90095.

E-mail address: smcdiarmid@mednet.ucla.edu

Currently, in the United States, a vascularized composite tissue allograft (VCA), such as a hand, is defined as a tissue; however, there is now debate as to whether VCAs should be recategorized as organs.[3] In many respects, the donation procedure required for hand transplantation is much more similar to that for a solid organ compared with tissue procurement. First, unlike tissue recovery, which is performed sometimes hours after donor asystole, a hand allograft is usually procured from a heart beating donor. It has already been emphasized in hand transplantation that limiting cold ischemia time preferably to less than 12 hours is important.[4] Therefore, coordination with other procurement teams, which often number as many as there are organs to be recovered, is paramount, as each team is under the same pressure to limit cold ischemia time. The other essential area of common interest between the recovery of a hand compared with a solid organ is donor assessment and management. In particular, determining the risk of disease transmission by the donor is critically important. In a relatively short time period, standardized screening tests must be obtained, judgments made on whether there are relative or absolute contraindications to offering organs, and communication made to transplant teams and candidates of a potentially high-risk donor.[5] In contrast, for tissue procurement, with the possible exception of corneas, the determination of risk for transmission of disease is just as rigorous but can proceed at a more measured pace. There are many published reports detailing the transmission of serious infectious diseases, including human immunodeficiency virus (HIV), to recipients of infected donors not identified using the standard screening tests.[6] These examples provide a chilling reminder of how compressed the timelines are in the donor recovery process. Although nucleic acid testing for hepatitis B and C and HIV has provided more accurate and rapid testing,[7,8] the need for highly trained personnel to meticulously perform and analyze these tests cannot be overemphasized. This is equally applicable to the procurement of a hand as it is to the procurement of a solid organ.

Another essential role fulfilled by the OPO for solid-organ procurement, which is equally important for hand procurement, is the ability to quickly communicate vital information regarding donor stability, biological compatibility, and details of donor management with surgical recovery teams. A further similarity between hand procurement and solid-organ procurement exists at the end of the procurement procedure. Under the duress of time, the organ or the hand must be safely and appropriately cooled, stored, packaged, labeled,

and set up for transportation. All these detailed procedures have already been developed for solid-organ donors and are directly applicable to the procurement of a VCA.

Despite the similarities between the procurement procedures needed for either a VCA or a solid-organ donation, and the ability of OPOs to provide this service, the established OPO infrastructure cannot be officially used for VCA donation while VCAs remain defined as tissues. As a consequence, each transplant center wishing to establish a hand transplant program is forced by necessity to establish self-styled protocols with their local, and sometimes, regional OPOs. Although no uniformity or standardization has been currently imposed on this process, in general, the protocols developed by hand transplant programs adhere closely to solid-organ procurement protocols. However, there are some important specific policies relevant to hand transplantation that are worthy of further discussion.

SPECIFIC REQUIRED ELEMENTS FOR HAND TRANSPLANT PROCUREMENT PROTOCOLS
Training Requirements

The OPO coordinators are essential to the donation process. Although hand transplantation is becoming more publicized, the number of procedures is still low in comparison to solid-organ transplantation. The life-saving benefits of solid-organ transplantation are easily appreciated, whereas hand transplantation is a life-enhancing procedure. The better informed the OPO requestors are about the benefits and outcomes of hand transplantation, the more effectively they can approach a donor family. In addition, the OPO coordinators need to know the operative aspects of the procurement procedure, and the logistics of coordinating the hand procurement team with other solid-organ procurement teams. Essential to this education process is the willingness of the transplant center team to interact personally with the OPO staff, providing didactic presentations as well as forums for interactive discussion.

Another important, but often overlooked, element is the training and education of the donor hospital staff. The donor hospital is often a small community hospital whose staff may not yet have had exposure to the success of hand transplantation and the increasing need for donors. Because there are many potential donor hospitals within a given OPO, disseminating this new information can be challenging. Some OPOs have used newsletters or online education materials to reach out to their potential donor hospital base.

Again, the time and input of the hand transplant center team are invaluable to provide appropriate educational materials. The effort is time well spent. A first-time hand procurement in a donor hospital in which staff are unprepared, or perhaps uncomfortable with the removal of a readily visible external body part, could set a negative precedent and hinder further procurement procedures.

The Consent Process

Much has been written about the consent process for solid-organ transplantation.[9] Currently in the United States, the conversion rate, that is, the number of actual donors recovered divided by the number of reported eligible deaths, is about 69.3% nationwide.[10] The environment in which consent is requested, the training and skill of the requestor, and the attitudes of the critical care team are paramount to the eventual likelihood that consent is obtained.[11] Cultural, religious, and educational factors are just some of the influences important in determining if individuals will indicate their wish to be donors[12,13] and if families will later respect that intent. However, despite the legally binding directives of individuals expressed on state registries, or on drivers' licenses, the consent or refusal of the donor family is generally respected. Family consent is perhaps even more important for these new requests for visible body parts. Persons who sign up to be a donor in response to well-publicized pleas to give the gift of life may not be thinking that they are also signing up for the possibility that their hands might be donated. We should anticipate that donor families may well view the request to donate a part of a limb quite differently than, for example, the request for donation of a heart. As individuals, we view our hands as intimate body parts performing complex and highly individualized tasks, and an extension of our own personality. For this reason, the barrier to consent for such a visible identifiable part of a loved one's physical presence is likely to be substantially higher than for a solid organ.[14] From the perspective of the donor family, another unique aspect to hand donation is that the physical integrity of the body is visibly altered in what may seem a startling way. Funeral arrangements, including the offer to provide a cosmetic prosthesis of a similar skin tone and size for families, should be part of the conversation.

Most importantly, requestors must approach the subject of possible donation of a hand(s) with great delicacy and in such a way that it does not risk derailing obtaining consent for life-saving solid organs for which more than 100,000 patients in the United States are currently waiting.[15] In developing hand donation procurement protocols, obtaining consent for solid-organ donation should be secured first. The request for a potential hand donation should be made separately at the discretion of the requestor, and, if successful, a second consent signed.

The other aspect of the consent process, which has always been held as an important principle in solid-organ donation, is protecting the confidentiality of the donor family and the anonymity of the donor. However, the hand may have identifying features, and of course has its own unique set of fingerprints. The requestor also needs to inform the donor family that despite the OPO's best efforts, protection of confidentiality may not always be assured. This is partly secondary to the intense media interest that these transplants are generating, as well as the possibility that surface features on the hand itself could identify the donor.

These unique and unusual aspects of the request process for donation of a hand will require that requestors, usually highly trained OPO coordinators, will need to be specifically trained to address the donor family's perceptions and encourage their understanding of the benefit of a hand transplant.

REQUIREMENTS FOR RECIPIENT AND DONOR DATA

The OPO requires explicit inclusion and exclusion criteria developed by the hand transplant team to initiate donor screening. As an example, in our program we use the inclusion and exclusion criteria shown in **Boxes 1** and **2**. The hand transplant team must also provide the OPO with donor characteristics that would allow an appropriate match with the proposed recipient. These include the usual parameters, such as gender, age, ethnicity, and ABO type. To date, HLA matching has not been shown to be necessary. The unique recipient characteristics that the OPO also requires relate to the hand size and skin color of the recipient. For unilateral hand transplantation, photographs of the other hand are helpful. The OPO requires a range of the recipient's acceptable skin tones as designated on standardized color cards so that a potential donor's skin tone can be matched with the recipient. Also, detailed measurements of the hand and digits of the recipient are needed by the OPO and the OPO staff will need training in the method to perform these standardized measurements. **Fig. 1** shows the standardized measurements for the hand and digits used by the UCLA hand transplant team.

During the donor assessment process, it is also important that efficient communication channels

---

Box 1
Extremity/hand transplant donor selection criteria

Inclusion Criteria

- Consent for donation/recovery of limb(s) (single or bilateral)
- Compatible or identical ABO blood type to the intended recipient
- Comparable age with intended recipient (at the discretion of transplanting surgeon)
- Same/similar ethnicity to the intended recipient
- Skin tone similar to the intended recipient, as defined by color chart range and/or photograph
- Hair pattern similar to the intended recipient (at the discretion of transplanting surgeon)
- No identifying marks on the hand/limb to be transplanted, including distinguishing birthmarks and tattoos

---

Box 2
Extremity/hand transplant donor selection criteria

Absolute Exclusion Criteria

- Risk for donor transmission of disease as determined by the physician based on the Centers for Disease Control guidelines for high-risk donors as used for solid transplantation and FDA guidelines for tissue donation
- Evidence of HIV, hepatitis B, or hepatitis C infection
- Current malignancy
- Paralysis of the hand/limb intended for transplant
- Inherited peripheral neuropathy
- Infectious, postinfection, or inflammatory (axonal or demyelinating) neuropathy
- Systemic disease with associated neuropathy (including diabetes, alcoholism, amyloidosis)
- Toxic neuropathy, ie, heavy metal poisoning, drug toxicity, industrial agent exposure
- Rheumatoid arthritis or extensive/severe osteoarthritis
- Significant trauma to the hand/limb intended for transplant
- Connective tissue disease

Relative Exclusion Criteria

- Viral encephalitis
- Paralysis of the hand/limb intended for transplant
- Uncontrolled hypertension
- System disease with associated neuropathy (including diabetes, alcoholism, amyloidosis)
- Hypertension requiring 2 or more medications for control
- Vasculopathy

Final determination of donor suitability is made at the discretion of the transplant physician(s).

---

between the OPO and the hand transplant team have been previously established. For solid-organ recoveries, OPO staff are now very familiar with the Internet-based data-sharing system made possible by technology provided by UNOS. However, for a hand transplant recovery, which is outside the UNOS system, alternate communication methods, including the ability to transmit data and images, are required. Because most hand transplant donors will also likely be solid-organ donors, OPO staff, already under pressure to place multiple organs under time constraints, will need an efficient and streamlined communication system to avoid delay in the placement of other organs.

DONOR MANAGEMENT AND OPERATING ROOM PROCEDURES

For the most part, the principles of donor management for solid-organ retrieval are applicable for hand recovery. The exception is the placement of arterial and venous lines in the upper extremity(s) to be procured. At the time the OPO coordinator considers hand donation likely, specific instructions should be given to the critical care and donor management teams to avoid placing such indwelling catheters. Also, emphasis should be placed on protecting perfusion to the extremity to be procured.

Donor operating room procedures require careful planning and discussion not only with OPO coordinators but also with the surgical teams in the area that procure solid organs. The overriding principle that both the hand and organ recovery teams should all agree to is that the successful recovery of life-saving solid organs always takes precedence over the hand recovery process. Adhering to this principle becomes of critical importance if the donor becomes unstable, requiring the solid-organ recovery teams to act quickly, unencumbered by any other considerations. However, in a stable donor, there is considerable benefit to the quality of the donor limb if

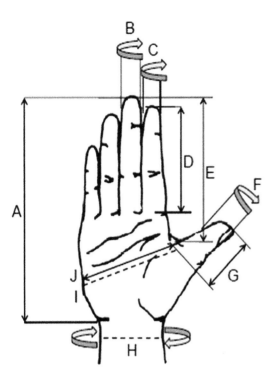

Fig. 1. Measurements for the hand and digits used by the UCLA hand transplant team. A, length of hand from fold to tip of middle finger; B, circumference of middle finger; C, circumference of index finger; D, length of index finger; E, length from first web space to middle finger; F, circumference of thumb; G, length of thumb from first web space; H, wrist circumference; I, hand circumference at Kaplan's cardinal line; J, Kaplan's cardinal line; K, ulnar length from the olecranon process to the styloid process.

procured first, before peripheral perfusion is compromised and cold ischemia time increased during the longer organ recovery process.[16] Limb recovery, as outlined in detail elsewhere, is a straightforward and rapid process. Because the amputation is done under tourniquet control, there is minimal blood loss and very little chance that the limb procurement will destabilize the donor. However, to avoid confrontation and confusion in the donor operating room, clear guidelines and a detailed sequence of events must have been previously agreed on by all parties. In developing our protocol with our local OPO, we developed a 2 scenarios. In scenario A, after 1 thoracic team and 1 abdominal recovery team arrive at the donor hospital, the patient is transported to the operating room. The hand recovery team asks if they can begin the arm recovery before the incision for the solid organs. If all transplant teams and centers agree, the hand recovery commences before the incisions for organ

recovery. If any transplant team opposes, all teams proceed with scenario B. In scenario B, the abdominal and thoracic teams begin the organ donation process and dissection. All applicable vessels are isolated. Just before heparin is given and cannulation is started, the recovery teams pause the organ recovery. The arm is then set up for procurement by the hand recovery team. The arm is recovered usually within 30 to 40 minutes. Once the recovery is completed, the tourniquet remains intact until after cross clamping. The organ recovery teams then proceed with cross clamping and procuring the organs.

The OPO and hand transplant team also need to develop a standardized basic instrument list for the donor hospital to provide for the limb recovery. Specialized instruments and devices need to be prepacked and brought to the hospital by the hand recovery team. After recovery of the disarticulated limb, the additional back table preparation requires the hand recovery team to bring their own solutions, instruments, and perfusion catheters.

The hand recovery team is also responsible for donor reconstruction, including tying off all vessels and appropriately closing the incision at the stump. If it has been established previously that the family requests a prosthesis, this should also be provided by the hand recovery team before departing the donor hospital.

The OPO and hand transplant team also need to establish procedures for appropriate labeling wrapping, packaging, and transportation of the recovered extremity. The labeling needs to differentiate whether the extremity is right or left; if bilateral extremities are recovered, separate labeling is required for each. The labeling also needs to include a donor identification number. Because labeling, wrapping, packaging, and cold storage of extremities have not yet been standardized, these details are an important aspect of the protocol developed for limb recovery.

Developing such extensive and detailed policies and procedures for hand procurement requires a significant commitment of time and effort between the OPO and the hand transplant team. In our experience, this was time well spent and resulted in an efficient procurement for our first hand transplant. The protocol that we developed with our local OPO has now been readily shared with neighboring OPOs without any further modifications.

LISTING AND ALLOCATION

In the United States, there are no listing criteria for potential hand transplant recipients; neither is there a national database for listing all approved candidates. This is in sharp contrast to the well-established listing criteria for solid-organ transplant candidates. It is a specific role of the OPTN/UNOS to maintain the list, and collect the data required to meet the allocation policies for each organ. Without any similar infrastructure to support hand transplantation (or VCA transplantation in general), it is up to individual centers and OPOs to forge relationships that will allow for the procurement and distribution of VCAs. Allocation policies to determine which candidate receives an organ do not exist for VCA. Up to now the number of candidates awaiting hand transplantation has been small, and competition for donors between centers is minimal. Hand transplant programs and the OPO community have cooperated to create their own local and regional sharing understandings. However, these ad hoc arrangements do not provide the best access for candidates waiting to find suitably matched hand donors. To date, the donor pool for hand transplantation has been small. This is more likely a reflection of infrequent requests for donation rather than an inherent lack of suitable donors. As the number of hand transplant centers in the United States increases, the number of candidates will also increase. The likely barrier to finding an appropriate donor will be the need to closely match donor and recipient skin tone and hand size. The traditional allocation algorithm for solid-organ transplantation has favored a tiered system in which donors are allocated preferentially to local candidates, followed by regional and then national sharing. Inequities based on this arbitrary geographic division into local units and regions have resulted.[17] This system is poorly suited to hand transplantation in which broad sharing of donors to find the right match will be necessary. Without policies to promote broad sharing of potential hand donors, there will be little incentive for OPOs that do not have a nearby hand transplant program to initiate requests for hand donors. If organized on a national system, it could be envisioned that the only geographic boundary limiting allocation would be the estimated cold ischemia time. However, until a national, unbiased organization is appointed to provide the infrastructure that would make possible broad sharing of available hand donors, growth in this new field of transplantation will be stalled.

Another important issue not yet addressed is how to prioritize who will receive a specific donation that matches for more than one candidate. Because there is no apparent advantage to more precise biological matching beyond blood type, and given that these are not life-saving

transplants, waiting time would seem to be the most logical tiebreaker. However, without a method to list patients and therefore calculate time waiting on the list, even this simplest of allocation principles cannot be instituted.

The national organization most suited to provide the emerging field of hand transplantation with a mechanism to list and fairly allocate organs already exists. The OPTN was specifically created to do just this. However, whereas VCAs are still officially designated as tissues, the OPTN/UNOS system, by federal regulation, is not authorized to fulfill this role. The FDA, which does have jurisdiction over VCA donations, has no strategies in place to address the specific donation and allocation needs of VCAs.

OVERSIGHT OF HAND DONATION

As already discussed, in the United States there is no entity that is charged with oversight regarding the practice of hand transplantation. For solid-organ transplantation, the OPTN/UNOS bears this responsibility and has put in place a rigorous system that not only strives to develop fair and safe allocation policies but also provides oversight to ensure these policies are adhered to. In addition, the OPOs, so essential to advancing the field of hand transplantation, are already under the jurisdiction and oversight of the OPTN. It seems an unnecessary and costly redundancy to create a new parallel universe to oversee VCA donation. Based on years of experience in trying to ensure appropriate donation and allocation policies for organ transplantation, transplant physicians and surgeons have clearly stated that they believe that the appropriate overseer for VCA donation is the OPTN/UNOS.[18] Leaders in the OPO community have made similar statements and the growing number of surgeons and physicians involved in VCA transplant programs have also come to the same conclusion. In response, the HRSA asked for public comment in a notice published in the Federal Register in May 2008. However, to date there has been no action taken.

The urgency to resolve this issue is that there are several potentially serious consequences if donation practices for hand transplantation continue to operate in a vacuum. We, as a transplant community, are open to 4 potential vulnerabilities. The first is the loss of public trust should there be a situation in which a hand transplant procurement does not go smoothly. The public expects us to perform organ and tissue recovery in an ethical manner, and, to this end, it is essential that we provide oversight and transparency.

Our second vulnerability is the possibility that real or perceived inequities in donor allocation will occur if there is no independent, nontransplant center–driven entity responsible for the development and oversight of allocation policies. Our third vulnerability is our inability to track outcomes without a database. As related to donation, this is particularly important for understanding the impact of donor factors on allograft function and for tracking donor-transmitted disease. Our fourth vulnerability is the undermining of the donor hospital, OPO, and transplant center relationship when there is no standardization of procedures linking these entities. This three-partner relationship is vital to the success of donation and to preserve the ethical standards of donation practices. Oversight is needed to protect all 3 parties, without which all 3 partners are at risk of censure. Just one negative press release involving a hand transplant procurement could not only be highly detrimental to the advancement of our field but also have a significant impact on donation rates for life-saving solid-organ transplants.

The obvious solution to the lack of oversight of donation for hand and other VCAs is to incorporate this function into the role of the OPTN. The same oversight mechanisms already established by the OPTN for solid-organ transplantation can easily be adapted to provide the same level of oversight for hand and other VCA donations. The experience the OPTN/UNOS bring to this field would be invaluable to us in the future.

SUMMARY

Hand transplantation is an exciting new frontier in transplantation. To advance the field, we need to increase the number of hand donors and improve access to potential recipients. To achieve this, developing standardized protocols for hand donation and officially empowering our OPOs to coordinate this essential function are vitally important. Also essential to the effectiveness of hand donation is the establishment of a national waiting list and a donor and candidate database that will allow the development of allocation polices with broad sharing within the limits of safe cold ischemia time. Transparency, public accountability, and oversight of this new field are expected by the public, on whom we depend for our donors, and by our patients, who depend on us.

REFERENCES

1. McDiarmid SV, Pruett TL, Graham WK. The oversight of solid organ transplantation in the United States. Am J Transplant 2008;8(4):739–44.

2. McAllister DR, Joyce MJ, Mann BJ, et al. Allograft update: the current status of tissue regulation, procurement, processing, and sterilization. Am J Sports Med 2007;35(12):2148–58.

3. Pondrom S. What's in a name? HRSA and the FDA consider adding vascularized composite allografts to their definition of "organs". Am J Transplant 2010;10(9):1953.

4. Gordon CR, Siemionow M. Requirements for the development of a hand transplantation program. Ann Plast Surg 2009;63(3):262–73.

5. Halpern SD, Shaked A, Hasz RD, et al. Informing candidates for solid-organ transplantation about donor risk factors. N Engl J Med 2008;358(26): 2832–7.

6. Ison MG, Hager J, Blumberg E, et al. Donor-derived disease transmission events in the United States: data reviewed by the OPTN/UNOS Disease Transmission Advisory Committee. Am J Transplant 2009;9(8):1929–35.

7. Pruss A, Caspari G, Kruger DH, et al. Tissue donation and virus safety: more nucleic acid amplification testing is needed. Transpl Infect Dis 2010;12(5): 375–86.

8. Humar A, Morris M, Blumberg E, et al. Nucleic acid testing (NAT) of organ donors: is the 'best' test the right test? A consensus conference report. Am J Transplant 2010;10(4):889–99.

9. Rey MM, Ware LB, Matthay MA, et al. Informed consent in research to improve the number and quality of deceased donor organs. Crit Care Med 2011;39(2):280–3.

10. Wynn JJ, Alexander CE. Increasing organ donation and transplantation: the U.S. experience over the past decade. Transpl Int 2011;24(4):324–32.

11. DuBois JM, Anderson EE. Attitudes toward death criteria and organ donation among healthcare personnel and the general public. Prog Transplant 2006;16(1):65–73.

12. Siminoff L, Mercer MB, Graham G, et al. The reasons families donate organs for transplantation: implications for policy and practice. J Trauma 2007;62(4): 969–78.

13. Salim A, Malinoski D, Schulman D, et al. The combination of an online organ and tissue registry with a public education campaign can increase the number of organs available for transplantation. J Trauma 2010;69(2):451–4.

14. Siemionow MZ, Rampazzo A, Gharb BB. Addressing religious and cultural differences in views on transplantation, including composite tissue allotransplantation. Ann Plast Surg 2011;66(4):410–5.

15. Anker AE, Feeley TH. Asking the difficult questions: message strategies used by organ procurement coordinators in requesting familial consent to organ donation. J Health Commun 2011;16(6): 643–59.

16. Schuind F, Abramowicz D, Schneeberger S. Hand transplantation: the state-of-the-art. J Hand Surg Eur Vol 2007;32(1):2–17.

17. Ellison MD, Edwards LB, Edwards EB, et al. Geographic differences in access to transplantation in the United States. Transplantation 2003;76(9):1389–94.

18. Cendales L, Granger D, Henry M, et al. Implementation of vascularized composite allografts in the United States: recommendations from the ASTS VCA Ad Hoc Committee and the Executive Committee. Am J Transplant 2011; 11(1):13–7.

Ethical, Financial, and Policy Considerations in Hand Transplantation

Jeff Chang, MS, MD, David W. Mathes, MD*

KEYWORDS

- Hand • Transplantation • Ethics • Immunosuppression
- Financial • Program

In 1964, surgeons in Ecuador attempted the first hand transplant. However, this transplant was performed without the availability of modern immunosuppression, and the allograft was rejected in approximately 2 weeks. Although the next attempt to transplant a human hand was 34 years later, interest in the transplantation of composite tissue allografts continued in the laboratory. Advances in understanding of the immunology related to composite tissue allotransplantation and improved immunosuppressive medications, coupled with success in the clinical transplantation of organs such as lung and intestine, led surgeons to believe that the time was right to revisit clinical transplantation of the human hand.

The first successful hand transplant was performed on September 23, 1998, in Lyon, France. The recipient was a 48-year-old man who, in 1984, lost his right forearm in a saw accident.[1,2] Although initially the transplant was a success, the patient was noncompliant with his immunosuppression, resulting in multiple episodes of rejection, and he ultimately sought to remove the rejected allograft in 2001. This incident highlighted the importance of improving the selection process and revealed the psychological stresses experienced by a hand transplant recipient. Despite this initial setback, there have now been, according to the International Registry on Hand and Composite Tissue Transplantation, 49 hands transplanted onto 33 recipients.[3]

The 1-year graft survival on current immunosuppression has been excellent, and long-term survival is promising, with the longest surviving hand transplant now greater than 12 years.[3] In addition to allograft survival, reports have documented the return of varying degrees of motor function and sensation, and functional magnetic resonance imaging studies have shown cortical reintegration of the transplanted hand. The early success of hand transplantation has led some to consider hand transplantation as a standard of care for bilateral hand amputees. Hand transplants have now been performed at multiple institutions around the world and there is increasing evidence of the therapeutic and psychological advantages of these transplants compared with traditional options for upper limb amputees.

The success of the emerging field of reconstructive transplantation, in general, and hand transplantation, in particular, depends on the continued reevaluation of the critical nonsurgical issues such as the ethical and financial viability of hand transplantation. There are still critics who argue the ethics of transplanting a nonlifesaving organ such as the human hand. In addition, some investigators have suggested that hand transplantation may not be a cost-effective treatment of hand amputees (especially in unilateral cases). This article examines the critical issues surrounding the ethical justification and financial support for transplantation of the human hand. In addition, the importance of establishing rules and regulations to ensure the safety and continued viability of this exciting area of surgery is discussed.

ETHICAL CONSIDERATIONS

Hand transplantation, like any operation, is subject to a set of ethical guidelines. The ethical discussion for hand transplantation focuses on the following principles: risks versus benefits, nonmaleficence

Division of Plastic and Reconstructive Surgery, Department of Surgery, University of Washington, Seattle, WA, USA
* Corresponding author.
E-mail address: dwmathes@u.washington.edu

Hand Clin 27 (2011) 553–560
doi:10.1016/j.hcl.2011.07.006

versus beneficence, paternalism versus autonomy, and informed consent.

Risk Versus Benefit

One of the central arguments against hand transplantation is that the risks of transplantation imposed on the recipient exceed its benefits. To truly grasp this concept, the risks and benefits of the procedure must be clearly defined and delineated.

In solid organ transplantation, such as liver, heart, and lung transplantation, the graft is essential for survival. Physicians rarely hesitate when faced with these life-sustaining operations. However, making decisions about hand transplantation is more complicated. The patient without a hand is not faced with the choice of receiving a transplant or dying, unlike potential recipients of solid organs such as liver. Transplantation of the hand is not essential for survival, and the act of undergoing hand transplantation has the potential to increase the recipient's chance of mortality. In addition, the value of hand transplantation can only be determined based on the quality of life derived from the procedure rather than the quantity of life added after a life-sustaining transplant.[4]

Thus, the critics of hand transplantation maintain that, given the level of risk, the mere improvement of the quality of life without the addition of quantity of life may not be an ethical bargain. Proponents acknowledge that hand transplantation is not lifesaving, but point out that other transplants, such as renal and pancreas, may also not be lifesaving.[5] Renal patients can be maintained on dialysis and, hence, do not absolutely require a renal transplant to preserve their quantity of life. Most physicians express few ethical concerns about transplanting a kidney to improve quality of life despite the risks. However, some of these same physicians question the validity of hand transplantation despite it being based on a similar exchange of risk for improvement of quality of life. What can account for this difference in attitude?

The defined risk to the recipient of a hand transplant is largely based on the need for long-term immunosuppression. The surgery itself carries particular risks, but most of the risk results from the patient's exposure to lifelong multidrug maintenance immunosuppression. Clearly, the transplant literature has shown that immunosuppression predisposes recipients to infection and malignancy. Along the same lines, reports also show development of malignancy and unique transplant-related problems such as posttransplant lymphoproliferative disease (PTLD). The medications themselves have side effects including hypertension, diabetes, nephrotoxicity, and Cushing syndrome.[6] Thus, some argue that administration of immunosuppression after hand transplantation is more likely to shorten life rather than prolong it.[7] These critics argue that potential hand recipients are, at baseline, generally healthier than solid organ transplant recipients and that subjecting them to the risks of immunosuppression does more harm than good.

The risks derived from the use of chronic immunosuppression may be more significant when an operation is performed that does not result in prolongation of life. This increase in risk rather than benefit may make the operation unethical, which is best illustrated by a case report published by Benatar and Hudson[8] where 2 children, aged 3 and 4 years, both lost their hands. After careful deliberation, it was decided not to perform hand transplantation in these 2 children. The surgeons believed that, although these children would benefit from hand transplantation from a functional standpoint, the chronic exposure and complications of immunosuppression at such a young age posed too much of a risk to justify the operation. However, this example is problematic because it complicates the calculation of risk and benefit by introducing the issue of performing these transplants in children.

The supporters of hand transplantation have argued that the risks of immunosuppression can be minimized with careful monitoring in the adult population. Remarkable progress and understanding in transplant immunology has taken place in the past several years. Newer immunosuppressive agents continue to expand the arsenal of medications and replace older, more risky agents. Combining and adding different medications may allow a decrease in the overall concentration of a single drug, effectively limiting its potential toxicity.[9] In addition, the good health status of hand transplant recipients may be a benefit when they are followed for possible side effects. The process of extrapolating the risks facing patients receiving hand transplants from those seen in solid organ studies where recipients are much sicker likely overestimate the risks.[9] Proponents of hand transplantation point out that the transplant does offer benefit in the restoration of self and the presence of a sensate hand. These benefits allow a hand recipient to integrate back into society and, in some cases, successfully return to work.[10]

Principles of Nonmaleficence Versus Beneficence

Given these risks, who ultimately chooses: the patient or the surgeon? This introduces the second critical concept of the principles of nonmaleficence versus beneficence. Surgeons follow the principle of primum non nocere, or that of nonmaleficence, because they do not want to harm patients who request a procedure that imposes too much risk compared with benefit. However, as health care providers, they also want to do what is best for their patients, which may include transplanting a hand, thereby fulfilling the obligation of beneficence. Critics of hand transplantation point out that, given the risks of immunosuppression, alternatives to hand transplantation, such as prosthesis, should be offered upper extremity amputees. In this situation, those physicians believe that the use of a prosthesis is best for the patient to prevent the inevitable harm that would occur from the complications of immunosuppression. The principle of nonmaleficence supports the position of not offering a hand transplant.

Supporters of hand transplantation argue that the rule of beneficence cannot be solidly adhered to in nonlifesaving situations, such as in cases of hand transplantation. For example, this principle is straightforward in solid organ transplantation, where a heart transplant is essential for patient survival. There is little disagreement among clinicians that transplantation is the treatment of choice. However, because hand transplants are not lifesaving, it is difficult for the physician alone to assess what is best for the patient, which has led some to argue that the only surgeon who can accurately assess whether hand transplantation is best for the patient is a double amputee surgeon.

Paternalism Versus Autonomy

However, if the physician alone cannot properly assess whether or not the patient will derive benefit after hand transplantation despite the known possible complications with immunosuppression, then who should make this decision? If the principle of beneficence is followed, then hand transplants would simply be denied to minimize all harm to the patients regardless of their wishes. This position would satisfy the basic principle of causing no harm. Although such an approach is appealing in its simplicity, it relies on the concept of paternalism. Although the medical establishment once relied on paternalism to guide decision making in medicine, it has fallen out of favor because of the increase in respect for patient autonomy.

Patient Autonomy

This principle recognizes that patients with capacity have a right to determine what is done to their bodies. In many medical scenarios, the decisions that are based on paternalism and patient autonomy will be similar. For example, in a case of a treatable malignancy, both the patient and the physician will agree to initiate treatment. However, in other cases, paternalism and patient autonomy are split. This split is exemplified in right-to-die cases, where the patients can decide not only to cease treatment but also to actively end their lives. Supporters of hand transplantation stress that, given the rights of the recipients, autonomy should be the deciding factor in deciding whether to transplant a hand. It is impossible for people who have 2 hands to understand the potential benefit that hand transplantation can have for an individual. Therefore, it must be acknowledged that, provided the potential recipients seeking hand transplantation can understand the risks, they should be allowed to make the individual decisions. Studies have shown that the potential benefits after hand transplantation include the following 3 essential desired effects: (1) restoration of functional status, (2) restoration of normal body image, and (3) potential elimination of phantom limb phenomenon.[11] To these patients, a better quality of life is valued more than quantity of life. According to published reports, both motor and sensation recovery, as well as restoration of self, occur after hand transplantation.[12–17] These favorable outcomes are similar to replantation of an amputated hand, which is far superior to that of prosthesis.[18]

Opponents of hand transplantation recognize the importance of patient autonomy, but argue that, because this procedure is still considered experimental, the principle of patient autonomy cannot be strictly adhered to.[19] Because of the experimental nature of these transplants, the patient cannot decide on the treatment because of a paucity of data in terms of outcomes. Given the lack of information pertaining to the procedure and immunosuppression, a potential recipient is unable to fully weigh the risks, and is therefore unable to make an informed decision. This principle of informed decision making is discussed later.

Double Effect

The second factor that led to the abandonment of the principle of paternalism is the double effect. This means that, regardless of the harm caused as a consequence of the operation, it is ethical to proceed as long as our primary intent is to cause good. The rule of double effect requires that the nature of a hand operation is good, the surgeon intends to achieve a good effect and not the bad effect (complications of immunosuppression), and, lastly, the good effect outweighs the bad effect, thereby justifying the operation.

Although the first 2 criteria are easily met from a surgical perspective, the third criterion is not so straightforward. As discussed earlier, proponents of hand transplantation state that, given patient autonomy, potential recipients decide on the benefit of the operation. They can accurately assess whether the good effect of hand transplantation exceeds its bad effect. Opponents state that, given the lack of informed decision making secondary to insufficient information presented by the clinician, recipients cannot accurately assess whether the risks would outweigh the benefits of hand transplantation. However, this concern has been mitigated by the increased amount of information derived from the outcomes of more than 40 hand transplants. As more outcome information is derived from the clinical hand transplantations, the ability to address the risks and benefits of the surgery becomes more accurate and this should allow for increased patient autonomy in the decision-making process. However, in order for patients to be able to follow the principle of autonomy, they must be able to obtain informed consent.

Informed Consent

First, to be autonomous, a potential recipient must be presented with a sufficient amount of information regarding hand transplantation, including its operation, recovery, and immunosuppression. From this information, the potential recipient must process such information, weigh the benefits and risks, and ultimately make an informed decision. Opponents of hand transplantation argue that this informed decision-making process is flawed because the patient does not have enough information presented to fully weigh the pros and cons.[7] Some question whether it is even possible to obtain true consent for a procedure that is experimental, complex, and emotional.[19] Critics of hand transplantation further argue that, because hand transplantation is a new and evolving field, a patient would be unable to fully comprehend the overall risks compared with a more established operation. In addition, there may even be a lack of experience on the part of the surgeon regarding the complications of hand transplantation.[4] Others state that hand transplantation fails to provide definite information on functional outcome and the likelihood of future rejections.[4]

Conversely, supporters of hand transplantation argue against these claims, pointing out that the risks from immunosuppression have well been documented in the solid organ transplant literature, and the current published complications of chronic immunosuppression after hand transplantation have been no different than those experienced by, for example, renal transplant recipients. Consequently, the potential recipient does have enough information regarding its risks to properly and accurately assess a risk/benefit ratio. In addition, some argue against the view that hand transplantation is considered experimental or research driven.[7] The surgical technique is not new or experimental because the replantation of the human hand is a common procedure, but the application of these techniques to hand transplantation is novel. Even if hand transplantation is documented as experimental, with increasing numbers of transplants performed, surgeons can now present the patient with adequate information including all published complications in addition to all other possible complications.

Studies have shown that potential recipients with no experience in transplantation can understand the complications of immunosuppression enough to perceive a risk value. For example, a survey inquiring about attitudes on immunosuppression would suggest that a person without prior experience as a recipient and taking chronic immunosuppression is similar to an actual recipient who received a transplant and is currently on immunosuppression.[20] The survey targeted 3 groups: the general public, potential recipients on the waiting list for a kidney, and those who had undergone renal transplantation. Results suggest that all 3 groups accepted the same amount of risk for certain unique transplants, namely face and double hand transplantation, regardless of whether or not the person surveyed had experience with immunosuppression. A similar survey performed on healthy individuals, organ transplant recipients, and upper and lower extremity amputees found similar results.[21] All groups perceived risk similarly despite their differences with immunosuppression or amputation, and all would accept the risk for a double hand transplant.

Identity

In addition to the principles discussed earlier, the concept of identity and intimacy is a rapidly emerging issue in hand transplantation. Although these topics did not play a significant role in solid organ transplantation, they need to be addressed with composite tissue allotransplantation, such as a hand transplantation.

In solid organ transplantation, the allograft is not subject to external visualization by either the recipient or society. In turn, solid organ transplants do not carry a stigma of identity. However, a hand transplant remains in full view and consequently plays a significant role in the identity of the recipient. Because the transplanted hand is in constant view, there is a strong psychological component such that recipients are constantly aware, and may even acknowledge, that the transplanted hand is not theirs. The recipient views the hand graft as if another person's personal qualities were transferred and may, consequently, psychologically reject these qualities.[7]

This issue was believed to be the cause of failure for the first Lyon recipient after his hand transplantation. The recipient became increasingly dissociated from his allograft and consequently became noncompliant with his immunosuppression. At the end, this recipient wished to have his graft removed and subsequently, in 2001, surgeons removed the transplant.

This incidence shows the importance of self-identity in hand transplantation. Opponents of hand transplantation question whether a recipient will perceive the transplanted hand as a violation of his or her body. Will patients perceive someone else's hand touching another part of their bodies? What if the hand becomes discolored or does not match the recipient's natural skin tone? What if the hand changes in size after transplantation? Some investigators make an important and underrepresented point: what about fingerprints?[22] In today's society, personal identity is paramount, especially given the increased frequency of identity theft. Donor fingerprints show little change after transplantation.[23] One Polish hand recipient received his hand allograft from a donor with a criminal record. Fingerprinting 40 months after transplantation showed no significant change from the time of transplant. Until now, there have been no issues with recipient-donor identity mismatch according to his transplant team. However, potential scenarios exist where fingerprinting the recipient could lead to confusion and problems. This serves as an early reminder for errors in identity after hand transplantation. As more hand transplants are performed each year, there will need to be more regulation to protect not only the identity of the donor, but to maintain the recipient's original identity.

Given how paramount identity is after hand transplantation in maintaining acceptance or rejection of the graft, as shown by the French recipient, hand transplant centers around the world now perform an extensive psychiatric evaluation to screen potential recipients. For example, Louisville has a mandatory formal psychiatric evaluation in order select which potential recipients would be ideal candidates from a psychological perspective to undergo hand transplantation.[24] This article discusses their program in more detail later. Screening for select candidates is important, as shown by another study.[25] The team interviewed 213 potential hand recipients and found only 9 who were eligible to undergo hand transplantation. During their evaluation, these 9 recipients stated that they would have a sense of physical and psychological ownership after a hand transplant, and that hand transplantation could make them whole again. Similarly, of 534 patients interviewed, the Italian hand program chose only 4 potential recipients to transplant.[26]

FINANCIAL CONSIDERATIONS

Given the limited numbers of hands transplanted, the economic and financial impact of this procedure is currently unclear. As health care costs are more closely monitored, the cost-effectiveness of a new operation is becoming increasingly important, especially if it is not lifesaving. Because of the small number of cases, few objective long-term data exist to determine the financial impact of hand transplantation on a health care system. Multiple financial factors must be considered, including costs of the operation, hospital stay, hand therapy, office visits, immunosuppression, and time off work. This cost must be offset by the benefit of returning a patient to the workforce.

A recent study by Chung and colleagues[27] analyzed the financial aspect of hand transplantation. The investigators surveyed 100 medical students and their preferences in using prosthesis, undergoing a single hand transplant, and undergoing a double hand transplant compared with baseline (2 normal functioning hands). Transplantation took into consideration the complications of immunosuppression. From the students' responses to the different scenarios, the investigators were able to translate the answers to quality-adjusted life years (QALY), a measure of the usefulness of a medical procedure. The QALY also took into account the value of direct and indirect operational costs, such as costs of the operation, hospital stay, immunosuppression, treatment of diabetes and hypertension resulting from immunosuppression, and time off work. After these costs were factored into the QALY, it was then converted to financial costs, defined as the increment cost/usefulness ratio (ICUR). ICUR measures the additional cost per QALY gained by using 1 treatment rather than another. Depending on the set cost threshold ($50,000/QALY was the defined threshold in this study), when the ICUR value exceeds the thresholds, it is considered not to be cost-effective. However, if the ICUR value is less than the set cost threshold, then it is deemed to be cost-effective.

The investigators estimated that the lifetime costs for a single or a double hand transplant is between $528,000 and $530,000. The lifetime cost for use of a single prosthesis is slightly more than $20,000 and, for use of a double prosthesis, it is slightly more than $41,000. The ICUR for double hand transplantation (single hand transplant was not calculated because, currently, use of a prosthesis is the preferred method) is $318,961/QALY. In their study, the threshold was set at $50,000, which is the approximate cost of a kidney. Thus, the ICUR for a double hand transplant far exceeds the threshold set by the investigators.

Given these findings, the investigators concluded that the use of prosthesis is the preferred treatment of amputation of an extremity rather than a single hand transplant, given its usefulness and financial advantage. Although the double hand transplantation provided greater usefulness than the use of a double prosthesis, the costs per QALY were deemed to exceed the traditionally accepted cost-effectiveness threshold. Therefore, according to this analysis, from an economic standpoint, the continued use of prosthesis for both single and double amputees is the preferred and optimal choice.

That study was based on a conservative scenario because it did not take into account other factors associated with hand transplantation. For example, the price of hand transplant rehabilitation, an essential part of postoperative treatment, was not included. From the Louisville center, total costs for unilateral hand transplantation averaged a total of 226 hours and amounted to $53,336. These costs were higher for a bilateral hand transplant, which averaged more than 260 hours and amounted to $63,360.[28] Had this been considered in the study discussed earlier, the cost of the ICUR might have been higher. Although the cost analysis is important, it is difficult to place a value on quality of life. The calculation of the QUALY is based on medical student time trade-off surveys that may not accurately estimate the true benefit derived from a unilateral or bilateral hand transplant.

RULES AND REGULATION

Hand transplantation, with its ethical considerations, possible self-identity issues, and financial complexity, must exist in a highly structured program to be properly overseen and follow the necessary regulations. As discussed earlier, the Louisville group developed a stringent screening process that each potential recipient must go through to be considered for hand transplantation. This article discusses Louisville's hand transplant program and how it can serve as a model for regulation of the way a team performs hand transplantation.

Founded in 1996, the University of Louisville, Kentucky's hand transplantation program consists of plastic surgeons, hand surgeons, transplant surgeons, and psychiatrists. Early on, the program was overseen by medical ethicists Dr Mark Siegler and Dr Paul Simmons.[24] Based on the novelty of hand transplantation, Louisville decided to structure its program to follow Dr Francis Moore's[29,30] standpoint on innovative surgery. Dr Moore[29,30] suggested that, with any new procedure, the following 6 factors must be considered: adequate scientific background and evidence to support the procedure, a knowledgeable and skillful team, a well-established ethical climate of the institution, full disclosure to the public, public evaluation of the procedure, and discussions regarding the proposed procedure with the public and the team.

Louisville has successfully integrated Moore's[29,30] 6 proposed criteria in its hand transplantation program. To show adequate scientific background and evidence in support of hand transplant, the center performed multiple studies showing feasibility in a swine model. Their investigators have attended and presented at multiple meetings. In addition, they established dedicated members of the psychiatric department to work in conjunction with the hand and transplant surgeons at Louisville. To address any ethical issues, they expanded the group of ethicists to include additional input from others outside Louisville. For public awareness, the program presented at multiple conferences and held open debates.

Given the potential identity conflicts that may arise after hand transplantation, each potential recipient must undergo a rigorous psychiatric evaluation to evaluate which candidate would benefit after hand transplantation. This screening emphasizes body image adaptation, level of realistic expectations, anticipated comfort with a cadaver hand, and potential for psychological regression and ultimate rejection of the hand. In addition, the team requires the recipient to name a personal advocate. This patient advocate is someone without relation to Louisville and any of its physicians participating in the care of the patient. The group strongly believes that patient advocacy ensures patient autonomy and enhances the informed consent.

SUMMARY

Since the first successful hand transplantation performed in 1998, multiple centers have followed, increasing the number of hand transplantations to 49 according to the 2010 publication by the International Registry on Hand and Composite Tissue. Since then, more than 65 hand transplants have been performed. Given its favorable long-term follow-ups with greater than 90% graft survival, hand transplantation is now being recognized as a procedure to salvage a lost limb and restore functionality. Studies show superiority of hand transplantation compared with prosthesis. Imaging shows cortical reintegration of the transplanted limb. There is increasingly favorable evidence to support hand transplantation and, if growth continues, hand transplantation may become the gold standard for treatment of a double amputee.

However, hand transplantation is still in its infancy and, as such, is subject to scrutiny from clinicians, patients, and society. Ethical debates regarding risks and benefits to this nonlifesaving procedure continue to split the transplantation community. In a survey conducted by Mathes and colleagues[31] consulting hand surgeons about their views on hand transplantation, 24% were in favor of hand transplantation, 45% were against such a procedure, and the rest (31%) were undecided. Issues of self-identity can cause significant problems in recipients and may have contributed to the loss of the first French hand transplant. Complete analysis of the financial impact of hand transplantation is currently not available, but studies translating the costs from replantation cases suggest that hand transplantation may not be a cost-effective alternative compared with the use of prosthesis, despite findings that functionality is better after a hand transplant.

Because hand transplantation is viewed as a quality of life rather than a lifesaving procedure such as many other solid organ transplants, careful discussion regarding the risks and benefits need to be thoroughly discussed with the patient. The clinician should disclose to the potential recipient that, despite the growing number of hand transplants performed around the world, the procedure itself is still novel and long-term follow-up data are still limited. Patient autonomy should be respected, keeping in mind the physician's duty of primum non nocere, or nonmaleficence. A psychiatric evaluation should be performed discussing concepts such as bodily image, acceptance of a cadaveric hand, and realistic expectations. Currently, all the centers performing hand transplantation mandate a comprehensive psychiatric evaluation to screen potential recipients before transplantation. Hand transplant centers must be well structured to allow for coordination of multiple teams including surgeons, ethicists, and psychiatrists. In addition, other centers require that recipients are seen by the Infectious Diseases department given the higher incidence of opportunistic and latent infections that develop after immunosuppression.

Until transplant tolerance becomes a clinical reality,[32,33] hand transplantation will continue to be limited by its need for chronic immunosuppression. Some hand centers currently attempt to minimize/wean immunosuppression using cell-based immunomodulatory approaches, showing encouraging initial results. Although this paper discusses many of the ethical principles of hand transplantation, one important issue that is not discussed is that of unilateral hand transplantation. This topic has been debated for a long time by both surgeons and ethicists, and some countries still regard unilateral hand transplantation as contraindicated. It will be worthwhile to see whether these countries' preferences change in any way after more centers perform unilateral hand transplantation and long-term follow-up data with these recipients are made more available.

What was once considered a failure in 1964 is now a clinical reality. Given the improved understanding in transplant physiology and new discoveries in immunosuppressive therapies, more hand transplants will be performed around the world. Because there is no other physiologic alternative that is equivalent to a hand transplant, this so-called experimental operation will likely become the standard of care for amputees. However, before medicine, society, and patients can accept this fact, there must first be agreement on whether hand transplantation is ethical and affordable. In addition, hand transplantation must be performed in dedicated centers that provide integration of multiple medical specialists, ethicists, pharmacists, and rehabilitationists.

REFERENCES

1. Dubernard JM, Owen E, Herzberg G, et al. The first transplantation of a hand in humans. Early results. Chirurgie 1999;124(4):358–65 [discussion 365–67].
2. Dubernard JM, Owen E, Lefrançois N, et al. First human hand transplantation. Case report. Transpl Int 2000;13(Suppl 1):S521–4.
3. Petruzzo P, Lanzetta M, Dubernard JM, et al. The International Registry on Hand and Composite Tissue Transplantation. Transplantation 2010;90(12): 1590–4.
4. Jones NF. Concerns about human hand transplantation in the 21st century. J Hand Surg Am 2002;27(5): 771–87.
5. Lanzetta M, Nolli R, Borgonovo A, et al. Hand transplantation: ethics, immunosuppression and indications. J Hand Surg Br 2001;26(6):511–6.
6. Hatrick NC, Tonkin MA. Hand transplantation: a current perspective. ANZ J Surg 2001;71(4):245–51.
7. Dickenson D, Widdershoven G. Ethical issues in limb transplants. Bioethics 2001;15(2):110–24.

8. Benatar D, Hudson DA. A tale of two novel transplants not done: the ethics of limb allografts. BMJ 2002;324(7343):971–3.

9. Breidenbach WC 3rd, Tobin GR 2nd, Gorantla VS, et al. A position statement in support of hand transplantation. J Hand Surg Am 2002;27(5):760–70.

10. Kaufman CL, Blair B, Murphy E, et al. A new option for amputees: transplantation of the hand. J Rehabil Res Dev 2009;46(3):395–404.

11. Lees VC, McCabe SJ. The rationale for hand transplantation. Transplantation 2002;74(6):749–53.

12. Brandacher G, Ninkovic M, Piza-Katzer H, et al. The Innsbruck hand transplant program: update at 8 years after the first transplant. Transplant Proc 2009;41(2):491–4.

13. Breidenbach WC, Gonzales NR, Kaufman CL, et al. Outcomes of the first 2 American hand transplants at 8 and 6 years posttransplant. J Hand Surg Am 2008; 33(7):1039–47.

14. Kvernmo HD, Gorantla VS, Gonzalez RN, et al. Hand transplantation. A future clinical option? Acta Orthop 2005;76(1):14–27.

15. Lanzetta M, Petruzzo P, Vitale G, et al. Human hand transplantation: what have we learned? Transplant Proc 2004;36(3):664–8.

16. Ravindra KV, Buell JF, Kaufman CL, et al. Hand transplantation in the United States: experience with 3 patients. Surgery 2008;144(4):638–43 [discussion: 643–44].

17. Brenneis C, Löscher WN, Egger KE, et al. Cortical motor activation patterns following hand transplantation and replantation. J Hand Surg Br 2005;30(5): 530–3.

18. Graham B, Adkins P, Tsai TM, et al. Major replantation versus revision amputation and prosthetic fitting in the upper extremity: a late functional outcomes study. J Hand Surg Am 1998;23(5):783–91.

19. Andrew Lee WP. The debate over hand transplantation. J Hand Surg Am 2002;27(5):757–9.

20. Brouha P, Naidu D, Cunningham M, et al. Risk acceptance in composite-tissue allotransplantation reconstructive procedures. Microsurgery 2006; 26(3):144–9 [discussion: 149–50].

21. Majzoub RK, Cunningham M, Grossi F, et al. Investigation of risk acceptance in hand transplantation. J Hand Surg Am 2006;31(2):295–302.

22. Agich GJ. Extension of organ transplantation: some ethical considerations. Mt Sinai J Med 2003;70(3): 141–7.

23. Szajerka T, Jurek B, Jablecki J. Transplanted fingerprints: a preliminary case report 40 months posttransplant. Transplant Proc 2010;42(9):3753–5.

24. Tobin GR, Breidenbach WC, Klapheke MM, et al. Ethical considerations in the early composite tissue allograft experience: a review of the Louisville Ethics Program. Transplant Proc 2005;37(2):1392–5.

25. Klapheke MM, Marcell C, Taliaferro G, et al. Psychiatric assessment of candidates for hand transplantation. Microsurgery 2000;20(8):453–7.

26. Lanzetta M. The Italian experience. Atlanta (GA): International Hand and Composite Tissue Allograft Society (IHCTAS); 2011.

27. Chung KC, Oda T, Saddawi-Konefka D, et al. An economic analysis of hand transplantation in the United States. Plast Reconstr Surg 2010;125(2):589–98.

28. McGill S, Emrich AB, Newsome L, et al. Hand transplant rehabilitation financial considerations. Atlanta (GA): International Hand and Composite Tissue Allograft Society (IHCTAS); 2011.

29. Moore FD. Three ethical revolutions: ancient assumptions remodeled under pressure of transplantation. Transplant Proc 1988;20(1 Suppl 1):1061–7.

30. Moore FD. The desperate case: CARE (costs, applicability, research, ethics). JAMA 1989;261(10): 1483–4.

31. Mathes DW, Schlenker R, Ploplys E, et al. A survey of North American hand surgeons on their current attitudes toward hand transplantation. J Hand Surg Am 2009;34(5):808–14.

32. Lee WP, Rubin JP, Bourget JL, et al. Tolerance to limb tissue allografts between swine matched for major histocompatibility complex antigens. Plast Reconstr Surg 2001;107(6):1482–90 [discussion: 1491–92].

33. Mathes DW, Randolph MA, Lee WP. Strategies for tolerance induction to composite tissue allografts. Microsurgery 2000;20(8):448–52.

BONUS ARTICLE:
Arthroscopic Dorsal Capsulo-ligamentous Repair in Chronic Scapholunate Ligament Tears

Christophe L. Mathoulin, MD, Nicolas Dauphin, MD,
and Abhijeet L. Wahegaonkar, MBBS, D.Ortho, MCh (Ortho),
Diplomate in Hand Surgery

Edited by David J. Slutsky, MD

Arthroscopic Dorsal Capsuloligamentous Repair in Chronic Scapholunate Ligament Tears

Christophe L. Mathoulin, MD[a],*, Nicolas Dauphin, MD[b],
Abhijeet L. Wahegaonkar, MBBS, D.Ortho, MCh (Ortho)[c,d]

KEYWORDS

- Scapholunate ligament • Dorsal capsuloplasty
- Dorsal capsulodesis • Wrist arthroscopy

The rupture of the scapholunate (SL) ligament occurs most often after a fall on an outstretched hand. Arthroscopy is the most valuable tool for the diagnosis and treatment of acute SL dissociation. In chronic lesions, treatment options are more controversial than in the acute cases. Most forms of treatment recommended in the literature consist of an open repair or alternative reconstruction techniques that can improve pain and grip strength, but often lead to stiffness in the wrist joint.[1] Furthermore, there is scant evidence that these interventions prevent or, at a minimum, delay posttraumatic carpal arthritis. Open techniques seem to result in some degree of wrist stiffness. The authors' hypothesis is that this complication is due to the extensive dissection of the wrist capsule. Therefore, we have developed our arthroscopic dorsal capsuloplasty technique to avoid open dissection of the wrist capsule.[2] We use the Geissler[3] arthroscopic classification and the Garcia-Elias[4] classification to assess the stage or grade of SL tear and treat the SL dissociation arthroscopically. In cases where the ligament is partially or completely ruptured, and where the

scaphoid is well aligned or can be reduced, we propose the new technique of arthroscopic dorsal capsuloplasty, which may be combined with K-wire fixation of the scapholunate and the scaphocapitate joints where the scaphoid seems malaligned. Our series of 36 patients shows encouraging preliminary results even with highly demanding patients in a short-term follow-up. Pain relief and recovery of grip strength were observed as with the other techniques. A low incidence of postoperative wrist stiffness was noted. Postoperative improvement of mean wrist motion was observed in all planes and all professional athletes returned to their preinjury level of sports training and competition.

INDICATIONS

Thirty-six consecutive patients with a suspected SL ligament tear underwent an arthroscopically assisted dorsal capsuloligamentous repair, with or without percutaneous pinning, at a mean age of 38.5 years (25–58 years). Of 25 men and 11 women, the dominant hand was involved in 21

[a] Institut de la Main, 6 Square Jouvenet, 75016 Paris, France
[b] Service de Chirurgie Plastique, Reconstructrice et Esthétique, Centre Hospitalier de, Luxembourg 4, Rue Ernest Barblé, L-1210 Luxembourg
[c] Department of Upper Extremity, Hand and Microvascular Reconstructive Surgery, Sancheti Institute for Orthopedics & Rehabilitation, 16 Shivajinagar, Pune 41105, India
[d] Department of Orthopedics and Traumatology, B.V.D.U. Medical College & Hospitals, Katraj-Dhankawdi, Pune 411043, India
* Corresponding author.
E-mail address: cmathoulin@orange.fr

Hand Clin 27 (2011) 563–572
doi:10.1016/j.hcl.2011.07.003
0749-0712/11/$ – see front matter © 2011 Elsevier Inc. All rights reserved.

cases (63.6%). The mean delay from trauma to surgery was 9.8 months (3–24 months). Thirteen patients had a fall or an accident and 23 patients suffered sport injuries, including tennis (5), cycling or motorcycling (5), ball games (6; volleyball, basketball, handball, football), fighting sports (4; boxing, judo, fencing), Golf (2), and gymnastics (1). Seven of them were high level or professional athletes (30.4% of the patients).

PREOPERATIVE ASSESSMENT
Clinical Assessment

Bilateral ranges of movement of all 36 patients were measured preoperatively. Tenderness in the affected wrist was noted and the Watson test performed. Radiographic assessments were standard posteroanterior and lateral; and oblique radiographs were performed on all patients. Both the SL gap and the SL angles were measured. MRI-arthrography was performed on each patient for further evaluation of the radiocarpal, midcarpal, and distal radioulnar compartments.

SURGICAL TECHNIQUE

The procedures were performed on an outpatient basis, using regional anesthesia and an upper arm tourniquet. The elbow was flexed to 90° on an arm table and the hand was suspended by means of a hand holder with traction of 3 to 5 kg.

We used the standard arthroscopic 3 to 4 and 6R portals for the radiocarpal joint (RCJ) and midcarpal radial and midcarpal ulnar for the midcarpal joint (MCJ). The joints were first insufflated with normal saline. A small transverse incision was made with a number 15 blade scalpel followed by blunt dissection with a mosquito forceps. The 2.4 mm arthroscope was introduced through the 3 to 4 portal and the instruments through the 6R portal—these two portals are interchangeable according to need. The MCJ was explored through the midcarpal ulnar portal. Exploration and palpation of the structures in the two joints confirmed the lesion and allowed for staging.

INTRAOPERATIVE STAGING

To evaluate the extent of SL dissociations, we used two classification systems that stage the cartilage status and the SL ligament lesion under arthroscopic vision. Geissler and Haley[3] describe four stages of arthroscopic SL lesions (**Box 1**). Garcia-Elias and colleagues[4] subdivide SL dissociations into six stages based on five questions answered during the clinical and arthroscopic assessment (**Table 1**).

Box 1
Arthroscopic Geissler classification of cartilage lesions

Stage 1. Attenuation or hemorrhage SL in RCJ; no incongruity in MCJ

Stage 2. Attenuation or perforation of SL in RCJ; small incongruity in MCJ

Stage 3. Perforation of SL in RCJ or incongruity and step-off in MCJ (> probe)

Stage 4. Incongruity and step-off in RCJ and MCJ; gross instability with manipulation

---

According to Garcia-Elias, only stages 2, 3, and 4 were treated with this technique. In these three stages the ligament is amenable to repair (stage 2) or irreparable (stage 3). As for the carpal alignment it was noted as either being preserved (stage 2 and 3) or amenable to correction where malalignment was present (stage 4). If the lesion coincided with one of the three stages, then the procedure of dorsal capsule-ligamentous repair was performed. Usually, the SL ligament was detached from the scaphoid and remained attached to the lunate. However, on the dorsal aspect, close to the normal insertion of the SL ligament to the capsule, there are remaining parts of SL ligament on the dorsal horn of lunate and the scaphoid. Usually, it was difficult to see the dorsal SL ligament (particularly its scaphoid portion) from a 6R portal, when the wrist was in traction, and the dorsal capsule was compressed against the ruptured ligament. We never had a problem, using correct triangulation with a 30° oblique scope in 6R, after releasing the traction. A needle inserted under visual control through the 3 to 4 portal. Instead of penetrating the RCJ, it was inserted through the dorsal capsule and used to spear the radial remnant of the SL

Table 1
Garcia-Elias staging system

Stages	I	II	III	IV	V	VI
Dorsal SL Ligament Intact?	Yes	No	No	No	No	No
Repairable SL Ligament?	Yes	Yes	No	No	No	No
Scaphoid Alignment Normal?	Yes	Yes	Yes	Yes	No	No
Carpal Malalignment Reducible?	Yes	Yes	Yes	Yes	No	No
Cartilage in RCJs and MCJs Normal?	Yes	Yes	Yes	Yes	Yes	No

ligament obliquely from dorsal to palmar, directed in a proximal to distal direction, with the needle tip coming out in the MCJ. The scope was then changed to the midcarpal ulnar portal and a 3.0 polydioxanon suture thread was passed through the needle and pulled out through the midcarpal radial portal with a forceps under visual control from the midcarpal ulnar portal (**Fig. 1**). A second suture was then passed parallel to the first one in the lunate-ulnar remnant of SL ligament and brought out through the same portal (**Fig. 2**). A knot was tied between the two sutures. Next, proximal traction was applied to both proximal ends of the sutures to place the first knot into the MCJ between the scaphoid and the lunate, volar to the dorsal part of the SL ligament (**Fig. 3**). A second knot was tied between the two proximal ends and introduced in the 3 to 4 portal incision, dorsal to the capsule. This knot lies outside the RCJ on the dorsal capsule. The net effect of this is to achieve a capsule ligamentous repair between the SL ligament and the dorsal capsule overlying the ligament (**Fig. 4**). If the SL ligament has been completely avulsed from the bone instead of being torn this procedure cannot be performed. The procedure for stage 4 cases is modified. In such instances, the scaphoid was reduced and stabilized in relation to the lunate and capitate. This is done by external and internal maneuvers under fluoroscopic control. Once the reduction is

confirmed, the capsuloplasty was performed. The scaphoid was stabilized by inserting 1.2 mm parallel K-wires through the scaphoid into the lunate and the capitate (**Fig. 5**). The final dorsal knot was tied down after the SL fixation. The two joints were thoroughly rinsed before instrument retrieval. The portal incisions were not sutured. The dressing consisted of gauze and a simple volar splint.

POSTOPERATIVE PROTOCOL

The wrist was immobilized in a splint for two months. After eight weeks, passive wrist motion was commenced under the supervision of a physiotherapist. The K-wires, where used (ie, in stage 4), were removed after two months and the patients underwent the same physiotherapy protocol.

POSTOPERATIVE ASSESSMENT
Clinical Assessment

The operating surgeon reviewed all patients at regular intervals. At final follow-up, patients were evaluated by the Disabilities of Arm, Shoulder, and Hand (DASH) outcome questionnaire. This was performed by an independent reviewer. The score predominantly consisted of a 30-item disability symptom scale, scored from 0 (no disability) to 100 (full disability). Forearm range of motion was

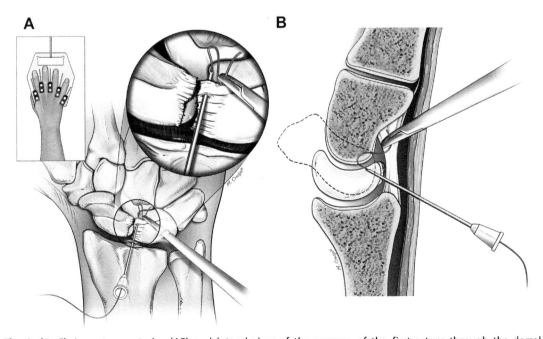

Fig. 1. (*A, B*) An anteroposterior (AP) and lateral view of the passage of the first suture through the dorsal capsule with a remaining dorsal fragment of the SL ligament attached to the dorsal horn of lunate. The passage is made from the RCJ to MCJ.

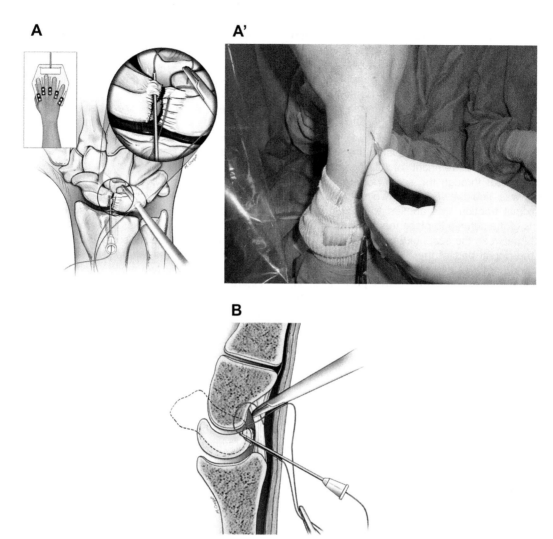

Fig. 2. (*A*, *A'*, *B*) An AP and lateral view of the passage of the second suture through the dorsal capsule with a remaining dorsal fragment of the SL ligament attached to the dorsal scaphoid. The passage is made from the RCJ to MCJ.

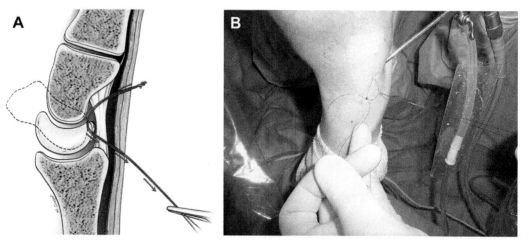

Fig. 3. (*A*, *B*) After a first knot is tied between the two sutures, proximal traction is applied to the proximal ends of the sutures to seat the first knot into the MCJ between the scaphoid and the lunate, volar to the dorsal part of SL ligament.

A

B

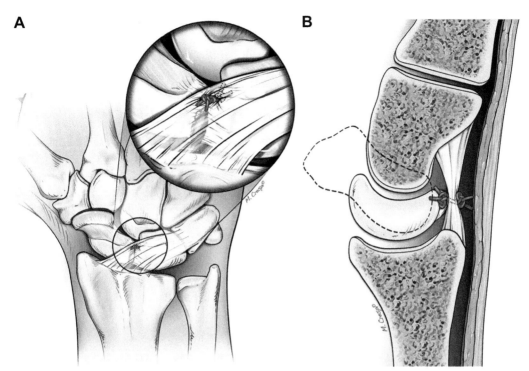

Fig. 4. (*A, B*) An AP and lateral view of the second knot tied between the two proximal ends and introduced in the 3 to 4 portal incision, dorsal to the capsule. This knot lies outside the wrist joint on the dorsal capsule. The net effect of this produces a capsuloplasty between the SL ligament and the dorsal capsule overlying the ligament.

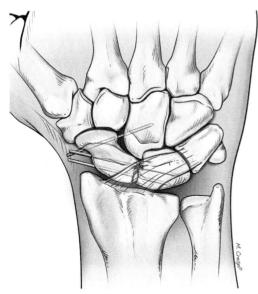

Fig. 5. An AP view of the stabilization of the scaphoid by1.2 mm parallel K-wires applied through the scaphoid into the capitate in only stage 4 according to the Garcia-Elias staging. The final dorsal knot is tied after the SL fixation.

recorded in flexion, extension, and radial-ulnar deviation.

Grip strength was measured using the JAMAR dynamometer (Preston, Cambridge, MA, USA) and compared with the opposite side. Furthermore, patient satisfaction was assessed by asking the patients to grade their postoperative result as excellent, good, fair, or poor.

Radiographic Assessment

Standard posteroanterior, lateral, and oblique radiographs were obtained for all patients at 8 weeks after surgery, then regularly until the last follow-up. The SL angle was determined by the operating surgeon and an independent examiner. MRI was routinely performed at 6 months postoperatively (**Fig. 6**).

Statistical Analysis

Data of paired groups were compared using the Mann-Whitney test. Results were considered significant for $P<.05$.

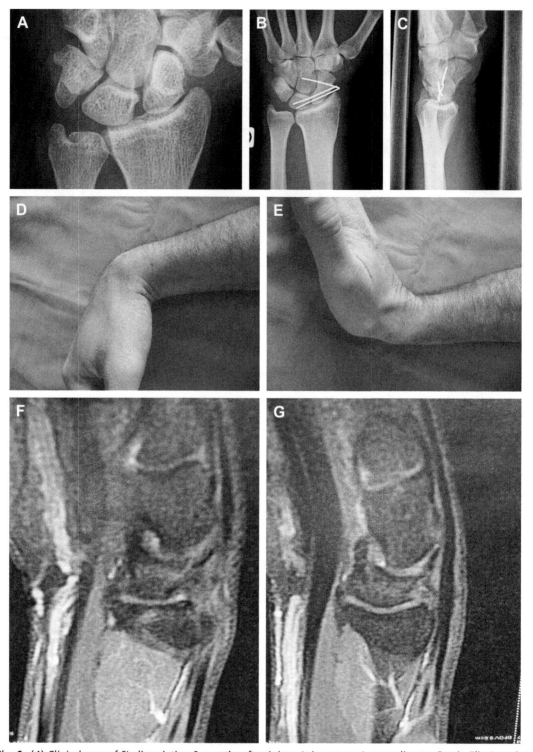

Fig. 6. (*A*) Clinical case of SL dissociation 9 months after injury. It is a stage 4, according to Garcia-Elias' staging. (*B, C*) Radiographs showing the correct reduction and stabilization of SL space after an arthroscopic dorsal capsuloplasty. (*D, E*) 12 month follow-up, recovery of excellent range of motion in both extension and flexion sectors. (*F, G*) MRI after 12 months showing a well reduced lunate and the effect of the dorsal capsuloplasty with a thickening of the capsule over the dorsal pole of the lunate with a tightening of the capsule toward the lunate.

RESULTS

Clinical Results

All patients were reviewed at a mean follow-up of 11.4 months (7–19 months). According to Geissler classification, 6 patients were at stage II, 22 patients at stage III, and 8 patients at stage IV. Using Garcia-Elias's staging system, 3 patients were classified at stage 2, 17 patients at stage 3, and 16 patients at stage 4. In these 16 cases, temporary K-wire fixation was necessary. Seven patients had associated triangular fibrocartilage complex lesions, which were treated arthroscopically in the same operative session. The average wrist flexion was 63° (40°–80°), extension was 71° (40°–90°), radial deviation was 24° (10°–40°), and ulnar deviation was 34° (25°–40°). The average grip strength of the injured wrists as measured with the JAMAR dynamometer was 39.3 kg (20–60 kg), which was 92% of the contralateral side. The results in terms of pain relief were excellent. Using the visual analog score, the mean preoperative pain was 3.3 (3 to 4). Pain symptoms improved significantly in the postoperative period and the mean postoperative Visual Analog Scale was 0.5 (0 to 3). Only six patients had occasional slight pain. All the patients returned to work at an average time of 9 weeks (1–12 weeks) and the seven professional athletes continued practicing at the same level as before the injury. Thirty-five patients (97.2%) were very satisfied or satisfied with their result. One patient had a fair result and was unsatisfied, mainly due to postoperative wrist stiffness. The mean preoperative DASH score was 34.5 (16.4–47.6). The mean postoperative DASH score was 9.5 points (0 to 40.1).

Radiographic Results

Preoperatively, 16 patients (44.4%) had a dorsal intercalated segmental instability deformity with a mean SL angle of 56.9° (40°–90°). Postoperatively, the mean knee SL angle was 49.2° (40°–65°). The deformity remained uncorrected in nine patients (25%).

DISCUSSION

Dissociation of the SL joint is due to a failure of the SL ligament and at least one of its secondary soft-tissue restraints.[3,5] Studies of patients suffering from pain and accustomed to wrist instability show that a long-standing SL dissociation may lead to carpal deterioration starting with the radial styloid-scaphoid articulation and gradually progressing to the radioscaphoid and then the capitolunate joint with relative sparing of the radiolunate joint. This feature is called the Scapholunate Advanced Collapse (SLAC)- wrist.[6,7] The goals of the many procedures described to address the SL dissociation are improvement of wrist pain and function in addition to addressing the possibility of preventing or delaying the onset of post-traumatic carpal arthritis.[1] The best outcomes from treatment of SL dissociation are obtained with treatment in the acute phase or in the first 2 months after the lesion, especially with partial tears. Whipple[8] introduced the idea of arthroscopically controlled K-wire fixation of the scaphoid to the lunate to create a fibrous ankylosis along the K-wires to reinforce the SL ligament.[3] Direct suture repair of the SL ligament with dorsal capsular augmentation is the most commonly used technique to treat acute lesions. Concerning chronic lesions without carpal arthritis, the treatment is still controversial. Numerous techniques have been described to treat lesions without articular cartilage compromise in the carpus. The options here include dorsal capsulodesis, ligament reconstructions using tendon grafts, and intercarpal arthrodesis techniques. Most of the techniques are effective for pain relief but lead to restriction of wrist motion, which can be significant. Furthermore, none of these modalities of treatment can prevent the posttraumatic arthritic changes leading to SLAC-wrist changes.[1] Hence, the authors developed a minimally invasive technique to stabilize the scaphoid to the lunate without extensive dissection, thus preserving maximum wrist movement. Decision-making was based on the Garcia-Elias classification of SL dissociation.[4] We do not completely agree with the Garcia-Elias suggestion because, in our own experience, stage 5 is almost never certain. Either we can reduce the scaphoid after opening the wrist and releasing surrounding fibrosis so stage 5 becomes stage 4 or we cannot. In these cases, often the cartilage status is not good and it becomes a stage 6. In his description, Garcia-Elias explained that some of stage 5 could be reduced to become stage 4. In other stages, he proposed a partial arthrodesis, as in stage 6 treatment.[4] We propose a modification of this classification or suggestion: modifying stage 5 as reducible by open surgery and stage 4 remaining reducible but only arthroscopically (**Table 2**). We, therefore, propose our arthroscopic technique of dorsal capsuloplasty in stages 2, 3, and 4 of the modified Garcia-Elias classification in chronic SL dissociation.[2] Furthermore, we no longer use K-wire to stabilize the scaphoid against the lunate and capitate in stage 2 and 3 lesions. The K-wire fixation is only used for stage 4 patients in whom the scaphoid has to be reduced. Stage 1 represents a partial tear of the SL ligament with its dorsal part being still

Table 2
Modified Garcia-Elias staging system

Stages	I	II	III	IV	V	VI
Dorsal SL Ligament Intact?	Yes	No	No	No	No	No
Repairable SL Ligament?	Yes	Yes	No	No	No	No
Scaphoid Alignment Normal?	Yes	Yes	Yes	No	No	No
Carpal Malalignment Reducible?	Yes	Yes	Yes	Yes (arthroscopy)	Yes (open approach)	No
Cartilage in RCJs and MCJs Normal?	Yes	Yes	Yes	Yes	Yes	No

intact. Watson and Ballet[6] describe this as a predynamic instability. In acute cases, this injury pattern can be treated by percutaneous K-wire fixation,[9] eventually under arthroscopic control. We also excluded stage 5 patients from the discussion because we think that they can be transformed in stage 4 by scaphotrapeziotrapezoid arthrolysis. Stage 6 lesions are genuine SLAC-wrists for which palliative treatments are commonly used to preserve a certain amount of wrist motion.[1] If the lesion is considered chronic, numerous investigators describe a K-wire fixation of the scaphoid to the lunate and/or to the capitate combined with open dorsal capsulodesis techniques as a complement.[10–14] The capsulodesis techniques are also used as an adjuvant in Garcia-Elias stage 2 lesions, in which the ligament is completely ruptured but can be repaired with a fair potential to heal. They represent the most frequently used treatment for this type of injury.[1] Open capsulodesis techniques with or without SL ligament repair try to advance a strip of dorsal capsule across the radiocarpal interval or they shift a part of the dorsal intercarpal ligament proximally.[9,13]

Gajendran and colleagues[15] did a retrospective review on dorsal intercarpal ligament capsulodesis and noted the following results. The mean wrist flexion dropped from 66° preoperatively to 50° in the long-term follow-up (24.3% loss). Extension dropped from 62° to 55° (11.3%), radial deviation from 24° to 17° (29.2%), and ulnar deviation from 45° to 36° (20.0%) postoperatively. Grip strength was nearly completely restored with 95.5% of the unaffected side. Unfortunately, 50% of the patients had SLAC-wrist changes at 5 years follow-up. Tendon grafts, such as the Brunelli technique or its modifications, can be used to stabilize the scaphoid.[4,16–21] One of the modifications is the three-ligament tenodesis proposed by Garcia-Elias and colleagues.[4] On short-term and midterm follow-up, the results are comparable to the capsulodesis procedures.[1,16] They can improve wrist

pain relief with up to 25% loss of motion in the wrist. Furthermore, SLAC-wrist changes are noted in 5% to 24% of the cases at a mean follow-up of 3 to 4 years.[4,15,17] In the recent literature, other alternatives, such as bone-ligament-bone graft techniques for SL interval reconstruction,[22] four-bone-weave techniques,[23] dynamic tendon transfers,[17,24,25] or the reduction and association of the scaphoid and lunate (RASL)-procedure[26] are described. However, these are less commonly used and only small series are reported with no long-term follow-up.[1]

In the Zarkadas and colleagues[27] survey article on the surgical management of SL instability by 468 hand surgeons of the American and Canadian associations with different soft-tissue and/or bone-tissue reconstructions, 99% expect a postoperative limitation of wrist motion, 66% expect only recovery of 40% to 60% of normal wrist motion, 33% consider that 61% to 80% could be restored, and only 1% expect 81% to 100% recovery. Grip strength of over 75% of normal value is only expected by 18% of the surgeons in chronic lesions. Furthermore, 84% consider that patients will end up with occasional pain on moderate use of the injured wrist. Deshmukh and colleagues[11] published a prospective study on 44 cases of SL dissociations treated by a Blatt capsulodesis. Wrist extension was restricted from 60° to 38° (36, 7% loss) compared with the unaffected side, flexion dropped from 71° to 40° (43, 7%), radial deviation from 17° to 4° (76.5%), and ulnar deviation from 16° to 13° (50%). Postoperative grip strength reached only 75.1% of the unaffected side in this series. Pain relief measured by the Visual Analog Scale improved from 7.9 preoperatively to 4.1 postoperatively, but only 21 patients (47.7%) had good or excellent relief of pain, whereas 52.3% had only fair-to-poor relief. Moran and colleagues[16] compared a modified Brunelli technique to the Berger capsulodesis. Thirty percent of loss of motion between the preoperative and postoperative values was noted in the tenodesis group and 27% loss was noted in the capsulodesis group. A statistically significant decrease of flexion-extension arc was seen in both groups. Grip strength was not significantly changed in either group. Links and colleagues[21] showed overall better results with the Brunelli technique compared with a four-bone-weave technique in 44 patients. Weiss and colleagues[28] noted a loss of wrist motion, improved grip strength, and good satisfaction in 14 patients with a bone-retinaculum-bone technique.

All of the techniques fail to show that they can prevent arthritic deterioration of the wrist joint. None of them prevented the wrist stiffness in flexion.[29,30] The authors' patients show similar or better results with the grip strength than in most of the other studies. Average postoperative improvement of grip strength compared with the preoperative measurements is 40.5% (25–42 kg). Average postoperative strength reached 95.5% of the unaffected side. Postoperative mobility was improved in all directions compared with the preoperative measurements. Pain relief was excellent and patient satisfaction was very high. The results on wrist motion are remarkable even in a high-demand patient group. We conclude that our technique seems to stabilize stage 2, 3, and 4 SL dissociations without the issue of wrist stiffness due to the extensive open dissection techniques that was used in most cases.

The arthroscopic dorsal capsuloplasty seems to stabilize stage 2, 3, and 4 SL dissociations without the typical problem of wrist stiffness. These results are promising in these difficult clinical cases. Our technique is a single, minimally invasive procedure with a low complication rate and excellent short-term results. With respect to pain relief, grip strength, and (especially) wrist motion, further evaluation is required in a larger cohort of patients and with a longer follow-up to confirm these results. The good results obtained in our series with respect to pain relief and wrist motion are encouraging. Not surprisingly, athletes develop dynamic stabilizing mechanisms for their wrists in a higher proportion than the normal population, which may be relatively successful in the short run. This may have been a factor behind the good clinical outcomes. Of course, this series is not representative of the normal population. Should the technique be used in heavy manual workers? Would the results be the same? This question cannot be answered now, but if the technique proves to be effective in pain relief in the midterm to long-term follow-up, then it would become a valuable addition to our armamentarium of management of chronic reducible SL dissociations.

REFERENCES

1. Kalainov M, Cohen MS. Treatment of traumatic scapholunate dissociation. J Hand Surg Am 2009;34(7): 1317–9.
2. Mathoulin CH, Dauphin N, Sallen V. Capsulodèse arthroscopique dorsale dans les lésions chroniques du ligament scapho-lunaire. Chir Main 2009;28(6): 398 [in French].
3. Geissler WB, Haley T. Arthroscopic management of scapholunate instability. Atlas Hand Clin 2001;6(2): 253–74.
4. Garcia-Elias M, Lluch AL, Stanley JK. Three-ligament tenodesis for the treatment of scapholunate dissociation: indications and surgical technique. J Hand Surg Am 2006;31:125–34.
5. Berger RA, Imeada T, Berglund L, et al. Constraint and material properties of the subregions of the scapholunate interosseus ligament. J Hand Surg Am 1999;24(5):953–62.
6. Watson HK, Ballet FL. The SLAC wrist: scapholunate advanced collapse pattern of degenerative arthritis. J Hand Surg Am 1984;9(3):358–65.
7. Pilny J, Kubes J, Hoza P, et al. Consequence of nontreatment of scapholunate instability of the wrist. Rozhl Chir 2006;85:637–40 [in Czech].
8. Whipple TL. The role of arthroscopy in the treatment of scapholunate instability. Hand Clin 1995;11(1):37–40.
9. Blatt G. Capsulodesis in reconstructive hand surgery. Dorsal capsulodesis for the unstable scaphoid and volar capsulodesis following excision of the distal ulna. Hand Clin 1987;3(1):81–102.
10. Busse F, Felderhoff J, Krimmer H, et al. Scapholunate dissociation: treatment by dorsal capsulodesis. Handchir Mikrochir Plast Chir 2002;34:173–81.
11. Deshmukh SC, Givissis P, Belloso D, et al. Blatt's capsulodesis for chronic scapholunate dissociation. J Hand Surg Br 1999;24(2):215–20.
12. Slater RR, Szabo RR, Bay BK, et al. Dorsal intercarpal ligament capsulodesis for scapholunate dissociation: biomechanical analysis in a cadaver model. J Hand Surg Am 1999;24:232–9.
13. Szabo RM, Slater RR, Bay BK, et al. Dorsal intercarpal ligament capsulodesis for chronic static scapholunate dissociation: clinical results. J Hand Surg 2002;27:978–84.
14. Wintman BI, Gelberman RH, Katz JN. Dynamic scapholunate instability: results of operative treatment with dorsal capsulodesis. J Hand Surg Am 1995;20:971–9.
15. Gajendran VK, Peterson B, Slater RR Jr, et al. Long-term outcomes of dorsal intercarpal ligament capsulodesis for chronic scapholunate dissociation. J Hand Surg Am 2007;32(9):1323–33.
16. Moran SL, Ford KS, Wulf CA, et al. Outcomes of dorsal capsulodesis and tenodesis for treatment of scapholunate instability. J Hand Surg Am 2006; 31(9):1438–46.

17. Brunelli F, Spalvieri C, Bremner-Smith A, et al. Dynamic correction of static scapholunate instability using an active tendon transfer of extensor brevi carpi radialis: preliminary report. Chir Main 2004;23(5): 249–53.

18. Chabas JF, Gay A, Valenti D, et al. Results of the modified Brunelli tenodesis for treatment of scapholunate instability: a retrospective study of 19 patients. J Hand Surg Am 2008;33:1469–77.

19. Talwalkar SC, Edwards AT, Hayton MJ, et al. Results of tri-ligament tenodesis: a modified Brunelli procedure in the management of scapholunate instability. J Hand Surg Br 2006;31:110–7.

20. De Smet L, Van Hoonacker P. Treatment of chronic static scapholunate dissociation with the modified Brunelli technique: preliminary results. Acta Orthop Belg 2007;73:188–91.

21. Links AC, Chin SH, Waitayawinyu T, et al. Scapholunate interosseous ligament reconstruction: results with a modified Brunelli technique versus four-bone weave. J Hand Surg Am 2008;33(6):850–6.

22. Harvey EJ, Berger RA, Osterman AL, et al. Bone-tissue-bone repairs for scapholunate dissociation. J Hand Surg Am 2007;32(2):256–64.

23. Almquist EE, Bach AW, Sack JT, et al. Four-bone ligament reconstruction for treatment of chronic complete scapholunate separation. J Hand Surg Am 1991;16:322–7.

24. Bleuler P, Shafighi M, Donati OF, et al. Dynamic repair of scapholunate dissociation with dorsal extensor carpi radialis longus tenodesis. J Hand Surg Am 2008;33:281–4.

25. Ogunro O. Dynamic stabilization of chronic scapholunate dissociation with Palmaris longus transfer: a new technique. Tech Hand Up Extrem Surg 2007; 11:241–5.

26. Rosenwasser MP, Miyasajsa KC, Strauch RJ. The RASL procedure: reduction and association of the scaphoid and lunate using the Herbert screw. Tech Hand Up Extrem Surg 1997;1(4): 263–72.

27. Zarkadas PC, Gropper PT, White NJ, et al. A survey of the surgical management of acute and chronic scapholunate instability. J Hand Surg Am 2004; 29(5):848–57.

28. Weiss AP. Scapholunate ligament reconstruction using a bone-retinaculum-bone autograft. J Hand Surg Am 1998;23:205–15.

29. Siegel JM, Ruby LK. A critical look at intercarpal arthrodesis: review of the literature. J Hand Surg Am 1996;21(4):717–23.

30. Pomerance J. Outcomes after repair of the scapholunate interosseous ligament and dorsal capsulodesis for dynamic scapholunate instability due to trauma. J Hand Surg Am 2006;31(8): 1480–6.

Index

Note: Page numbers of article titles are in **boldface** type.

A

Allograft(s), composite tissue, vascularized, 546
    versus nerve allograft, 496–498
        migration of Schwann cells in, 496–498
    nerve, versus composite tissue allograft, 496–498
        migration of Schwann cells in, 496–498
Allotransplantation, bilateral hand, 412–414
    vascular complications of, 416
    composite tissue, 481
        candidates for, 423–424
        nerve regeneration in, clinical strategies to
            enhance, **495–509**
            optimizing surgical technique for, 502–504
    first hand, 411–412
    hand, 443
        dissection and identification of structures for,
            525–526
        donor limb for, 523
        forearm length and, 523
        goal of, 522
        muscle/tendon repair for, 527–528
        nerve repair for, 528
        osteosynthesis and, 526–527
        postoperative care in, 529
        preoperative planning for, 523–524
        skin closure and dressing for, 528–529
        skin incisions for, 524–525
        surgical techniques for, 522–529
        team coordination for, 523–524
        timing of, 524
        vessel repair for, 526–527
    nerve, information learned from, 496
        Schwann cell migration in, 496, 497
    upper extremity, benefit versus risk, 512
    vascularized composite, 405
        societies and monitoring, 407
Arthroscopic dorsal capsuloligamentous repair, in
    scapholunate tears. See *Scapholunate ligament
    tears.*
Axonal regeneration, speeding of, quality of
    regeneration and, 499–500

B

Bone marrow, donor, infusion/augmentation of, in
    solid organ transplantation, 513–514
    chimerism and operational tolerance in, 514–515

C

Chen functional score, 445, 447, 450, 451
Composite tissue allografts. See *Allotransplantation,
    composite tissue.*

D

Disabilities of Arm, Shoulder and Hand (DASH)
    measure, 444, 450–451
Donor, algorithm and transplant logistics, for hand
    transplantation, 536
    issues related to, in hand transplantation, **545–552**
    limb, for hand allotransplantation, 523
    management and operating room procedures, for
        hand transplantation, 548–549
    retrieval for hand transplantation, 536–537

F

FK-506, 499–500
French program, clinical hand transplantation,
    bilateral, functional recovery of, 415
        cases of, 411–416
        donor and recipient characteristics for, 412
        update of, **411–416**

H

Hand, allotransplantation of. See *Allotransplantation,
    hand.*
    donation of, oversight of, 550–551
    forearm, and arm transplantation, Spanish
        experience with, **443–453**
Hand and forearm transplantation, Innsbruck
    program, functional outcomes after, **455–465**
Hand transplant, recipients, Louisville hand
    transplant program, 418–421
        complications of, 419, 420, 421
        psychological aspects in, 424–426
Hand transplant psychology, 407–408
Hand transplant team, 532
    core organization of, 531–532
    dealing with media, 537–538
    occupational/physical therapist for, 533–534
    psychiatrist for, 533
    transplant coordinator for, 533
    transplant physician for, 532

Hand Clin 27 (2011) 573–575
doi:10.1016/S0749-0712(11)00098-9

hand.theclinics.com

Hand transplantation, American experiences
    in, 407
    anatomic evaluation for, 540
    Asian experience in, 407
    clinical, update from Louisville hand transplant
        program, **417–421**
        update from Polish program, **433–442**
        update on French program, **411–416**
        update on Innsbruck program, **423–431**
    consent process and, 547
    critical breakthroughs in 1980s and 1990s, 406
    donor algorithm and transplant logistics for, 536
    donor management and operating room
        procedures for, 548–549
    donor-related issues in, **545–552**
    donor retrieval for, 536–537
    double effect and, 555–556
    early developments in 1950s and 1960s, 406
    ethical, financial, and policy considerations in,
        553–560
    ethical considerations in, 553–557
    European experience in, 407
    financial considerations for, 557–558
    functional screening for, 540
    graft monitoring for rejection in, 427–428
    history of, 521–522
        and evolution of, **405–409**
    immunologic screening for, 541
    immunosuppression in. See *Immunosuppression,
        in hand transplantation.*
    immunosuppressive data in, summary of,
        473–477
    immunosuppressive protocols and immunological
        challenges related to, **467–479**
    in Louisville, KY, USA, 406
    in Lyon, France, 406
    in Pittsburgh, PA, USA, 406–407
    in US Department of Defense, 407
    informed consent for, 556
    medical screening for, 540, 541
    modern era of, 406–407
    motivation for, 425
    nonmaleficence versus beneficence of,
        554–555
    paternalism versus autonomy of, 555
    patient autonomy in, 555
    patient initial visit for, 540
    patient screening visit for, 540–542
    patient selection for, 542–543
    postoperative care and long-term management
        in, 537
    procurement protocols, specific required
        elements for, 546–547
    protocol for, preparation of, 534
    psychiatric screening for, 541–542
    psychological screening for, 542
    recipients for, evaluation of, 534–535

    listing and allocation of, 549–550
    procedure for, 537
    recruitment of, 534
    screening and selection of, to select right
        candidate, **539–543**
    screening of, as multistage process, 539–540
    transplant committee approval for, 535–536
    rejection in, 482–490
        acute cellular, 482–485
        antibody-mediated, 485–486
        chronic, 486–490
    risk versus benefit of, 554
    rules for, and regulation of, 558
    social screening for, 542
    surgical and technical aspects of, **521–530**
    world experience in, 482

I

Immunology of transplantation. See *Transplantation
    immunology.*
Immunomodulatory therapies, novel, bidirectional
    paradigm and, 515–516
Immunosuppression, in hand transplantation, 408
    challenges of, 473
    complications of, 473, 474–475, 476
    side-effect profile in, 476–477
    minimizing and weaning, premise and implications
        of, 512–513
    optimal, importance of, 513
Immunosupressive agents, induction agents, 471–472
    maintenance, 472
    mechanism of action of, 471–472
Immunosupressive protocols, 472–473
Innsbruck program, clinical hand transplantation,
    complications and side efects, 429
        functional outcome and, 428
        immunosuppression and immunologic
            complications in, 428
        rejection episodes in, 428–429
    clinical hand transplantation in, 424
        bilateral transplantation versus unilateral,
            425–426
        psychological evaluation of candidates for, 425
        psychological screening program,
            psychometric instruments for, 425, 426
        surgery for, 426–427
        update on, **423–431**
    hand and forearm transplantation, clinical
        outcome of, factors of importance in, 455
        functional outcomes after, **455–465**
            factors influencing, 456
            goals of, 456
            patients for, 456
            rehabilitation protocol following, 457
International Registry on Hand and Composite Tissue
    Transplantation, 407

L

Louisville hand transplant program, clinical hand transplantation, update on, **417–421**

M

Microsurgical reconstructive ladder, 405–406
Muscle/tendon repair, for hand allotransplantation, 527–528

N

Nerve allotransplantation, information learned from, 496
    Schwann cell migration in, 496, 497
Nerve regeneration, critical window of time for, 498–499
    in composite tissue allotransplantation, clinical strategies to enhance, **495–509**
Nerve repair, for hand allotransplantation, 528
Nonmyeloablative depletional induction, and prope tolerance, 515

O

Occupational/physical therapist, for hand transplant team, 533–534
Operational tolerance, in solid organ transplantation, 514–515
Organ procurement organization, requirements for recipient and donor data for, 547–548
    transplant program and, 536, 545, 546
Organ Procurement Transplant Network (OPTN), 545

P

Peripheral nerve, injury to, and regeneration, 495–496
Pittsburgh protocol, risk-benefit balance for upper extremity transplantation and, **511–520**
Polish program, clinical hand transplantation, cases evaluated for, 433–434
    donor acquisition for, 434
    inclusion criteria for, 433
    patient 1: 32-year-old man, 434–435
    patient 2: 42-year-old man, 435
    patient 3: 29-year-old man, 435–437
    patient 4: 30-year-old man, 437–438
    patient 5: 33-year-old man, 439–440
    update from, **433–442**
Psychiatrist, for hand transplant team, 533

R

Reconstructive Transplantation Innsbruck, 424

S

Scapholunate ligament tears, chronic, arthroscopic dorsal capsuloligamentous repair in, **563–572**
    indications for, 563–564
    intraoperative staging for, 564–565

postoperative assessment of, 565–568
postoperative protocol for, 565
preoperative assessment for, 564
results of, 569
surgical technique for, 564
Schwann cell(s), migration of, in composite tissue allograft versus nerve allograft, 496–498
    in nerve allotransplantation, 496, 497
of host, alternative sources for, 501–504
support of, ensuring of, 500–501
Skin antigenicity of, 482
Skin immune system, 481
Spanish experience, with hand, forearm, and arm transplantation, **443–453**
    analysis of outcomes of, 447
    anesthesia management in, 444–445
    measurement of function and disability in, 445–446
    patients and methods in, 444–447
    rehabilitation following, 446–447
    results of, 447–449
    surgical technique for, 445, 446

T

Tacrolimus, 499–500
Transplant program, financial clearance and insurance negotiations for, 535
    identification of multidisciplinary group of surgeons/clinicians/ancillary staff for, 532–534
    upper extremity, development of, **531–538**
    working with organ procurement organization, 536, 545, 546
Transplantation, reconstructive, immunomodulation versus immunosuppression, 516–517
    solid organ, infusion/augmentation of donor bone marrow in, 513–514
        chimerism and operational tolerance in, 514–515
    upper extremity, acute and chronic rejection in, **481–493**
        risk-benefit balance for, in Pittsburgh protocol, **511–520**
Transplantation immunology, 467–471
    activation of T cells: signals 1, 2, and 3, 469–470, 471
    basics of, 468–469, 470
    immunological challenges of composite tissue, 470–471

U

Upper extremity, transplant program, development of, **531–538**
Upper extremity transplantation, acute and chronic rejection in, **481–493**
    risk-benefit balance for, in Pittsburgh protocol, **511–520**

United States Postal Service

Statement of Ownership, Management, and Circulation
(All Periodicals Publications Except Requestor Publications)

1. Publication Title	2. Publication Number	3. Filing Date
Hand Clinics	0 0 0 - 7 0 9 9	9/16/11

4. Issue Frequency	5. Number of Issues Published Annually	6. Annual Subscription Price
Feb, May, Aug, Nov	4	$338.00

7. Complete Mailing Address of Known Office of Publication (*Not printer*) (*Street, city, county, state, and ZIP+4®*)

Elsevier Inc.
360 Park Avenue South
New York, NY 10010-1710

Contact Person
Amy S. Beacham
Telephone (Include area code)
215-239-3687

8. Complete Mailing Address of Headquarters or General Business Office of Publisher (*Not printer*)

Elsevier Inc., 360 Park Avenue South, New York, NY 10010-1710

9. Full Names and Complete Mailing Addresses of Publisher, Editor, and Managing Editor (*Do not leave blank*)

Publisher (*Name and complete mailing address*)

Kim Murphy, Elsevier, Inc., 1600 John F. Kennedy Blvd. Suite 1800, Philadelphia, PA 19103-2899

Editor (*Name and complete mailing address*)

David Parsons, Elsevier, Inc., 1600 John F. Kennedy Blvd. Suite 1800, Philadelphia, PA 19103-2899

Managing Editor (*Name and complete mailing address*)

Barbara Cohen-Kligerman, Elsevier, Inc., 1600 John F. Kennedy Blvd. Suite 1800, Philadelphia, PA 19103-2899

10. Owner (*Do not leave blank. If the publication is owned by a corporation, give the name and address of the corporation immediately followed by the names and addresses of all stockholders owning or holding 1 percent or more of the total amount of stock. If not owned by a corporation, give the names and addresses of the individual owners. If owned by a partnership or other unincorporated firm, give its name and address as well as those of each individual owner. If the publication is published by a nonprofit organization, give its name and address.*)

Full Name	Complete Mailing Address
Wholly owned subsidiary of	4520 East-West Highway
Reed/Elsevier, US holdings	Bethesda, MD 20814

11. Known Bondholders, Mortgagees, and Other Security Holders Owning or Holding 1 Percent or More of Total Amount of Bonds, Mortgages, or Other Securities. If none, check box ☐ None

Full Name	Complete Mailing Address
N/A	

12. Tax Status (*For completion by nonprofit organizations authorized to mail at nonprofit rates*) (*Check one*)
The purpose, function, and nonprofit status of this organization and the exempt status for federal income tax purposes:
☐ Has Not Changed During Preceding 12 Months
☐ Has Changed During Preceding 12 Months (*Publisher must submit explanation of change with this statement*)

PS Form **3526**, September 2007 (Page 1 of 3 (Instructions Page 3)) PSN 7530-01-000-9931 **PRIVACY NOTICE**: See our Privacy policy in www.usps.com

---

13. Publication Title	14. Issue Date for Circulation Data Below
Hand Clinics	May 2011

15. Extent and Nature of Circulation			Average No. Copies Each Issue During Preceding 12 Months	No. Copies of Single Issue Published Nearest to Filing Date
a. Total Number of Copies (*Net press run*)			1717	1726
b. Paid Circulation (By Mail and Outside the Mail)	(1)	Mailed Outside-County Paid Subscriptions Stated on PS Form 3541. (*Include paid distribution above nominal rate, advertiser's proof copies, and exchange copies*)	942	865
	(2)	Mailed In-County Paid Subscriptions Stated on PS Form 3541 (*Include paid distribution above nominal rate, advertiser's proof copies, and exchange copies*)		
	(3)	Paid Distribution Outside the Mails Including Sales Through Dealers and Carriers, Street Vendors, Counter Sales, and Other Paid Distribution Outside USPS®	312	232
	(4)	Paid Distribution by Other Classes Mailed Through the USPS (e.g. First-Class Mail®)		
c. Total Paid Distribution (*Sum of 15b (1), (2), (3), and (4)*)			1254	1097
d. Free or Nominal Rate Distribution (By Mail and Outside the Mail)	(1)	Free or Nominal Rate Outside-County Copies Included on PS Form 3541	29	33
	(2)	Free or Nominal Rate In-County Copies Included on PS Form 3541		
	(3)	Free or Nominal Rate Copies Mailed at Other Classes Through the USPS (e.g. First-Class Mail)		
	(4)	Free or Nominal Rate Distribution Outside the Mail (Carriers or other means)		
e. Total Free or Nominal Rate Distribution (Sum of 15d (1), (2), (3) and (4))			29	33
f. Total Distribution (Sum of 15c and 15e)			1283	1130
g. Copies not Distributed (See instructions to publishers #4 (page #3))			434	596
h. Total (Sum of 15f and g)			1717	1726
i. Percent Paid (15c divided by 15f times 100)			97.74%	97.08%

16. Publication of Statement of Ownership
☐ If the publication is a general publication, publication of this statement is required. Will be printed in the **November 2011** issue of this publication. ☐ Publication not required

17. Signature and Title of Editor, Publisher, Business Manager, or Owner

[signature]   Date
Amy S. Beacham – Senior Inventory Distribution Coordinator   September 16, 2011

I certify that all information furnished on this form is true and complete. I understand that anyone who furnishes false or misleading information on this form or who omits material or information requested on the form may be subject to criminal sanctions (including fines and imprisonment) and/or civil sanctions (including civil penalties).

PS Form **3526**, September 2007 (Page 2 of 3)

Moving?

Make sure your subscription moves with you!

To notify us of your new address, find your **Clinics Account Number** (located on your mailing label above your name), and contact customer service at:

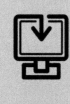

Email: journalscustomerservice-usa@elsevier.com

800-654-2452 (subscribers in the U.S. & Canada)
314-447-8871 (subscribers outside of the U.S. & Canada)

Fax number: 314-447-8029

Elsevier Health Sciences Division
Subscription Customer Service
3251 Riverport Lane
Maryland Heights, MO 63043

*To ensure uninterrupted delivery of your subscription, please notify us at least 4 weeks in advance of move.

Printed and bound by CPI Group (UK) Ltd, Croydon, CR0 4YY

03/10/2024

01040348-0010